The Hypomania Handbook

THE CHALLENGE OF ELEVATED MOOD

Christopher M. Doran, MD

Associate Clinical Professor of Psychiatry
University of Colorado Health Sciences Center
Englewood, Colorado

 Wolters Kluwer | Lippincott Williams & Wilkins
Health

Philadelphia · Baltimore · New York · London
Buenos Aires · Hong Kong · Sydney · Tokyo

Publisher: Charles W. Mitchell
Managing Editor: Sirkka Howes Bertling
Project Manager: Nicole Walz
Senior Manufacturing Manager: Benjamin Rivera
Associate Director of Marketing: Adam Glazer
Art Director: Risa Clow
Cover Designer: Melissa Walter
Production Service: Laserwords Private Limited, Chennai, India

© 2008 by LIPPINCOTT WILLIAMS & WILKINS, a Wolters Kluwer business
530 Walnut Street
Philadelphia, PA 19106 USA
LWW.com

Printed in the USA

Library of Congress Cataloging-in-Publication Data

Doran, Christopher M., 1946-
  The hypomania handbook : the challenge of elevated mood / Christopher M. Doran.
    p. ; cm.
  Includes bibliographical references and index.
  ISBN-13: 978-0-7817-7520-5
  ISBN-10: 0-7817-7520-5
  1. Hypomania—Handbooks, manuals, etc. I. Title.
  [DNLM: 1. Bipolar Disorder—diagnosis. 2. Bipolar Disorder—therapy. WM 207 D693h 2007]
  RC516.D67 2007
  616.89′5—dc22

                                                      2007017486

Care has been taken to confirm the accuracy of the information presented and to describe generally accepted practices. However, the authors, editors, and publisher are not responsible for errors or omissions or for any consequences from application of the information in this book and make no warranty, expressed or implied, with respect to the currency, completeness, or accuracy of the contents of the publication. Application of the information in a particular situation remains the professional responsibility of the practitioner.

The authors, editors, and publisher have exerted every effort to ensure that drug selection and dosage set forth in this text are in accordance with current recommendations and practice at the time of publication. However, in view of ongoing research, changes in government regulations, and the constant flow of information relating to drug therapy and drug reactions, the reader is urged to check the package insert for each drug for any change in indications and dosage and for added warnings and precautions. This is particularly important when the recommended agent is a new or infrequently employed drug.

Some drugs and medical devices presented in the publication have Food and Drug Administration (FDA) clearance for limited use in restricted research settings. It is the responsibility of the health care provider to ascertain the FDA status of each drug or device planned for use in their clinical practice.

To purchase additional copies of this book, call our customer service department at (800) 638–3030 or fax orders to (301) 223–2320. International customers should call (301) 223–2300.

Visit Lippincott Williams & Wilkins on the Internet: at LWW.com. Lippincott Williams & Wilkins customer service representatives are available from 8:30 am to 6 pm, EST.

10 9 8 7 6 5 4 3 2 1

To My Wife Maureen
My Friend
My Love
And
My First Editor

Contents

Preface

The Hypomania Handbook is challenging. It is challenging in that it is written about elevated mood, a rapidly changing subject. The very concepts of elevated mood, hypomania, and bipolar disorder have been evolving even as this text is being written. Some of the subjects discussed are ones about which even well-respected experts in the field of psychiatry have significant disagreements. The author has attempted to look at the concept of elevated mood from the perspective of hypomania. This is divergent from most works that focus on mania. Since this is not simply a treatment guide, some of the material, by necessity, touches on the evolving development in neurofunctioning, normal mental processes, and mental illness.

The genetic revolution is upon us, yet even as we unravel the genetic code we begin to see the complexity of regulatory, expressive, and transformative processes that occur between genetic coding and the entities that we now label as mental illness including disorders of elevated mood.

This book is also challenging because it is in fact three texts in one. First, it traces *the evolution of the concept of elevated mood* including the recent reemergence of the bipolar spectrum model. This model includes the historical perspectives of Kraeplin and others from the 18th century. Such a review reminds us of how our current conceptualizations fit into a much larger picture. Nowhere is this more important than in our understanding of the nature of elevated mood and bipolar disorder. In the latter portions of Chapter 1, new graphic representations of the spectrum of elevated mood within the fabric of mood disorders in general will be presented. From this background, Chapter 2 presents a new model to organize psychiatric data called the *GEnES Fingerprint*, which incorporates bodies of new evidence such as genetics and endophenotypes. In addition to being a model of elevated mood disorders, it provides a framework for the future organization of psychiatric data.

Second, this is a book about *the many faces of elevated mood* and how it is diagnosed. Since many of the elements of the GEnES Fingerprint are yet to be elucidated, we continue to diagnose hypomania and elevated mood using phenotypic data with all its limitations. This information begins in Section II and continues in the chapters of Section IV. In Section IV, specific aspects of the diagnosis and treatment of elevated mood in special populations will be reviewed. Also, diagnostic situations and symptoms of elevated mood that present special challenges are discussed in more detail.

Lastly, this is a book about the *treatment of elevated mood*. Medication prescription for elevated mood has been a mainstay of treatment, and is covered extensively in the literature. This text reviews research data and provides up-to-date, evidence-based recommendations for clinicians in the use of medication to modulate elevated mood. Specific attention is given to milder forms of elevated mood in which medication may be effective, but where side effects and/or tolerability significantly affect treatment decisions. Features unique to this are discussed in Chapters 5 and 6 that focus on the principles and challenges in addressing elevated mood through nonpharmacologic treatment methodologies. Specific schools of thought, treatment approaches, analogies, and clinical dialogues are offered that clinicians can consider with any elevated mood patient, regardless of their therapeutic orientation.

This handbook is multifaceted in its use. It serves as a guide for intelligent clinical practice utilizing a full spectrum of resources including medication and other psychotherapeutic interventions. It serves as a reference text for ongoing review in treating the difficult elevated mood patients, including those with specific comorbid conditions. Lastly, it provides a stimulus to readers in expanding their thoughts about causality, not only in elevated mood disorders but also in mental illness and mental health in general. The GEnES Fingerprint model serves to focus our attention on the role of both neurocellular and environmental factors as they influence the causality of mood states. While the GEnES Fingerprint model is a flexible way of categorizing and organizing mental health data, it also serves as a stimulus for asking more specific questions and producing more refined data models about mental states.

Our understanding of the cause of elevated mood and hypomania will continue to evolve and become more precise. Our medications and other treatments will become more targeted, safer, and more tolerable. Psychological measures and treatment approaches to the patient with hypomania outlined in this text, in any regard, will remain helpful. The combination of biologic and psychological treatments together will continue to be the mainstay of our treatment armamentarium as we forge into the new frontiers of understanding human emotion and its disorders.

Christopher M. Doran, MD
University of Colorado Health Sciences Center
Denver, Colorado, 2007.

Acknowledgments

Many thanks to Sirkka Bertling and Charley Mitchell at Lippincott Williams & Wilkins for sheparding this work through the publishing process, and to Christine Hackett for her many laborious hours of typing. A very special thanks to Don Weule and Michelle LaCasse for their graphic designs and drawings that bring the text material to life.

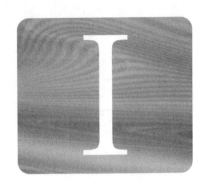

Elevated Mood—Past, Present, and Future Viewpoints

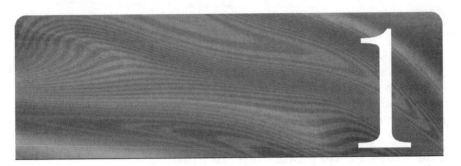

THE EVOLUTION OF ELEVATED MOOD

"... In the early stages, I feel good about the world and everybody in it ... I like it. All of a sudden I have the confidence that I could do what I set out to do. I take on more projects, largely because I'm not worried about running out of energy. I'm not grandiose, but I feel vigorous and active; accelerated, willing to take more risk. This feeling can last for days, sometimes weeks and it's wonderful. There's no other way of describing it." "... It's a very infectious kind of thing. We all have an appreciation for someone who's positive and upbeat. Others respond to the energy. People ... seem happy around me. It is very easy to make friends. There's also the personal sense...of an enhanced ability to act and reason." (1)

"When you're high, it's tremendous. The ideas and feelings are fast and frequent like shooting stars ... But, somewhere this changes. The fast ideas are far too fast and there are far too many ... Overwhelming confusion replaces clarity. Everything previously moving with the grain is now against—you are irritable, angry, frightened and uncontrollable ..." (2)

- The early history of elevated mood
- Why hypomania has been underappreciated
- The many definitions of hypomania
- Why is hypomania important?
- Consequences of misdiagnosis
- Definitions and parameters
- Elevated mood as part of bipolar disorder
- When does elevated mood constitute an illness?

- Devilishly vexing or heaven sent
- Traditional mood concepts
- Mood spectrum
- Back to the future
- Three-dimensional view of mood
- The bottom line
  References

Mania, derived from the Greek word for madness, has been described from antiquity. "Hypo" mania, again from Greek, is hierarchically below or beneath mania, and fills the gap between the full syndrome of mania and the more normal states of joy and elation. The formal term *hypomania* was first introduced by Mendel in 1891 (3).

The early history of elevated mood

The history of hypomania is long and intermingled with the concepts of mania, cyclothymia, bipolar disorder, and elevated mood in general. Elevated mood as a mental condition was identified as early as the 5th century BC by Hippocrates, who speculated on the biologic origin of mental disorders and felt that mania was attributed to an increase in yellow bile. Aristotle later speculated that the heart, rather than the brain, was the impaired organ responsible for elevated mood. In the 2nd century AD, Areteaus of Cappadocia was one of the first to suggest that elevated mood was an end-stage process of melancholia and described cyclothymia as a form of mental disease alternating between periods of depression and mania.

Nineteenth century scholars, including Falret and Baillarger, independently suggested that mania and depression were different expressions of the same disease occurring in a biphasic illness, dubbed *folie circulaire* or circular insanity. Hypomania was described as "that form of mania that typically shows itself only in the mild stages, abortively so to speak" (3). In the same century, Kahlbaum described cyclothymia as episodes of both depression and elevated mood that did not end in dementia. Emil Kraeplin, in his 1921 seminal work on what we now call *bipolar disorder*, described hypomania as one manifestation of the illness distinct from acute mania, delusional mania, and depressive or anxious mania.

More modern definitions of mania and hypomania derive from the studies of Clayton, Pitts, and Winokur whose published criteria were eventually incorporated into the *Diagnostic and Statistical Manual of Mental Disorders, Third Edition* (DSM-III) (4). These were further refined by Dunner et al. in 1970 into bipolar type I and bipolar type II disorders. The latter term described individuals with severe depression and milder manic symptoms, who did not appear to suffer from the disruption of the full mania of bipolar type I disorder. From this work, bipolar type II disorder became an official part of DSM-IV as well as the 10th revision of the International Classification of Diseases (ICD-10). It replaces "atypical bipolar disorder" to describe conditions characterized by depression and hypomania. The bipolar type II category was based in part on family pedigrees and follow-up studies suggesting a distinct subgrouping of persons with milder elevated mood. This group was also characterized by increased rates of suicide and suicide attempts, as well as a high risk of bipolar disorder in their relatives (5,6). Of particular note to this text and current diagnostic criteria is the proposal of Dunner et al. that a period of 3 or more days of hypomania is necessary for bipolar type II disorder to be

TABLE 1.1
DSM-IV criteria for a hypomanic episode

A. A distinct period of persistently elevated, expansive, or irritable mood, lasting through at least 4 days, that is clearly different from the usual nondepressed mood

B. During the period of mood disturbance, three or more of the following symptoms have persisted (four if the mood is only irritable) and have been present to a significant degree:
  1. Inflated self-esteem or grandiosity
  2. Decreased need for sleep (e.g., feels rested after only 3 hours of sleep)
  3. More talkative than usual or pressure to keep talking
  4. Flight of ideas or subjective experience that thoughts are racing
  5. Distractibility (i.e., attention too easily drawn to unimportant or irrelevant external stimuli)
  6. Increase in goal-directed activity (either socially, at work, or at school) or psychomotor agitation
  7. Excessive involvement in pleasurable activities that have a high potential for painful consequences (e.g., the person engages in unrestrained buying sprees, sexual indiscretions, or foolish business investments)

C. The episode is associated with an unequivocal change in functioning that is uncharacteristic of the person when not symptomatic

D. The disturbance in mood and change in functioning are observable by others

E. The episode is not severe enough to cause marked impairment in social or occupational functioning, or to necessitate hospitalization and there are no psychotic features

F. The symptoms are not due to the direct physiologic effect of a substance or a general medical condition

diagnosed. ICD-10 later included a 4-day or longer period of hypomania as the minimal duration of hypomanic symptoms necessary for the diagnosis. As we shall see, these time frames have recently been challenged by several authors, carrying potentially significant ramifications.

According to the DSM-IV criteria (see Table 1.1) hypomania is characterized by less intense, manic-like symptoms including elevated, expansive, or irritable mood during which time the person experiences inflated self-esteem or grandiosity. There is a decreased need for sleep, pressure to talk, flight of ideas, or racing thoughts. These symptoms are increasingly distractible and result in an increase in psychomotor activity and/or agitation.

Hypomania is symptomatically and categorically distinguished (at least in theory) from full mania that has the criteria shown in Table 1.2.

Many textbooks have been written on mood disorders or elevated mood. Most of these focus on the most severe form of elevated mood—mania—and touch on hypomania as an afterthought. Theoretically, hypomania is often viewed as a milder form of mania or, in some cases, a benign precursor. Michael Stone's chapter in the American Psychiatric Association Publishing Textbook

TABLE 1.2

Diagnostic criteria for a manic episode [a]

A. A distinct period of abnormally and persistently elevated, expansive, or irritable mood, lasting at least 1 week (or any duration if hospitalization is necessary)

B. During the period of mood disturbance, three (or more) of the following symptoms have persisted (four if the mood is only irritable) and have been present to a significant degree:
   a. Inflated self-esteem or grandiosity
   b. Decreased need for sleep (e.g., feels rested after only 3 hours of sleep)
   c. More talkative than usual or pressure to keep talking
   d. Flight of ideas or subjective experience that thoughts are racing
   e. Distractibility (i.e., attention too easily drawn to unimportant or irrelevant external stimuli)
   f. Increase in goal-directed activity (either socially, at work or school, or sexually) or psychomotor agitation
   g. Excessive involvement in pleasurable activities that have a high potential for painful consequences (e.g., engaging in unrestrained buying sprees, sexual indiscretions, or foolish business investments)

C. The symptoms do not meet criteria for a mixed episode

D. The mood disturbance is as follows:
   a. Sufficiently severe to cause marked impairment in occupational functions, usual social activities, or relationships with others
   b. Necessitates hospitalization to prevent harm to self or others, or
   c. Has psychotic feature

E. The symptoms are not due to the direct physiologic effects of a substance (e.g., a drug of abuse, a medication, or other treatment) or a general medical condition (e.g., hyperthyroidism)

[a] Adapted from DSM-IV TR; manic-like episodes that are clearly caused by somatic antidepressant treatment (e.g., medication, electroconvulsive therapy (ECT), light therapy) should not count toward a diagnosis of bipolar I disorder.

of Mood Disorders (3) lists 89 references to depression and melancholy, 60 references to mania and manic behavior, but only 8 references to hypomania, 2 to hyperthymic temperament, and 2 to bipolar spectrum disorder. As will be seen, hypomania is crucial to, and connected with the latter two concepts. Research literature is likewise centered on evaluating and studying acute mania, but underrepresented with research and articles about hypomania, although recent studies suggest that hypomania may be five to ten times as common as acute mania (7–12).

Until recently, hypomania has been seen as a minor condition, and potentially less worthy of study, and has been relegated to a less visible position in the hierarchy of psychiatric diagnoses. This text will take a new perspective and focus on elevated mood from the point of view of milder mood states, particularly hypomania. This information will serve as a bridge between the more severe states of manic mood and "normal" mood states. It is suggested that hypomania is, in fact, a significant and crucial diagnosis both for practical and theoretical reasons. Hypomania and subsyndromal elevated mood states will be seen as important elements in accurate diagnosis and quality mental health treatment. They will also be seen as holding a central position in a continuum of elevated mood. In order to advance these theses, we need to first understand why hypomania has been underappreciated and also the definitions of those conditions that border on hypomania in the spectrum of elevated mood.

Why hypomania has been underappreciated

There are a variety of reasons for this diagnosis being underappreciated or overlooked, as listed in Table 1.3.

The underappreciation of hypomania begins with its overlapping similarities with normal traits that are valued and appreciated in the human personality and society. High energy, work productivity, social jocularity, friendliness, and talkativeness are all traits which are often admired. As these are also traits associated with mild to moderate hypomania, it is no wonder that, for many individuals and their families, periods of hypomania are often not seen as an illness. Conversely, these periods are viewed as a strength and evidence of good mental health. Even when symptoms are exaggerated, elevated mood can be viewed as an expected result of circumstances (a promotion, receiving praise, completing a life goal, etc.). At other times, the patient is simply seen to be "feeling good" or "having a great day." When, on the other hand, the symptoms of hypomania are not euphoric and grandiose but angry and irritable, the patient may be seen as "grouchy," "moody" or the symptoms are viewed as a part of a patient's "touchy," "volatile" personality. Significant numbers of individuals with hypomania, therefore, never present

TABLE 1.3
The underappreciation of hypomania

Hypomania has been viewed or assessed as follows:

- A normal part of personality and not an illness
- A condition containing elements that are socially valued and encouraged
- A lesser form of mania, which is the condition of real importance
- Simply a "way station" to or from mania
- A welcome relief as a patient recovers from depression
- A condition categorized by overly rigid diagnostic criteria as noted in DSM-IV TR

to medical professionals for evaluation or treatment, and are seldom seen by mental health practitioners.

When hypomanic patients do present to mental health offices, there may also be a lack of spontaneous reporting of hypomania to clinicians because patients are embarrassed and reluctant to report elevated mood behaviors which may be viewed as indiscretions. Even when directly questioned, some patients will deny impulsive, reckless, or contradictory behaviors for fear of admonishment or disdain on the part of the clinician. On occasion, patient may even repress the memory of these behaviors unless confronted with irrefutable evidence.

Beyond embarrassment, some patients may fail to spontaneously report mild to moderate hypomanic behaviors/feelings because they do not see them as "symptoms" at all. Even detailed questioning by astute clinicians may fail to elicit hypomanic symptoms unless family members, employers, or others who know the patient can give a full picture of the patient's behavior.

Hypomania may also be seen by clinicians as simply a lesser form of mania, a transient phase on the "way up" to or on the "way down" from mania. When elevated mood and hypomania exist in the context of depressive bouts (which, as we shall see, are very common) hypomanic symptoms may be missed by the clinician *and* the patient, as they are seen as a welcome sign that depression is lifting. Many patients who have been treated for depression cease treatment shortly after they start feeling better and the hypomanic elements of their outcome are lost to evaluation and further treatment. Whether the depressed patient has reached a normothymic mood and subsequently experiences hypomania, or proceeds directly into hypomania, this hypomanic mood state is often not observed by the clinician. Even if patients present for subsequent episodes of depression, they may not report the presence of the intervening hypomanic symptoms unless specifically asked by the clinician.

More recently, another reason for underdiagnosis of hypomania has been pointed out by Akiskal, Angst, et al. (8–12). Although discussed in more detail later, suffice it to say that proposals from a growing group of international researchers suggest that the DSM-IV TR (text revision) criteria for hypomania are too rigid and overly narrow, resulting in lesser forms of hypomania and subsyndromal elements of elevated mood being clinically overlooked. Currently, in order to satisfy the DSM-IV criteria for hypomania, a person must have had 4 or more days of symptoms and three to four specific behaviors. With less rigid criteria, many patients with elevated mood may be seen to experience hypomanic intervals for shorter periods of time or of lesser severity, but are hypomanic nonetheless.

The many definitions of hypomania

One would think that with the criteria outlined previously in DSM-IV, most clinicians would have a standard conceptual and symptomatic understanding of hypomania. Unfortunately, this is not the case. Some professionals view hypomania only as a temporary state on the "way up" to or "way down" from mania whereas others see hypomania as a "final destination," that is, a state which can persist for lengthy periods of time. Even if the time course and symptoms of hypomania are agreed upon (which they are not), there are other factors that may complicate the diagnosis. The borderline dividing highly energetic (hyperthymic) personality traits and hypomania is not clearly defined. Purely symptomatic assessment does not reliably identify a distinct borderline between severe hypomania and true mania. Because hypomania can exist and persist with virtually no elements of depression (although this is relatively uncommon), hypomania presenting with episodes of depression (bipolar type II) may be different than pure hypomania without such depressive elements.

The approach taken by DSM-IV TR and previous editions of the DSM has at times been labeled as a *Chinese menu approach*, where the clinician selects one item from column A and several from column B in order to make the diagnosis. Staying with this analogy, such an approach would result in very different meals if, for example, a person selected a meal of three fish dishes, as compared to a meal with one pork dish and two with beef, or three vegetarian choices. Likewise, hypomania may appear quite different depending on the symptoms identified in any given individual. A pressured, driven, and irritable hypomanic will look and act differently than a person who presents with rapid speech, distractibility, and grandiose ideas. They may, in fact, not even have the same form of the illness. Chapter 2 will suggest that the term *hypomania* describes a heterogeneous group of symptoms and does not reflect a truly uniform population of patients.

Why is hypomania important?

If, as stated in the preceding text, the patient, the family, researchers, and some practitioners seem not to recognize or seemingly care about hypomania, why should the reader? It is perhaps one of the most important questions that makes this text necessary. In order to answer this question appropriately, one needs to look at the consequences of not recognizing hypomania. Beyond the possible philosophic and theoretic consequences of a wrong diagnosis, there are practical concerns that have direct and serious ramifications for the patient and for the practitioner. These elements are listed in Table 1.4.

Consequences of misdiagnosis

Bipolar disorder has long been linked to impaired quality of life and functional status. When compared with unipolar depression, bipolar disorder has also been associated with impaired occupational functioning, greater health care utilization, and increased medical costs. Two surveys of the members of the National Depressive and Manic Depressive Associations (DMDA), conducted 8 years apart, reveal that bipolar disorder misdiagnosis is a widespread problem. In 1992, when the first survey was conducted, 73% of the 500 bipolar

TABLE 1.4
Risks of hypomania misdiagnosis

- The presence of hypomania is a strong signal that an illness is moving toward the bipolar end of the spectrum of mood disorders and away from a unipolar disorder
- When compared with unipolar disorder, mood disorders with bipolar characteristics require different treatments and carry different risks
- Standard treatments for unipolar depression (e.g., traditional antidepressants) may worsen hypomanic and bipolar symptoms
- Misdiagnosis and inappropriate treatment of hypomania can lead to increased incidence of suicide

disorder patients surveyed reported receiving alternative explanations of their symptoms before being correctly diagnosed with bipolar disorder. Almost half the number of these patients had consulted at least three professionals before receiving the appropriate diagnosis. More than a third of patients had 10 years elapse between their first professional contact and being correctly diagnosed with bipolar disorder (13). The second survey in the year 2000 showed that 69% of the 600 patients surveyed said they had initially been misdiagnosed (14). Several other studies by Ghaemi et al. (15,16) and Dilsaver (17) further support evidence of frequent misdiagnosis in clinical patient populations.

There are practical consequences to missing the presence of hypomania or bipolar disorder. When bipolar disorder is misdiagnosed during an initial mental health evaluation prompted by depressive rather than manic symptoms, antidepressants are often used as monotherapy without a mood stabilizer, thereby delaying the most effective treatment for bipolar disorder (18). Treatment with antidepressants can worsen the prognosis for the patient by potentially inducing hypomania, mania, or increasing cycle frequency (15,19–22). Misdiagnosis results in increased direct and indirect health care costs and higher rates of psychiatric hospitalization (23,24). Of particular note is the increased suicidal ideation and attempts in these misdiagnosed patients (24). Suicidality has been noted to be particularly high in bipolar II disorder and hypomania, when compared with lower rates in bipolar I disorder patients with pure manic episodes (25).

If hypomania is missed and represents the first sign of an emerging full-fledged bipolar I disorder, full mania may ultimately result with all its social, personal, financial, and even life-threatening consequences. However, when hypomania is appropriately identified and treated, the patient's initial upward swing of mood, energy, and hyperactivity may be treated before a serious incident of manic episode ensues.

Misdiagnosis also clouds much of our research into affective disorders because studies of individuals with "bipolar" disorder, according to current definition, have eliminated a large number of patients with subsyndromal elevated mood. Inclusion of this cohort with less severe and shorter periods of elevated mood could substantially alter study outcomes. Similarly, research on individuals ostensibly with pure major depression may inadvertently have included persons with low-level bipolar spectrum disorder and subsyndromal hypomania (see subsequent text for definitions of these terms and their importance). Such studies normally attempt to exclude individuals with bipolar disorder, but those with mild bipolar spectrum disorder and/or subsyndromal elevated mood may have not been excluded from the study when restrictive DSM-IV definitions of elevated mood are used as exclusion criteria.

Definitions and parameters

In this text, hypomania takes a central position in the realm of elevated mood. As can be seen in Figure 1.1, there is a gradient of elevated mood. On the less severe end of the elevated mood range is normal mood blending into hyperthymic temperament, progressing to subsyndromal elevated mood, hypomania, and severe elevated mood states including mania and ultimately psychotic mania.

The reader should note that the material in this section refers to a range consisting solely of elevated mood. This is to be differentiated from "bipolar spectrum" disorders that are discussed later in the chapter. To avoid confusion, the spectrum of elevated mood states will be referred to as a range of elevated mood. Although it is tempting to arbitrarily separate these entities as distinct subgroups, this is difficult to accomplish on a symptomatic basis. It is assumed here that the boundaries between the elements of elevated mood are indistinct and blend with adjacent states.

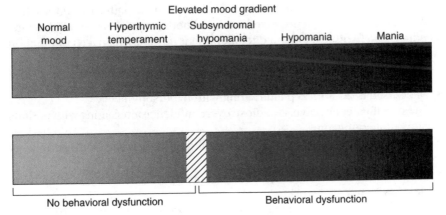

Figure 1.1 Elevated mood gradient.

The parameters of the range of elevated mood spectrum are defined as follows:

Temperament refers to stable behavior traits with strong affective coloring. By definition, temperament is within the realm of normal behavior and does not in itself indicate functional impairment. There is, however, an indistinct line between certain types of temperament and subsyndromal affective disorders. By definition, when functional impairment occurs, the patient moves from the category of temperament into a diagnosable disorder. The three temperamental types that are particularly important to mood diagnosis and treatment are as follows:

Hyperthymic temperament is characterized by a personality style or set of personality traits that include (26,27)

- increased energy and productivity,
- short sleep patterns,
- vivid, active, extroverted,
- self assured/self confident,
- strong willed,
- risk taking/sensation seeking,
- breaking social norms,
- generous and spendthrift,
- cheerful and jovial,
- unusual warmth,
- expansive,
- robust and tireless,
- irrepressible, infectious quality.

Individuals with hyperthymic temperament are often seen as strong, energetic, productive, and well respected. By definition, hyperthymic temperament does not have significant elements of dysfunction in mental, interpersonal, business, or social situations.

Cyclothymic temperament is characterized by a pattern of alternation between elevated and depressive/irritable moods, cognitions, and behaviors. The individual with cyclothymic temperament normally manages to function within societal norms albeit with varying consistency and success. This temperamental type evidences some of the following traits (adapted from 27,28):

- Decreased need for sleep alternating with hypersomnia
- Shaky self-esteem: naïve, grandiose overconfidence alternating with periods of mental confusion
- Periods of sharpened and creative thinking alternating with periods of apathy
- Marked unevenness in the quantity and quality of productivity, often associated with unusual working hours
- Uninhibited people-seeking alternating with more introverted self-absorption

- Excessive involvement in pleasurable activities without concern for potentially painful consequences alternating with restriction of involvement in pleasurable activities and guilt over past activities
- Alternation between overoptimism or exaggeration of past achievement and a pessimistic attitude toward the future, or brooding about past events
- Talkative with inappropriate laughing, joking, and punning; then, less talkative, even tearfulness or crying
- Frequent shifts in work, study, interest, or future plans
- Occasional financial extravagance
- Frequent changes in residence or geographic location
- Tendency toward promiscuity with repeated conjugal or romantic failure
- Alcohol or drugs used to control moods or to augment excitement

Depressed temperament features a pattern of depressive cognitions and behavior (adapted from 29,30). The depressive temperament type is

- complaining, humorless;
- critical, blaming, and derogatory toward self and others;
- brooding and given to worry;
- negativistic, critical, and judgmental toward others;
- pessimistic, preoccupied with failure;
- prone to feeling guilty and remorseful;
- sluggish, passive, and has few interests;
- a habitual long sleeper.

Persons with this temperament also have

- a mood often dominated by dejection, gloominess, cheerlessness, joylessness, or unhappiness;
- a poor self-concept that includes feelings of inadequacy, worthlessness, and low self-esteem.

Subsyndromal affective conditions are circumstances in which a patient may experience one or more affective symptoms, but the sum total of these symptoms does not reach the threshold of currently defined, diagnosable disorders. Such subsyndromal conditions may have a measure of functional impairment from one or more symptoms and, therefore, could be seen as needing treatment. Many individuals with subsyndromal elevated mood do not recognize this state as an illness, nor present for treatment. Usually from a diagnostic standpoint though, these conditions fall into nomenclature categories included under the term *not otherwise specified*.

Progressing along the range of elevated mood in Figure 1.1, the next most severe condition is hypomania, which has been discussed and defined by DSM-IV TR earlier in the chapter. For purposes of this text, hypomania has a constellation of core symptoms as listed in Table 1.1. Clinically, it is evident that there is also a range of severity *within* the diagnosis of hypomania stretching from mild hypomania, often manifesting as only one or two areas of functional impairment to significant hypomania that borders on mania and may have multiple areas of functional disability.

Lastly, along the range of elevated mood is the most severe form of elevated mood—mania—which has been characterized in DSM-IV TR as shown in Table 1.2. The most severe manifestations of mania include psychotic features, delusions, and hallucinations.

These elements of elevated mood form a continuum stretching from "normal" to nonpathologic hyperthymic temperament, to subsyndromal affective episodes to hypomania and, finally, to mania. Although it is tempting to assume that this spectrum represents a single condition with increasing severity of symptoms and a single pathologic underpinning, it is not at all clear that this is true. As will be seen with the analogy to diabetes in Chapter 5, the spectrum of hyperglycemia to type 2 diabetes to type 1 diabetes has, in fact, different mechanisms and different causal underpinnings for the various components. This structure may or may not apply to elevated mood. Therefore, although it is reasonable to assume that there is increasing severity and dysfunction as one progresses from left to right on this spectrum, one cannot assume that this represents unitary causality.

Elevated mood as part of bipolar disorder

Although this text is written from the perspective that hypomania holds a central position in the spectrum of elevated mood, it cannot be written without discussion of bipolar disorder as it is currently defined. As is well known, bipolar disorder is a mood disorder that is characterized by the occurrence of one or more manic, hypomanic, or mixed affective episodes. The presence of one manic episode, as defined in the phenomenologic terms in Table 1.2, places the condition into the bipolar type I category. The presence of one or more hypomanic episodes as in Figure 1.1, without the occurrence of a full manic episode, places the patient in the category of bipolar type II. The presence of mixed affective episodes *per se*, although signifying a bipolar disorder, does not specifically relegate the diagnosis into a type I or type II categorization (see Chapter 8). This distinction is made on the basis of the severity of other nonmixed elevated mood episodes. Therefore, mixed episodes that occur in a patient with at least one manic episode are labeled as bipolar type I. Mixed episodes without additional mania or solely with hypomania are labeled bipolar type II. Conditions with exclusively or predominantly mixed episodes are likely to be categorized as bipolar disorder not otherwise specified (bipolar NOS) in the current diagnostic scheme.

Owing to the multiple definitions associated with elevated mood, the rapidly evolving developments in the concept of hypomania, and the relatively few patients with purely elevated mood, we are confronted with a situation in which elevated mood research almost inevitably focuses on patients with some form of bipolar disorder; that is, conditions that have both elevated and depressed mood. Research subjects for these studies are not often separated into bipolar type I and bipolar type II disorders, so study populations are often a combined group. It is quite unclear what, if any, difference would be made if hypomanic subjects were studied as a single group rather than including them in research populations of bipolar type I patients who have full manic episodes. Although this may well limit the application of our current research, it is a fact of the current state of our knowledge. It is only as we elucidate more definable and explicit underlying characteristics of elevated mood (as described in the following chapter) that we may have more "pure," homogeneous research samples and improved data.

When does elevated mood constitute an illness?

For the purposes of this text, the assumption is made that when elevated mood causes functional impairment, illness is present. Theoretically, it should be simple to distinguish clinical situations that involve functional impairment and thereby diagnose a "psychiatric illness." In real-world clinical practice, however, this is not as easy as it might appear. Evaluating the presence of, or the extent of, functional impairment is not always obvious to the clinician assessing an individual patient with elevated mood. It may be necessary to receive feedback from family members or other patient observers in order to detect the presence or extent of day-to-day dysfunction in elevated mood cases. There may be differences between what the patient sees as "normal" (or even exceptional) and what other family members may believe to be a problem that interferes with daily functioning. It may also fall to the therapist's judgment to differentiate the degree of impact on the patient's life and what constitutes "impairment."

For example, demandingness, high expectations of employees, and intolerance for substandard performance may be considered good management style by some. If intense and unchecked, however, such behavior may fall into the category of functional "impairment." Similarly, when a person is significantly productive, but is so at the cost of family interaction or disruption, does this constitute functional impairment or not? As demonstrated in Figure 1.1, there is a progression of elevated mood that has indefinite boundaries and is subject to clinical interpretation. Similarly, interpretation of functional impairment or interference may have indistinct boundaries and be subject to judgment by a clinician. What is clear, however, is that patients who are at the high end of the scale are "sicker" and more likely to present for treatment, either through self-recognition or at the insistence of others.

Devilishly vexing or heaven sent

Depending on the severity, intensity, and frequency of hypomanic symptoms and their intrusion into the patient's individual or family life, hypomania may be seen as "devilishly vexing" or "heaven sent." Even if intermixed with areas of deficit, prominent symptoms of hypomania often include increased sociability, talkativeness, increased energy, and elements of self-confidence. Both the patient and the family may see these qualities as part of a personality that is easy to get along with, socially lubricating, and resilient to stress. When under control, such symptoms may be valued in the workplace or family. The individual may be seen as a "workhorse" or social catalyst with exceptional functional capacities, creativity, and productivity.

When hypomania is out of control and/or the prominent symptoms are being irritable, demanding, or impulsive, the condition may be seen as an indicator of personality deficits. These individuals have problems with coworkers and family members. Depending on the severity of functional impairment, therefore, the condition may be seen as a wonderful person's personality or as an illness needing treatment.

Traditional mood concepts

Most practitioners educated in the last 40 years have been significantly influenced by the formulation of the DSM and its revisions. An important concept as it relates to elevated mood, has been the artificial distinction between "unipolar" and "bipolar" disorders. These have been seen as distinct, separate entities with some potential overlapping symptoms. The presence of mania or hypomania, by definition, has been the hallmark of bipolar disorder. Depression is common to both conditions. Only rarely does mania or hypomania occur in isolation without depression.

Mental health education has often been illustrated with two-dimensional graphs similar to those shown in Figures 1.2, 1.3, and 1.4. In these graphs, the boundaries of normal mood are shown between the dotted lines. Distinct periods of mood that extend beyond the dotted lines are labeled as periods of abnormal mood. When these periods are significantly above the upper dotted line, they are manic and if they are mildly above the line, they are hypomanic. When mood is mildly below the lower dotted line, it is dysthymic and when significantly below the line, a major depression. These graphs conveniently illustrate the subtypes of bipolar disorder as they were defined in DSM-III and IV. Bipolar type I, as shown in Figure 1.2, has episodes of major depression and full mania. Episodes of hypomania may be present in bipolar type I disorder but there is at least one spontaneous full manic episode. The patterns and time course of these depressive and manic episodes is variable from person to person. They may show predominantly depressed episodes (A in Figure 1.2), predominantly elevated mood episodes (D), regularly alternating patterns of depression and elevated mood (B), or no apparent pattern at all (C).

Similarly, bipolar type II patients show patterns of full depressive episodes with solely hypomanic episodes as shown in Figure 1.3. As with bipolar type I, the time pattern of these episodes may be regular or irregular. The overall course may be dominated by depressive episodes, dominated by hypomania, or more evenly balanced.

Bipolar I variations

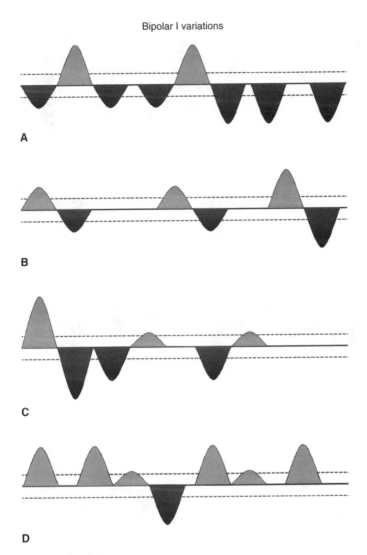

Figure 1.2 Bipolar I variations.

A third form of elevated mood diagnosis identified in DSM-IV is that of cyclothymia and is shown in Figure 1.4. In this case, the patient has hypomanic episodes and dysthymic episodes but does not have full-fledged manias or major depressive episodes. As with the two previous diagnostic patterns, the length of these episodes, as well as the pattern of their occurrence, is variable from individual to individual. Other episodes of mood swings, which do not fit succinctly into these three categories, are characterized as bipolar disorder NOS and cannot easily be illustrated in graph form.

Bipolar II variations

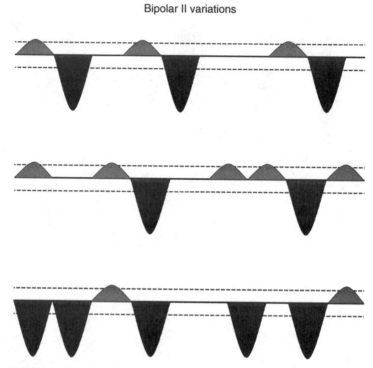

Figure 1.3 Bipolar II variations.

Cyclothymic variations

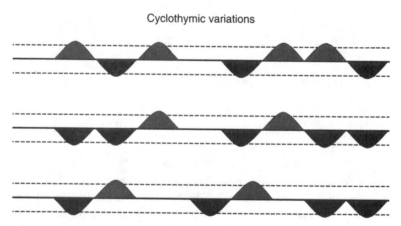

Figure 1.4 Cyclothymia variations.

These two-dimensional diagrams, while helpful in terms of identifying patterns of moods, also reinforce an apparent exclusivity of symptoms of elevated and depressed mood. The implication is that when a person is in a period of elevated mood, there is no element of depression, and when a person is depressed, there are no symptoms of elevated mood. Mixed affective states, in which both elevated and depressed mood symptoms coexist (a concept that will be discussed in more detail in Chapter 8), are not easily depicted. As will be seen later in this chapter, these two-dimensional drawings are outdated and reinforce stereotypes of mood disorders that are not consistent with our current understanding.

Mood spectrum

Utilizing mania as the primary measure of elevated mood is analogous to measuring the incidence of epilepsy primarily from the occurrence of grand mal seizures, while failing to assess complex partial seizures, temporal lobe epilepsy, and petit mal seizures. Similarly it is viewing diabetes solely from the point of view of diabetic ketoacidosis, disregarding prediabetes, milder hyperglycemia, and type 2 diabetes (the incidence of which actually surpasses type 1 diabetes). By including "softer signs" of elevated mood, the incidence of hypomania, and various forms of bipolar disorder are now seen to be potentially much greater than previously thought.

Traditionally, using the more restricted criteria in DSM-IV TR, the lifetime prevalence of bipolar type I disorder has been approximated as 1%. In the United States, the lifetime prevalence for bipolar type I disorder was reported to be 0.8% in the Epidemiological Catchment Area study (31) and 1.6% in the National Comorbidity Survey (32). Because bipolar disorder encompasses a much broader range of illness than just bipolar type I, the concept of a "bipolar spectrum disorder" (see subsequent text) has been proposed to include bipolar type I, bipolar type II, and other forms of elevated mood (33–35). Various subtypes have been proposed by Hirschfeld, Klerman, Ghaemi, Akiskal, and Pinto (20,35–38); however, there has been no universal agreement on the validity and reproducibility of these categories. What has been validated, however, is the presence of many milder forms of bipolar disorder when a wider dimension of diagnostic criteria has been used. Judd and Akiskal have reanalyzed the Epidemiological Catchment Area database taking into account subthreshold cases of subsyndromal manic symptoms, and show a 6.4% lifetime prevalence for bipolar spectrum disorders (39). *This would suggest that subthreshold cases are at least five times more prevalent than the current 1% estimate of bipolar disorder.* These cases, which included subsyndromal symptoms, show high rates of lifetime health service utilization, high need for welfare and disability payments, and higher prevalence of suicidal behavior when compared with a comparable group without mental disorder. Identification of this milder end of the bipolar spectrum, therefore, has significant economic and public health ramifications.

Most experts now agree that the DSM-IV TR categories are overly restrictive and artificially exclude a significant number of individuals who have briefer or "softer" periods of hypomania. Although there is disagreement as to the exact method for classifying these individuals, it is becoming universally accepted that recognition and possible treatment of such briefly appearing signs is important.

Back to the future

Professional writings have begun to challenge the exclusivity of unipolar and bipolar disorders, returning to the 19th century concepts of Emil Bleuler. Bleuler postulated that affective disorders existed on a spectrum but were aspects of a single entity. Within this spectrum, which he called *manic depressive illness,* he included various subtypes. Those who experienced only depressive episodes were said to have unipolar disorder, and those who experienced manic symptoms had bipolar disorder. It is only within the last 40 years that the empiric data used to support DSM-III again began to separate the concepts into separate illnesses.

Several major psychiatric clinicians/researchers have returned to the more unitary concept of mood disorders and introduced the concept of "bipolar spectrum disorder." This is a term in which there is a continuum of mood disorders that include both elevated and depressed mood episodes. There are four ways in which the term *bipolar spectrum* has been defined by various authors. These are listed in Table 1.5 and graphically depicted in Figure 1.5. As the concept of "bipolar spectrum" has become internationally used, many treatises, reviews, and journal articles refer to the term without defining which of the definitions is being used (37–49).

Whichever definition of bipolar spectrum emerges as the most valid, it is becoming clear that a sizable portion of patients, who have been currently diagnosed as having a major depressive episode, do in fact have some symptoms of bipolarity or mixed affective episodes. Therefore, they are more rightly categorized as "bipolar" in nature rather than strictly "unipolar" or "depressive."

Three-dimensional view of mood

The two-dimensional drawings shown earlier in this chapter significantly hamper any attempt to illustrate the bipolar spectrum, mixed affective states, rapid cycling, the potential relationship between depressed mood and elevated mood, and the relationship between bipolar disorder and other psychiatric diagnoses. Newer methods to illustrate mood disorders are required.

Assuming that there is a spectrum of bipolar disorders (and this text does make that assumption), a more useful diagrammatic view of mood is shown in Figure 1.6.

TABLE 1.5

Definitions of bipolar spectrum

1. All DSM categories of bipolar disorder including classic bipolar I disorder, bipolar II disorder, and bipolar NOS disorder. See A in Figure 1.5

2. Ghaemi and Goodwin have proposed that any form of bipolar disorder that is not bipolar I disorder is within the bipolar spectrum. This then covers bipolar II disorder and bipolar NOS diagnoses. They suggest that bipolar I disorder is separate from other types and could be referred to as *Cade's disease*, named for the pioneering work by John Cade in the use of lithium. See B in Figure 1.5. They further go on to propose operational criteria for this definition of bipolar spectrum disorder, which are shown in Table 1.6

3. Any form of bipolar disorder that does not conform to the bipolar I and bipolar II diagnoses. This refers then to the DSM diagnosis of bipolar NOS attempting to be more specific and detailed about this currently heterogeneous category. See C in Figure 1.5

4. In addition to bipolar types I, II, and NOS, the conceptualization favored by Hagop Akiskal (33,36) would include all of the following diagnostic categories: schizobipolar disorder, depressions with hypomania irrespective of duration, hypomania first experienced as a response to antidepressants, depression in association with hyperthymic, cyclothymic and dysthymic temperaments, and recurrent "pseudounipolar" depressions with a bipolar family history. See D in Figure 1.5

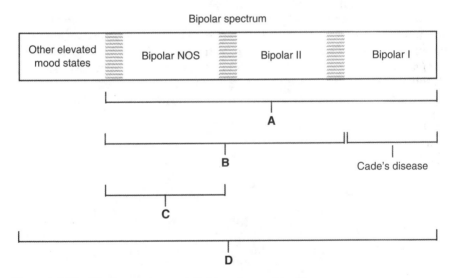

Figure 1.5 The Bipolar spectrum definitions in graphical form.

TABLE 1.6

Proposed criteria for operational spectrum disorder

A. At least one major depressive episode

B. No spontaneous DSM-IV hypomanic or manic episodes

C. Either of the following plus two from D, or both the following plus one from D:
   a. First-degree relative with bipolar disorder
   b. Antidepressant-associated mania or hypomania

D. If none from C, at least six of the following:
   a. Hyperthymic personality
   b. More than three depressive episodes
   c. Brief major depressive episodes (of duration <3 mo)
   d. Atypical depressive symptoms
   e. Psychotic major depressive episodes
   f. Early age at onset (<25 y old)
   g. Postpartum depression
   h. Antidepressant wear-off (acute but not prophylactic response)

From Ghaemi SN, Ko JY, Goodwin FK. "Cade's disease" and beyond: Misdiagnosis, antidepressant use, and a proposed definition for bipolar spectrum disorder. *Can J Psychiatry.* 2002;47:124–134.

This three-dimensional illustration shows a "fabric" of mood like the canvas of a tent with "tent poles" designating the area of depressed mood and elevated mood. Some might prefer to see this illustration as mountain peaks with valleys and plains. The higher the elevation, that is, the further up the slope, the more severe the symptomatology. A patient may be positioned on this graph closer to the depressed pole for primary depressive illness and nearer to the elevated mood pole when bipolar symptoms are more apparent.

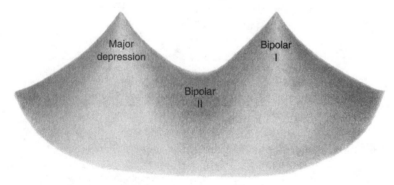

Figure 1.6 The bipolar landscape.

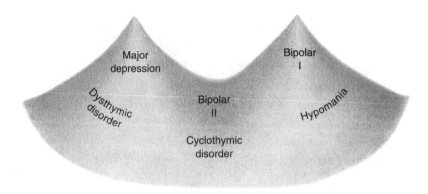

Figure 1.7 The landscape, including less severe mood conditions.

There could be many individuals in the "valley" between the two poles or more toward the depressive peak, who would still have some evidence of bipolarity of limited or subsyndromal intensity. Within this graphic it is difficult to define exact areas along the mountain slopes that are distinct bipolar type I, bipolar type II, and major depression. These form a contiguous area along both peaks that merge into one another. This conceptualization would explain some of the operational difficulties in using the DSM as discussed in this chapter and the next. Areas with firm boundaries are difficult to picture and define because they do not exist when the diagnoses are defined by purely phenomenologic symptoms.

Patients who have less intense symptomatology such as dysthymic disorder, cyclothymic disorder, and relatively pure hypomania would be shown as being further down the slope as shown in Figure 1.7. Again, distinct boundaries are absent as the diagnoses merge into one another rather than have sharp demarcations.

Figure 1.8 also shows an indistinct or overlapping boundary between mood diagnoses and nonpathologic affective temperaments (such as dysthymic, cyclothymic, and hyperthymic temperament). Because they do not, by definition, cause functional impairment, temperaments are on the plain and not truly up the slope. Subsyndromal mood episodes are not pictured, but would occur further "upslope" from temperaments, but not as elevated as diagnosable conditions.

This new conceptualization also suggests the possibility for there are other "mountains" visible in the landscape, as shown in Figure 1.9. Although it is as yet more speculative than proved, it suggests that there may be similar indistinct divisions between mood disorders and other psychiatric conditions including borderline personality disorder or schizophrenia.

Although an improvement over two-dimensional mood graphs, these illustrations do have limitations, particularly when attempting to delineate

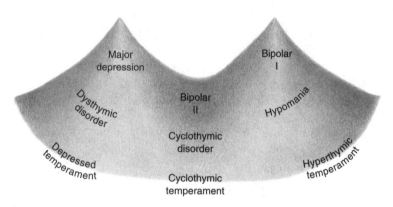

Figure 1.8 The landscape, including nonpathologic temperaments.

sharp differentiations between various psychiatric diagnoses. Attempting to rigidly diagram current diagnoses is inherently flawed since the diagnoses themselves are based on variable phenotypic symptoms that are observed and reported. These phenotypic symptoms are themselves heterogeneous, imprecisely defined, and likely to have multifactorial causes that are different in each individual. This three-dimensional conceptualization is, therefore, a step forward, but we must rapidly move to a further improved system of classification based on endophenotypes and genetics as described in Chapter 2.

The bottom line

- Hypomania has been underappreciated as a factor in the diagnosis of mood disorders.

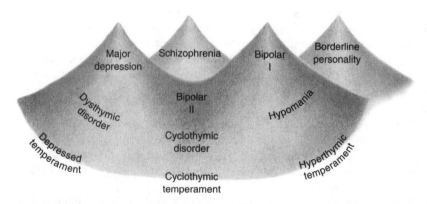

Figure 1.9 The landscape, including other diagnoses.

- The artificial separation of unipolar major depression and bipolar disorder is a relatively recent phenomenon in psychiatric classification, and may well not be a valid distinction.
- Bipolar disorder has likely been underdiagnosed whereas major depressive episodes have been overdiagnosed in contemporary psychiatry. This will be corrected as the definition of elevated mood:
  - Includes an emphasis on overactivation, not just elevated mood
  - Shortens the time necessary to qualify as an elevated mood episode
  - Requires fewer criteria to qualify as a subsyndromal elevated mood episode
- There is a range of elevated mood conditions that include hyperthymic temperament, subsyndromal hypomania, hypomania, and mania.
- The interface between affective temperaments and psychiatric illness is indistinct. It is unclear to what extent affective temperament and our currently defined mood disorders are causally or symptomatically connected.
- The term *bipolar spectrum disorder*, although likely valid, is defined differently by different authors.

REFERENCES

1. Whybrow PC. *A mood apart: A thinker's guide to emotion and its disorders.* New York: HarperCollins; 1997:44.
2. Jameson KR. *An unquiet mind: A memoir of moods and madness.* Random House; 1995:67.
3. Stein DJ, Kupfer DJ, Schatzberg AF. *Textbook of mood disorders.* American Psychiatric Association Press; 2006:14.
4. Clayton PJ, Pitts FN Jr, Winokur G. Affective disorder IV. Mania. *Compr Psychiatry.* 1965;6:313–322.
5. Dunner DL, Gershon ES, Goodwin FK. Heritable factors in the severity of affective illness. *Sci Proc Amer Psychiatric Assn.* 1970;123:187–188.
6. Dunner DL, Gershon ES, Goodwin FK. Heritable factors in the severity of affective illness. *Biol Psychiatry.* 1976;11:31–42.
7. Stallone FI, Dunner Dl, Ahearn J, et al. Statistical prediction of suicide in depressives. *Compr Psychiatry.* 1980;21:381–387.
8. Akiskal HS. Le spectre biopolaire: Acquisitions er perspectives cliniques [The bipolar spectrum: Research and clinical perspectives]. *Encephale.* 1995;21:3–11. spec no 6):
9. Akiskal HS. Validating "hard" and "soft" phenotypes within the bipolar spectrum: Continuity or discontinuity? *J Affect Disord.* 2003;73:1–5.
10. Akiskal HS, Hirschfeld RM, Yerevanian BI. The relationship of personality to affective disorders. *Arch Gen Psychiatry.* 1983;40:801–810.
11. Angst J, Marneros A. Bipolarity from ancient to modern times: Conception, birth and rebirth. *J Affect Disord.* 2001;67:2019.
12. Angst J, Perris C. Nosoligie endogener depressionen: Vergleich der ergebnissen zweier untersuchungen [On the nosology of endogenous depression: Comparison of the results of two studies]. *Arch Psychiatr Nervenkr.* 1968;201:373–386.

13. Lish JD, Dime-Meenan S, Whybrow PC, et al. The national depressive and manic-depressive association (DMDA) survey of bipolar members. *J Affect Disord.* 1994;31:281–294.

14. Hirschfeld RM, Lewis L, Vornik LA. Perceptions and impact of bipolar disorder: How far have we really come? Results of the National Depressive and Manic-Depressive Association 2000 survey of individuals with Bipolar Disorder. *J Clin Psychiatry.* 2003;64:161–174.

15. Ghaemi SN, Sachs GS, Chiou AM, et al. Is bipolar disorder still underdiagnosed? Are antidepressants overutilized? *J Affect Disord.* 1999;52:135–144.

16. Ghaemi SN, Boiman EE, Goodwin FK. Diagnosing bipolar disorder and the effect of antidepressants: A naturalistic study. *J Clin Psychiatry.* 2000;61:804–808.

17. Dilsaver SC, Akiskal HS. High rate of unrecognized bipolar mixed states among destitute Hispanic adolescents referred for "major depressive disorder". *J Affect Disord.* 2005;84:179–186.

18. Perugi G, Micheli C, Akiskal HS, et al. Polarity of the first episode, clinical characteristics, and course of manic depressive illness: A systematic retrospective investigation of 320 bipolar I patients. *Compr Psychiatry.* 2000;41:13–18.

19. Ghaemi N, Sachs GS, Goodwin FK. What is to be done? Controversies in the diagnosis and treatment of manic depressive illness. *World J Biol Psychiatry.* 2000;1:65–74.

20. Ghaemi SN, Ko JY, Goodwin FK. "Cade's disease" and beyond: Misdiagnosis, antidepressant use, and a proposed definition for bipolar spectrum disorder. *Can J Psychiatry.* 2002;47:124–134.

21. Goldberg JF, Whiteside JE. The association between substance abuse and antidepressant-induced mania in bipolar disorder: A preliminary study. *J Clin Psychiatry.* 2002;63:791–795.

22. Henry C, Sorbara F, Lacoste J, et al. Antidepressant-induced mania in bipolar patients: Identification of risk factors. *J Clin Psychiatry.* 2001;62:249–255.

23. Birnbaum HG, Shi L, Dial E, et al. Economic consequences of not recognizing bipolar disorder patients: A cross-sectional descriptive analysis. *J Clin Psychiatry.* 2003;64:1201–1209.

24. Shi L, Thiebaud P, McCombs JS. The impact of unrecognized bipolar disorders for patients treated for depression with antidepressants in the fee-for-services California Medicaid (Medi-Cal) program. *J Affect Disord.* 2004;82:373–383.

25. Rihmer Z, Pestality P. Bipolar II disorder and suicidal behavior. *Psychiatry Clin North Am.* 1999;22:667–673, ix–x.

26. Akiskal HS. *The evolutionary significance of affective temperaments.* http://www.medscape.com/viewwartical/457152. 2003.

27. Akiskal HS. Delineating irritable and hyperthymic variants of the cyclothymic temperament. *J Personal Disord.* 1992;6(4):326–342.

28. Chiaroni P, Hantouche EG, Gouvernet J, et al. The cyclothymic temperament in healthy controls and familially at risk individuals for mood disorder: Endopheno-type for genetic studies? *J Affect Disord.* 2005;85(1–2):135–145.

29. Akiskal HS. *Dysthymia, cyclothymia and related chronic subthreshold mood disorders.* In: Gelder M, Lopez-Ibor J, Andreasen N, eds. *New oxford textbook of psychiatry.* London: Oxford University Press; 2000:736–749.

30. Akiskal HS. The depressive temperament is adapted from Table 16.6-1, "Attributes of depressive and hyperthymic temperaments," Mood disorders: Clinical

features. In: Kaplan HaroldI, Saddock BenjaminJ, eds. *Comprehensive textbook of psychiatry/VI*, Vol. 1. Baltimore: Williams & Wilkins; 1995:1125.

31. Weissman MM, Bruce LM, Leaf PJ. Affective disorders. In: Robins LN, Regier DA, eds. et al. *Psychiatric disorders in america: The epidemiological catchment area study*. New York, NY: The Free Press; 1991:53–80.

32. Kessler RC, McGonagle KA, Zhao S, et al. Lifetime and 12-month prevalence of DSM-III-R psychiatric disorder in the United States: Results from the National Comorbidity Survey. *Arch Gen Psychiatry*. 1994;51:8–19.

33. Akiskal HS. The bipolar spectrum: New concepts in classification and diagnosis. In: Grinspoon L, ed. *Psychiatry update: The American Psychiatric Association Annual Review*, Vol. 2. Washington, DC: American Psychiatric Press; 1983:271–292.

34. Akiskal HS, Bourgeois ML, Angst J, et al. Re-evaluating the prevalence of and diagnostic composition with the broad clinical spectrum of bipolar disorders. *J Affect Disord*. 2000;59:S5–S30.

35. Hirschfeld RM. Bipolar spectrum disorder: Improving its recognition and diagnosis. *J Clin Psychiatry*. 2000;69:S5–S30.

36. Akiskal HS. The prevalent clinical spectrum of bipolar disorders: Beyond DSM-IV. *J Clin Psychopharmacol*. 1996;16(Suppl 1):4S–14S.

37. Akiskal HS, Pinto O. The evolving bipolar spectrum. Prototypes I, II, III, and IV. *Psychatr Clin North Am*. 1999;22:517–534.

38. Klerman GL. The spectrum of mania. *Compr Psychiatry*. 1981;22(1):11–20.

39. Judd LL, Akiskal HS. The prevalence and disability of bipolar spectrum disorders in the US population: Re-analysis of the ECA database taking into account subthreshold cases. *J Affect Disord*. 2003;73(1–2):123–131.

40. Dunner DL. Clinical consequences of under-recognized bipolar spectrum disorder. *Bipolar Disord*. 2003;5(6):456–463.

41. Kelsoe JR. Arguments for the genetic basis of the bipolar spectrum. *J Affect Disord*. 2003;73(1–2):183–197.

42. Angst J, Gamma A. A new bipolar spectrum concept: A brief review. *Bipolar Disord*. 2002;4(Suppl 1):11–14.

43. Klerman GL. The spectrum of mania. *Compr Psychiatry*. 1981;22:11–20.

44. Goodwin G. Hypomania: What's in a name. *Br J Psychiatry*. 2002;191:94–95.

45. Hirschfeld RM. Bipolar spectrum disorder: Improving its recognition and diagnosis. *J Clin Psychiatry*. 1001;62(Suppl 14):5–9.

46. Cassano GB, McElroy SL, Brady K, et al. Current issues in the identification and management of bipolar spectrum disorders in 'special populations'. *J Affect Disord*. 2000;59(Suppl 1):S69–S79.

47. Cassano GB, Dell'Osso L, Frank E, et al. The bipolar spectrum: A clinical reality in search of diagnostic criteria and an assessment methodology. *J Affect Disord*. 1999;54(3):319–328.

48. Papolos DF, Faedda GL, Veit S, et al. Bipolar spectrum disorders in patients diagnosed with velo-cardio-facial syndrome: Does a hemizygous deletion of chromosome 22q11 result in bipolar affective disorder? *Am J Psychiatry*. 1996;153(12):1541–1547.

49. Deltito JA. The effect of valproate on bipolar spectrum temperamental disorders. *J Clin Psychiatry*. 1993;54(8):300–304.

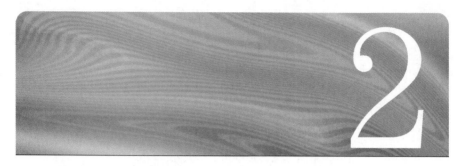

THE GEnES FINGERPRINT—
THE FUTURE

A framework to organize mental health data

For over a century, psychiatry has primarily utilized phenomenology—those occurrences and behaviors that are reported or are observed—as the basis for categorizing mental illness. Kraeplin organized the myriad presentations of mental conditions on the basis of what clinicians could observe and what patients described. Freud postulated mental forces and hypothetical constructs of mental functioning: the ego, id, and superego—entities that could not directly be observed. Psychoanalytic theory inferred their presence, but their loci could not be found. Observable symptoms of mental disorders were the result of interactions between these forces based on therapist observation and patient verbal report. These two major thinkers shaped our conceptualizations and thinking during most of the 20th century. Even as we began to see many mental conditions as "brain illnesses" and began to categorize the symptom lists that make up the *Diagnostic and Statistical Manual of Mental Disorders* (DSM), we continue to rely on phenomenology in formulating our diagnostic categories.

The age of tools

Three major advances—endophenotyping, neuroimaging, and genotyping— are changing our view of the brain, both literally and figuratively, and have begun to take center stage in the field of mental health. We now have the ability to observe neural structure and activity through an expanding series of brain-imaging techniques. We have also begun to genotype and categorize sequences of genetic material that occur with some predictability in both normal and abnormal mental states. Let us look at each of these issues more closely.

Endophenotypes

First used by Gottesman in 1991 and described in more detail by Gottesman and Gould in 2003 (1), the concept of endophenotypes makes a conceptual break with pure phenomenology by focusing on basic elemental concepts. *Endophenotypes*, which can be either biologic or psychological, are intermediate steps between genes and disease states. They are more precise than heterogeneous symptoms such as paranoia, hypomania, and mania, and more exact than symptom clusters or diagnoses such as bipolar I and II disorders or cyclothymia. Endophenotypes are specific, measurable biochemical elements such as the levels of serotonin in brain synapses or amygdala concentrations of catechol O-methyltransferase (COMT). They can also be measurable behavioral traits such as eye movement tracking, auditory startle response, and levels of risk avoidance. Endophenotypes, as more fundamental elements of brain functioning, are potentially *components of, and/or signals for*, diagnosable illnesses.

Critical endophenotypes are those processes related to a disorder but not necessarily symptoms of the disorder. They serve as proxy measures of the trait or disorder being studied, by connecting the external manifestation of the illness to underlying neural circuitry and genetic mechanisms. In order to satisfy criteria that are useful to clinical practice as well as research, critical endophenotypes must be *reliable, stable, narrowly defined, and readily identifiable*. Critical endophenotypes must also have phenotypic and genetic correlations, that is, they are specific to a particular disease (*phenotypic correlation*) and must be connected to underlying genetic mechanisms (*genetic correlation*). Lastly, these genetic and phenotypic correlations must relate to causality.

The concept of endophenotypes is immensely useful in virtually all areas of mental functioning, both normal and abnormal. As we focus on more basic elements of neural functioning, neurocircuitry, neurochemistry, and neurophysiology, there will be less direct focus on phenotypes and phenomenology.

Neuroimaging

Historically, the study of the physical brain was limited to viewing cadaver tissue. Newer processes of imaging the brain have given us *in vivo* methods to view brain structure and functioning. To use magnetic resonance imaging (MRI) as an example, we can noninvasively measure the size of neural tracts and brain centers in both normal and diseased individuals. We are able to statistically compare shapes and sizes of various brain loci between individuals, and in aggregate, between groups of individuals. It is possible to observe changes in brain structure and function over time, either in a quiescent state or when stimulated by biological and environmental perturbations. Functional magnetic resonance imaging (fMRI), single positron emission computerized tomography (SPECT), positron emission tomography (PET), blood oxygen–level–dependent magnetic resonance spectroscopy (BOLD), and other techniques provide us a glimpse of the brain as it operates normally, in disease, or in response to chemical and environmental stimuli. We are able to see what areas "light up" or "turn off" in response to tasks, stresses, and/or restriction of specific stimuli. By combining the images of multiple individuals, we can discern patterns of response and make hypotheses about neural functioning as it relates to disease. As we become more sophisticated in our imaging techniques, procedures such as diffusion tensor imaging (DTI), voxel-based morphometry (VBM), cortical surface–based analysis, and spherical harmonic (SPHARM) detection will explore specific circuits and fiber pathways more deeply and microscopically.

Genetic sequencing

Much work has occurred over the last decade in the area of human genomics. This painstaking $2.7 billion process culminated in 2003 in the accomplishment of the virtual, complete sequencing of the human genome. With the pattern of the genetic code established, processes such as positional cloning (linkage) and allelic association (linkage disequilibrium) as well as other techniques, are now unraveling the roles of specific genes. These roles include protein synthesis, gene regulation, and the downstream effects of gene products on other genes, neural circuits, and end organs in both normal and diseased individuals.

The need for a new system of data organization

Despite endophenotypic and genomic advances, the focus on phenomenology has persisted in our nosology. Although we are no longer constrained to live behind the wall of phenomenology, we continue to categorize psychiatric data with outdated methodology. Although precise phenomenological nosology may be useful, it is hardly sufficient. *No amount of phenomenological precision alone will directly provide precise information about the causality of mental illnesses.* Even laboratory measurement of biochemical endophenotypes and neuroimaging are only likely to be intermediate steps in understanding the causes of mental disorders. *Genetic testing of family inherited patterns and associated linkages as modified by exogenic and epigenetic phenomena, which are then correlated to biochemical endophenotypes and diagnostic syndromes, is a more rapid and accurate path to understanding the causes of mental disorders.* We have spent decades obsessing about minor elements of phenotypic differences. We have clustered our symptoms into "diagnoses." Although perhaps it has been the best that could have been accomplished at the time, this preoccupation is the slowest road to precise causality and symptomatic treatment. It may be less helpful to wrangle about whether a person has bipolar I or bipolar II disorder, or is cyclothymic than to separate and validate target symptoms, especially as we understand critical underlying endophenotypes and neurocircuitry that lead to these symptoms.

Any new classification and model of mental illness will need to conform to the following:

1. Be based on data beyond pure phenomenology.
2. Link biopsychosocial information to genetic and neurophysiologic data.
3. Connect new research data to currently used diagnostic concepts.
4. Facilitate the redefinition and restructuring of current diagnostic concepts and symptoms into more basic elements.
5. Identify consistent data categories that can be organized into a standardized searchable database to identify connections between disparate forms of data regarding a particular disease entity or patient.

A new conceptualization of the continuum from genetics to diagnosis—the GEnES fingerprint

This chapter proposes a new framework for classifying psychiatric data that includes all current information sources in a simple, yet flexible model of mental processes called the *GEnES Fingerprint*. Beyond creating a system for organizing and collecting data on psychiatric *illnesses*, this model also easily adapts itself to providing a biologic and psychological understanding of variations of *personality traits*, both "abnormal" and "normal." It is a model that allows for the input of the effects of nongenetic sources such as environment, parenting, culture, medication, and nonmedication treatments such as psychotherapy and electroconvulsive therapy (ECT).

By spelling "GEnES" this way, the capital letters suggest the four primary types of data in a continuum—Genetics, Exogenic modifications, Endophenotypes, and Syndromes. Each data set is separate, and connects to the others in

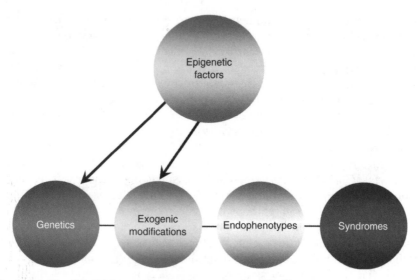

Figure 2.1 The GEnES fingerprint continuum in simplified form.

a linear manner shown in simplified form in Figure 2.1. As the model is elucidated, the GEnES Fingerprint of each psychiatric condition will ultimately be
found to be as unique as a person's fingerprint. This level of precision requires
sophisticated measurement tools. Some disease fingerprints will have more
specificity than others. It will take time to develop each data set and initially
there may be a complete absence of information or only hypothetical links
from one data set to the next.

Further refining of the four primary data types includes the development
of distinct subgroups within each type of data—Genes, Exogenic modifications, Endophenotypes, and Syndromes. These subgroups are labeled with
consistent numbering and abbreviations (see Tables 2.1, 2.2). By labeling data
with its category and subset number, a coherent stable system is created for
researchers, clinicians, and educators to collect, organize, analyze, and teach
mental health data. As information is ultimately connected to elements within
the other data sets, underlying causal mechanisms will be connected to the

TABLE 2.1

Genetic data sets

Genetic 1	Genetic data from genetic epidemiology (allelic association)
Genetic 2	Genetic data from positional cloning (linkage)
Genetic 3	Genetic data elucidated by other methodologies

TABLE 2.2
Endophenotypic data sets

Endophenotypes	
Endo 1	Biochemical
Endo 2	Infectious
Endo 3	Endocrinologic
Endo 4	Neurobehavioral
Endo 5	Inflammatory
Endo 6	Neuroanatomic
Endo 7	Neuropsychological
Endo 8	Cognitive
Endo 9	Immunologic

phenotypic expressions that we call personality traits, personality disorders, diagnoses, and mental illnesses. Although many elements of the fingerprint may not yet be known, the methodology will more clearly direct our thinking toward formulating more precise research, as well as more specific treatments and therapies.

Discussion of the model components
Type 1 data—genetics

In the article *Psychiatric Genetics: a Methodological Critique*, Kendler describes four paradigms of the role of genetic factors in the etiology of psychiatric disorders (2). He describes both basic and advanced genetic epidemiology, which are statistical analyses of an individual's risk or liability of psychiatric illness. These risks result from familial hereditary effects as measured in twin or adoption studies. Other researchers refer to this form of genetic study as *positional cloning* (linkage) in which chromosomal abnormalities located in genome-wide scans are "linked" to a disorder. In this methodology, there is a search for relationships between loci of deoxyribonucleic acid (DNA) nucleotide markers and diseases, as they present in high-risk families. Results yield large chromosomal regions of multiple nucleotide pairs that appear linked to a particular condition, thereby yielding data that is often relatively nonspecific. When further study on these lengthy DNA sequences is congruent (3,4) the genomic region for a particular disease such as bipolar disorder can be narrowed down to a smaller sequence or possibly an isolated nucleotide pair (see Figure 2.2).

Positional cloning (Linkage)
Multiple high-risk families (e.g., with bipolar disorder)

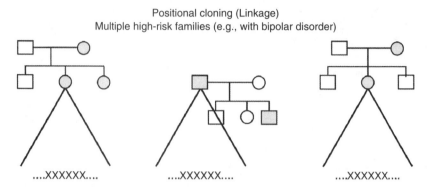

....XXXXXX....   ....XXXXXX....   ...XXXXXX....

Figure 2.2 XXXXXX—An abnormal sequence of DNA (which may be quite large) that appears in multiple families.

Kendler goes on to describe gene identification research that seeks to find more precise areas of genetic abnormality that can then be tied to neuroanatomic or neurophysiologic changes, and ultimately to phenotypes and psychiatric illness. Other researchers use the term *Allelic Association or Linkage Disequilibrium* to describe this type of genetic research. In this methodology, there is a search for relationships between specific changes in a genetic sequence (alleles) that code for the formation of neuroanatomic structures and specific neurophysiologic processes. It is hoped that these expressions of genetic material can be tied to disease phenotypes in general and/or specific psychiatric disorders in unrelated individuals. This data can be potentially exact, but in order to be clinically useful, the data needs to be correlated to endophenotypes and symptoms through the identification of neural circuits related to the disorder (see Figure 2.3).

Each of these paradigms has strengths and weaknesses, and results in different forms of data. They are shown in Table 2.1 in the subsequent text.

Allelic association

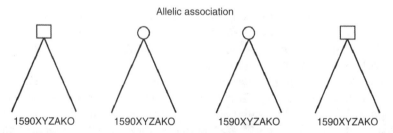

1590XYZAKO   1590XYZAKO   1590XYZAKO   1590XYZAKO

Figure 2.3 After scanning multiple unrelated individuals, gather a group, each of whom has the same allelic abnormality 1590XYZAKO, then hopefully find a disease, endophenotype or trait related to this abnormal sequence.

Genetic 1 and 2 data are useful in understanding the ultimate causality of psychiatric illnesses, neurophysiologic deficits, and strengths. Other methodologies to identify genetic contributions to mental illnesses may be elucidated, and as genetic investigation progresses, further categories will likely be created.

It is tempting to assume that once the genetic coding is elucidated using the methodologies described in the preceding text we will have a clear biologic explanation of bipolar disorder and other psychiatric illnesses. This assumes a rather simplistic genetic model that Kendler has termed *the essentialist gene model* (5). As was put forth in the model of Mendelian genetics, this postulates a very strong connection between disruption of gene function and the ultimate illness. There are, however, many other factors beyond simple genetic coding that may influence the ultimate syndromal outcome of genetic sequences. Although the role of these processes is only rudimentarily understood, the model can account for them.

Gene products are not always consistent—exogenic modifications

As we now know, a variety of influences may impact the ultimate output of genetic DNA. These can include regulation of the quantity of protein made by a gene, modification of the genetic transcription process, and effects of messenger ribonucleic acid (RNA) to name a few. These processes, in different ways, alter the proteins created from the underlying genetic sequencing. If these processes emerge as significant links in the chain from DNA to endophenotypes and syndromes (and it is probable that they do), simply identifying abnormal genetic sequencing may only be part of the causal chain to psychiatric illnesses.

The elements of gene regulation and expression, as well as elements of design, exist "downstream" of the genetic coding itself; that is, beyond DNA. We now know that the "one gene equals one enzyme" hypothesis is untrue. In the human genome, 75% of human genes are alternatively spliced, leading to alternative forms of each gene (6). Because of this, the same gene (i.e., the same nucleotide sequence) can produce different messenger RNA transcripts that can result in different proteins (7).

Gene sequences at a distance and separate from an individual gene locus can regulate the amount of protein produced and the actual nature of the protein produced by that locus. Because of multiple promoters and regulators of gene activity, different protein variants can emerge from a single gene at different times in different tissues. Some of these alterations occur because of different splicing of DNA sequences and others occur because of RNA editing. In the latter activity, the posttranscriptional RNA sequence is edited from that originally encoded by the DNA and can, in some cases, alter the structure of the expressed protein (8).

The impact of RNA in relation to the ultimate expression of proteins adds another layer of complexity to the overly simplistic "one gene–one protein" theory. There are at least two forms of RNA that are noncoding. The first is housekeeping RNA involved in splicing and translation. The second is regulatory RNA that alters gene expression through transcriptional and posttranscriptional mechanisms. In at least one species of plants (9), elements of design reside outside DNA in ancestral RNA. If such elements were found to be present in humans, an entirely new level of information would emerge, which could be further factored into the ultimate explanation and understanding of mental health phenotypes, and would introduce novel sites for mental health treatments.

In the GEnES Fingerprint, these chemical processes that occur "downstream" from DNA sequencing and transcription are combined under the rubric of "exogenic modifications." We are just beginning to understand the role of these various processes in the development of endophenotypes and ultimately in mental health syndromes, but the pictorial model shown in Figures 2.4 and 2.6 highlight the likelihood that a strict gene-to-endophenotype path is unlikely. Although it remains purely speculative at this time in our understanding, one can postulate that the epigenetic factors shown in this diagram exert their influence at least in part through these exogenic mechanisms that modify the protein output from DNA. In this way, the epigenetic factors influence the emergence of endophenotypes and ultimately syndromes.

Scientific advancement is dependent on expanding the current purely phenomenologic model to one that incorporates the other factors. There

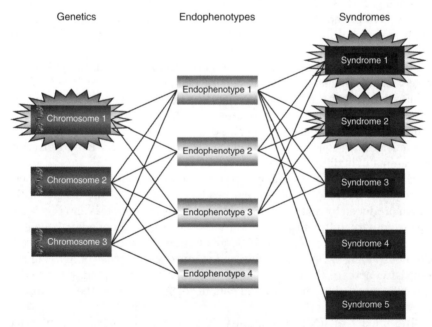

Figure 2.4 Multiple gene–endophenotype—syndrome connections.

is little doubt that as we collect, organize, compare, and connect various elements of biologic and psychological data, refinements of the GEnES model or other novel models will emerge. The flexibility of the GEnES Fingerprint model is that it allows for input and refinement that can easily be incorporated as new information is uncovered.

Endophenotypes

As defined in the preceding text, endophenotypes are intermediate, more basic steps between genes and diseases. This type of data is further broken down into subtypes as shown in Table 2.2 and discussed in the subsequent text. This section presents examples of potential endophenotypes with some current research validity; however, no attempt is made to suggest that these are, in fact, criteria which will ultimately have clinical, heuristic, or therapeutic usefulness. As discussed later, there are relatively few endophenotypes that specifically relate to elevated mood. Therefore, illustrative examples are presented from other various mental conditions and research.

It is predictable that data will fit several endophenotypes and will be catalogued in more than one location within the model. One would expect that as data sources are entered, recorded, and connected, further refinements and subtyping of endophenotypes will occur.

Biochemical endophenotypes

Examples include COMT activity in patients with rapid cycling bipolar disorder (10) or basal and stimulated cortical gamma-aminobutyric acid (GABA) and calcium levels in olfactory receptor neurons of individuals with bipolar disorder (11). Here, the levels of serotonin resulting from a mutation in the gene for human tryptophan hydroxylase-2 (12) and the pituitary response of adrenocorticotropic hormone (ACTH) in the brain to dexamethasone are also catalogued (13).

Infectious endophenotypes

Although in its infancy, PITAND (pediatric infectious triggered autoimmune neuropsychiatric disorders) data (14,15) and data that relates to the possibility of an infectious cause for autism (16) are categorized here.

Endocrinologic endophenotypes

This subcategory includes all data regarding the effects of endocrine systems in the body such as the thyroid, adrenal glands, and other hormone-secreting systems. The effects of insulin deficiency on Alzheimer's disease (17), the psychological effects of excess glucocorticoids on psychological states in Cushing's syndrome (18), and research on psychosexual development and androgen insensitivity syndrome (19) can also be categorized here.

Neurobehavioral endophenotypes

Examples of information in this category include data on the behavioral effects of sleep deprivation and recovery sleep (20), tic frequency in Tourette's syndrome (21) and behavioral reactions to anhedonia (22).

Inflammatory endophenotypes

This category includes data such as the effect of omega-3 fatty acids and uridine as potential protectors against mood disorders (23) and research associating the CRH-1 receptor genotypes with antidepressant response and stress-inflammatory pathways (15).

Neuroanatomic endophenotypes

Data here includes gross measurement of brain structures such as hippocampal and superior temporal gyrus volumes, as well as measurement of dopamine and serotonin transporter densities. Also included are the effects of neurologic and non-neurologic illnesses (e.g., cancer, multiple sclerosis, blunt brain trauma, and others). Also listed are the neuroanatomic correlates of the psychopathologic components of major depressive disorder (24), the amount, distribution and ratio of complexin I and II in the hippocampi of schizophrenics (25), and the balance between excitatory parietal cell firing and GABA-mediated inhibition (26).

Neuropsychological endophenotypes

Examples here include assessment of P50 suppression and prepulse inhibition of startle response (27) and measurements of emotional processing such as performance on the Affective Go/No Go test in the face of chronic methylenedioxymethamphetamine (MDMA "ecstasy") use (28). This subgroup also includes configured self-reports such as reports of subjective experiences (29), the effect of personality traits on other endophenotypes or behaviors such as suicidal actions (30,31) and using a self-report depression scale to identify remission (32). Data on neuropsychological impairments in tasks measuring episodic memory, verbal fluency, psychomotor speed, and executive functioning in anxious patients (33) would be listed here as well as under the cognitive subtype.

Cognitive endophenotypes

Data here includes tests of visual executive processing and selective attention indicated by continuous performance tasks such as the forced choice visual oddball task (34). Additionally, cognitive testing results of individuals at high risk for schizophrenia or Alzheimer's disease, such as assessments of working memory, cognitive dysmetria, and the fMRI of persons performing working memory tasks (35) are categorized here. Information about the latter can include scores on the Boston Naming Test and the Block Design subtest of the Wechsler Intelligence Scale for children-Revised (36).

Immunologic endophenotypes

Here, information about the neural response to infectious agents, vaccinations, and autoimmune responses of the body are listed. Examples include data related to the PANDAS (psychiatric autoimmune neuropsychiatric disorders associated with streptococcal infections) and their possible connection to obsessive-compulsive disorder (OCD) and tic disorders such as Tourette's syndrome (37). Identifying GABAergic synapses in the brain using antisera to GABA (38), the possibility of "vaccinating" individuals against a neurodegenerative disorder such as Alzheimer's disease (39) and immunoglobulin treatment strategies for autism (40–42) are also categorized here.

Other endophenotypes

Before moving on to the concepts of syndromes as defined in this model, it must be mentioned that there are considerable psychiatric data that fall under the rubric of *measurement* of endophenotypes. These data are not endophenotypes *per se* but are data generated by tools that document the presence of, and quantify the extent of endophenotypes in humans and animals. There are five such data types, as shown in Table 2.3.

Imaging

These data include a variety of neuroimaging results from currently used and potentially new neuroimaging technology, such as SPECT, PET, fMRI, BOLD, VBM scans, and others. There can be scans of individuals, composite data from multiple scans of a group of individuals, or comparative scans of the same individual at different times and under differing conditions.

TABLE 2.3
Measurements of endophenotypes

Imaging
Electrophysiologic measurements
Data from pharmacologic intervention
Animal models
Other miscellaneous measurements

Specific examples are fMRI data related to smooth pursuit eye movement tasks in schizophrenia when nicotine is introduced (43), MRI hyperintensities in individuals with depression (44), PET scans during presleep wakefulness and non-REM (rapid eye movement) sleep (45), SPECT scans of dopamine transporter densities in patients with OCD (46), and voxel-based morphometry of gray matter in patients with bipolar disorder (47).

Electrophysiologic measurements

These data include baseline or sleep-deprived electroencephalogram (EEG) tracings, evoked potential, and other measurements of brain electrical activity in the resting or stimulated state. Examples could also include eye-tracking dysfunction and deficits in P50 event-related potential inhibition in the auditory-click-conditioning test paradigm and saccadic inhibition deficits (48) as well as measurement of auditory startle response through eye blink electromyograms and skin conductance response (49).

Effects of pharmacologic interventions

This subcategory contains information relating to the effects of specific pharmacologic agents on brain functioning, neurophysiologic or neuroanatomic substrates. It can be organized by both specific medications and groupings of medications (if the latter are shown to provide consistently similar neural effects). For example, impaired GABA neural response to acute benzodiazepine administration (50), the occurrence of tachyphylaxis (loss of effect) during antidepressant treatment (51) and the safety profile of various medications in the pregnant patient are categorized in this subtype. Also codified here would be the rates of response of anxiety and depression measures in patients to paroxetine (52) or the prediction of drug response based on genetic polymorphisms (53). This latter procedure connects pharmacologic response rates to genetic haplotypes.

Animal models

Information derived from examination of animal behavior, anatomy, and physiology are categorized here. Examples could include variable foraging demand (54), models of social subordination and dominance (55), and models of animal attachment (56–58). Information on the effects of green fluorescent protein in the neurons of simple animals such as the *Aequorea Victoria* jelly fish, allowing the observation of cellular processes as they occur (59) can also be listed here. These animal models could then be connected with other biochemical endophenotypes such as levels of corticotropin-releasing factor and *N*-acetyl aspartate (60).

Other measurements of endophenotypes

Once clearly identified, many endophenotypes will permit direct testing with current and as-yet-to-be-discovered measurement techniques. Other data sources are *indirect* measures of endophenotypes. For example, a test of blood or cerebrospinal fluid that reliably tracks and measures synthesis or degradation of a neural protein is categorized here. Another example would be the measurement of β arrestin-1 in leukocytes (61). Measurements of levels of COMT activity in red blood cells, the possible connection to COMT activity in the brain, and its role in schizophrenia, OCD, or other mental health illnesses would be categorized here. Other external measurements such as a glucose tolerance test, measurement of pulse and blood pressure, polysomnography, and serum reactivity to human immunodeficiency virus (HIV) would also be listed in this grouping. Similarly, broad-spectrum psychological measures such as the elements of a neuropsychological testing battery are listed under this category.

Syndromes

The fourth principle element in the GEnES Fingerprint is labeled as "syndromes." Medical practice has commonly come to identify the concept of "syndrome" with a disorder, abnormality, or illness. Specifically, we often define a syndrome as a group of signs and symptoms that are together characteristic or indicative of a specific disease (62). Used as its only meaning, however, this is an artificial narrowing of the term, which was derived from the original Greek root *syndrome*—meaning "concurrence" and *sundromos* meaning "running together."

When one looks at other definitions of "syndrome" or definitions from nonmedical dictionaries, one finds a broadening of meaning. For example, a syndrome is:

> *"A distinctive or characteristic pattern of behavior: the syndrome of conspicuous consumption in wealthy suburbs" or "the feast-or-famine syndrome of big business" (63),*

> *"A distinctive or characteristic pattern or behavior" (62).*

It is within the context of these latter definitions that the term *syndrome* is used in the GEnES Fingerprint model. Syndrome does not refer exclusively to an illness or diagnosis, but refers equally to a set of behaviors or characteristics that have a positive or neutral meaning. This is not to suggest that the term *syndrome* will not, or should not, be used in the context of mental health illnesses or conditions. The terms *Tourette's syndrome, Gulf War syndrome, fetal alcohol syndrome,* and Down's syndrome, to name a few, are all valid terms and will remain so. "Syndrome" is simply not *solely* used in this model with a negative or illness connotation.

Within the GEnES Fingerprint, therefore, concepts traditionally labeled as diagnoses, illnesses, personality traits, complex behaviors, and complex symptoms would all fall under a broadened definition of "syndrome." By doing so, the distinction between illness and normalcy is blurred. There are many traits, behaviors, and collections of traits that may have both positive and negative valence, or be seen as both assets and liabilities. Individuals may have a personality bias or predisposition that is not necessarily categorized as illness, but may in certain circumstances leave an individual vulnerable to illness or functional disability, given the presence of other circumstances or precipitants. A trait at one level of intensity could, in the absence of other factors, serve as a strength, but when carried to an extreme, become a liability. For example, the ability to attend to detail and insist on accuracy and completeness is a trait often associated with productive, high-achieving individuals. Taken to extreme or not held in check, this same trait is a common symptom of OCD.

Rather than refer arbitrarily to the concepts of "illness" or "disease" with all the associated negative connotations, and "normal" with its supposed positive connotations, this model views all individuals as a mix of unique biologic, behavioral, and psychological traits with underpinnings of genetic patterns and neural circuitry, modified by epigenetic factors. In removing automatic designations and assigned valences used in current phenotypic classifications, we can choose to identify specific traits or collections of traits by the presence of, and intensity of functional impairment. Without predetermined prejudice, syndromes include underlying traits that may lie dormant or become visible only under provocation, which could predict a higher likelihood of "disease" when coexisting with other vulnerabilities, or are brought into the open by environmental or internal precipitants.

There are, of course, other terms that could be used for this data such as "vulnerabilities," "assets," "strengths," "resiliency," "positive traits," "personality," "temperament," "tendencies," "outcomes," or others. In this model, these are all the phenotypic expressions of underlying biologic processes that need not be artificially separated into categories with positive or negative valence. For example, is there a connection between what we now call hyperthymic temperament, cyclothymia, or bipolar disorder? Where is the line of demarcation between a productive outcome and disease? What is the connection, if any, between intelligence, autism, and the "idiot-savant?" What distinction can be made between a person who, in a manic psychosis, mentally recalls the words and tone of his/her therapist for self-soothing, and the person who proclaims "Mary, the Mother of God is telling me what to do?"

By using the word syndrome in its broadest sense, we hopefully leave behind our arbitrary assessment of various traits and behaviors, which in many ways has hampered our understanding of the human brain processes, the changes that can occur in these processes, and how these changes can affect human behavior. Every behavior, mental trait, and activity begins as an underlying biologic mechanism initiated by genetic coding. The nature and quantity of protein output from genetic coding is modified by exogenic mechanisms that alter, stimulate, minimize, or silence genetic output and protein production. Epigenetic factors including culture, physical and psychological environment, gender, and treatment interventions can significantly affect the ultimate outcome of this process, likely through exogenic mechanisms. Proteins act on receptors, neurons, neural circuits, and other genes to produce intermediate neurophysiologic responses or traits that we label endophenotypes. When endophenotypic clusters show predictability and consistency, they are labeled as syndromes. Syndromes may be problematic, neutral and/or beneficial to the individual depending on whether they create mild, moderate, or significant functional impairment, are neutral and/or protect against impairment.

Syndromes that create functional impairment are labeled as illnesses or diseases and become the target for our psychiatric interventions. Some endophenotypic syndromes may signal vulnerability to functional impairment or illness, but only in the presence of one or more precipitating environmental or biologic events. Other syndromes that provide resistance to impairment or improve functioning are syndromes of strength and resiliency.

This model also leaves open the possibility that there are a variety of combinations of internal or external pathways from genes to circuits and endophenotypes that can produce similar-appearing outward, phenotypic syndromes, e.g., grieving and depression or hyperthymic temperament and hypomania. The relationships between phenotypes with similar outward appearances and the genetics/neural circuitry that underlie them need to be determined through research and clinical understanding.

The complexity of gene abnormalities, endophenotypes, and behavioral phenotypes has been outlined by deGeus (64). In this schematic drawing, shown in Figure 2.5, genetic abnormalities are listed as quantitative trait loci (QTL) and indicate that one genetic abnormality can lead to several endophenotypes. Multiple endophenotypes and abnormalities may be necessary for the development of a behavioral phenotype (i.e., a mental illness or other cognitive or affective dysfunction).

In Figure 2.4, we have seen a more generalized schematic diagram of this within the GEnES Fingerprint.

It is important to note that this model does not in any way diminish the effect of parenting, interpersonal support, psychotherapy, friendship, or a myriad other activities that may strongly affect mental and emotional functioning. The model simply postulates that once genetic coding is in place, certain neural and neurobiologic circuits and activities are set in motion. There may be many events—intrauterine, developmental, cultural, or experiential—that can modify the biologic structure and products of gene expression and the ultimate phenotypic expressions of these biologic processes. It is as yet unproved if these influences create their effects through specific exogenic modifications and/or other mechanisms.

Categorizing syndromes

It is tempting to leave the concept of phenotypic expressions broadly defined as *syndromes* because our understanding of the connection between neural

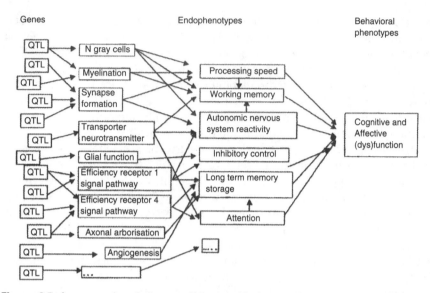

Figure 2.5 An example of the possible genetic interactions on a specific set of behaviors—cognitive and affective function/dysfunction (Used with permission).

behaviors, complex behaviors, psychological traits, temperament, personality, symptoms, and diagnoses is at best, rudimentary. However, this simplicity is not helpful because it isolates emerging genetic and endophenotypic data from the large body of phenotypic categorizations (e.g., "diagnoses") already created and organized.

Retaining a definition of syndromes that is overly broad, therefore, is not most helpful. Subcategorization of the "syndrome" portion of the model is necessary in order to relate newer forms of data to our current concepts of personality, temperament, symptoms, and diagnoses.

It might also be tempting to simply divide syndromes into three parts—syndromes with documented significant functional impairment (diseases); syndromes with no consistent, observable functional impairment (traits and personality); and syndromes that provide resilience. This separation, too, is limiting and assumes *a priori* that we know with certainty which traits and conditions are helpful to the individual and which are harmful or pathologic. Therefore, in this model, phenotypic syndromes are divided into six subtypes as shown in Table 2.4 and elaborated subsequently.

Behaviors

Behaviors can be simple or complex. Examples of simple behaviors might include actions such as nodding one's head, blinking one's eye, or reflex withdrawal from a painful stimulus. Complex human behaviors may be

TABLE 2.4
Syndromes

Syndrome 1	Behaviors
Syndrome 2	Neuropsychological activities
Syndrome 3	Diseases/diagnoses
Syndrome 4	Temperament and personality
Syndrome 5	Disease vulnerability
Syndrome 6	Resiliency and strengths

exemplified by multiple physical activities such as simultaneously gripping an object while balancing a plate on one's head or performing activities that simultaneously involve both physical and mental activities such as daydreaming while jogging. Additionally, unified activities with physical, cognitive, and emotional elements occur simultaneously with a wide variety of mental and physical skills. Examples include mentally composing and writing a poignant letter at a computer keyboard or enjoying the music produced as one plays the violin.

Even as some behaviors appear "simple," the line of distinction between simple and complex is likely to be indistinct. As our knowledge expands, it may prove true that there are few truly "simple" behaviors that cannot be broken down into more elemental components.

Neuropsychological activities

Neuropsychological activities are certain to be comprised of multiple elements from seemingly simple activities such as hearing a sound, visualizing an image, or remembering an experience, to apparently more complex activities such as assembling a jigsaw puzzle and dreaming. These functions require the interplay of a variety of brain systems and are presumably mediated through multiple endophenotypes. Even with our limited current information, it is likely that there is no such thing as a truly "simple" neuropsychological activity.

Diseases/diagnoses

The term *disease* remains as it has been defined both by scientific and common usage:

> *"An impairment of health or a condition of abnormal functioning"* (65).

> *"A pathological condition of the body that presents a group of clinical signs, symptoms, and laboratory findings peculiar to and setting the condition apart as an abnormal entity differing from other normal or pathological conditions"* (66).

The term *diagnosis* again remains consistent with our common usage:

"The name of a disease or condition" (67)

"Identification of a disease or disorder based on review of signs, symptoms, and laboratory findings" (68).

Temperament and personality

The concept of *temperament* is defined as follows:

"A person's typical way of responding to his or her environment" (69) or

"A conceptual term that categorizes a functionally significant component of an individual psychological structure. It is not immutable but it shows consistency over time and also a degree of cross-situational consistency" (70).

Personality is the distinctive constellation of relatively stable behaviors, thoughts, motives, and emotions which characterize an individual or

"The complex of all the attributes—behavioral, temperamental, emotional, and mental—that characterize a unique individual" (65).

There is considerable overlap between the terms *temperament* and *personality*. Many might use "personality" in a broader, more global sense. It is difficult to maintain a definitive boundary between these two concepts, if indeed one exists.

Disease vulnerability

When used in the context of the syndrome portion of the GEnES Fingerprint model, the term *disease vulnerability* describes behavioral or psychological traits that could be simple or complex, and indicate with replicable reliability a higher likelihood to develop symptoms or specific diseases. It is possible within the model that there may be basic, measurable neuroanatomic or neurophysiologic *endophenotypes* that can themselves mark vulnerability to disease. To the extent that these more basic endophenotypes become delineated, they are likely to be more reliable markers of disease vulnerability than the complex, perhaps heterogeneous, phenotypic syndromal observations recorded as disease vulnerabilities recorded in this portion of the model.

Resiliency and strengths

Although a broad generalization, data categorized under resiliency and strengths is the opposite of disease vulnerability. These behavioral or psychological traits could be simple or complex, and show replicable reliability to resist specific symptoms or diseases, or demonstrate a resistance to mental disorders in general. Traits such as genetic and learned self-regulation of emotion, attachment behaviors, positive self-concept, altruism, social support, the ability to disclose emotions, and the ability to convert helplessness into learned helpfulness are included under this category (71–73).

Epigenetic factors

Even with the assumption that there is a linear relationship between genetics and basic endophenotypes, almost certainly the ultimate phenotypic expressions of the conditions that we label as psychiatric illnesses are affected by other factors that cannot be easily explained linearly from genetics (Figure 2.2). The so-called "epigenetic factors" have a significant effect on the ultimate expression of mental health phenotypes. For purposes of this model, epigenetic factors are broad overlying factors that exist beyond the level of DNA coding. As is pictured in Figures 2.6 and 2.7, these factors envelop and surround the path from genes to syndromes. Although there is little data, it is reasonable to speculate that these epigenetic factors will ultimately be found to exert their influence through exogenic mechanisms. These epigenetic factors would therefore affect protein production through stimulation, regulation, or alteration of gene products.

There are at least five major epigenetic factors that can have significant effects on the prevalence or presentation of mental illnesses, listed in Table 2.5.

In the GEnES Fingerprint model, epigenetic factors may be facilitative, neutral, or preventative in the expression of illness. As can be seen in Figure 2.7, epigenetic elements can affect and join the linear expression from genes to endophenotypes to phenotypes.

In this model, there are few direct linear gene-to-phenotype mental health conditions that are not modified, at least in part, by other factors. There are "many-to-many" connections within the GEnES Fingerprint and these interconnecting pieces are surrounded and impacted by epigenetic factors. In pictorial representation, this model resembles the anatomy of a neuron with a series of axons and dendrites surrounded by a myelin sheath. At one end there are multiple genes with their potential recombinations. At the other end are multiple outputs or syndromes.

Culture

Cultural factors have a significant impact on the occurrence and presentation of various mental health phenotypes. Although recently questioned (74), a commonly accepted example has been the incidence of anorexia and bulimia in Western cultures as compared with non-Western cultures (75,76). Another example is culturally based differences in the incidence of suicide and assisted suicide (77,78).

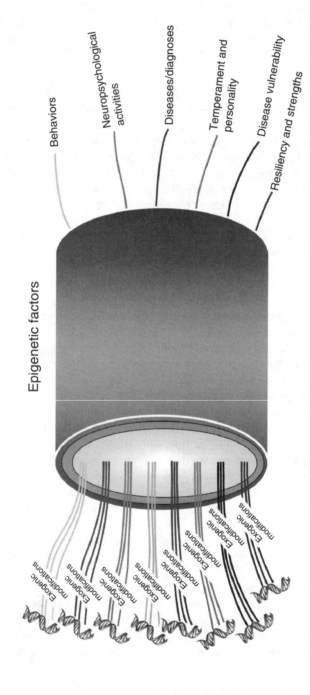

Figure 2.6 Epigenetic factors envelop the linear progression and likely exert their effects through exogenic modifications.

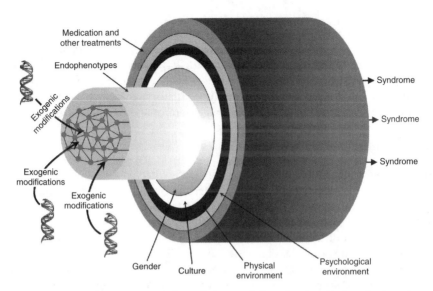

Figure 2.7 Magnified cross section of the model at the level of endophenotypes showing epigenetic factors.

Physical environment

The physical environment consists of multiple elements affecting mental illness. These include elements of infectious agents, environmental pollutants or other substances, both man-made and natural. These biologic agents and processes could be present in the womb or at any point throughout the course of the individual's history. Some of these events could be categorized under specific endophenotypes listed as infectious or biochemical, whereas some substances may affect multiple endophenotypes simultaneously or sequentially. Common examples are the effects of maternal alcohol abuse on fetal psychological outcome, the onset of an HIV infection, and the ingestion of a toxin or exposure to radiation. Such biologic factors could be one-time or chronic events.

TABLE 2.5
Epigenetic influences

Cultural factors
Physical environment
Psychological environment
Medication and other treatments
Gender

Psychological environment

An individual's psychological environment is enormously varied and may include negative elements, such as stressful life experiences, abusive parenting, or acute psychological trauma. Positive events also occur including praise and encouragement, empathy, understanding, supportive human relationships, meditation, prayer, and successful management of stressful situations.

Medication and other treatments

Although possibly subsumed under the rubric of physical environment, in this model the issues of medication and treatments are identified separately. Because of its importance in current psychiatry, medication is then identified and categorized as a separate factor when organizing data.

Other nonmedication forms of treatment are also categorized here. These include ECT, transcranial magnetic stimulation, vagal nerve stimulation, acupuncture, biofeedback, and psychotherapy. Also included are therapeutic use of music and sound, herbal treatments, diet, massage, and exercise.

Gender

Gender can be considered either genetic or epigenetic. Genetic coding determines gender and its corresponding hormone and endocrine differences. However, there are factors of gender that appear to be outside of the linear genes-to-phenotype sequence. For example, in Western culture, the incidence of anorexia and bulimia is markedly higher in women when compared with that in men (79). Although possible, it is not likely that this is a totally genetic issue, and may more likely reflect issues of Western emphasis on slimness and physical attractiveness of women.

Further examples of gender-based differences are cited in quotations from World Health Organization statistics.

> *"Gender-specific risk factors for common mental disorders that disproportionately affect women include gender-based violence, socioeconomic disadvantage, low income and income inequality, low or subordinate social status and rank, and unremitting responsibility for the care of others. The high prevalence of sexual violence to which women are exposed and the correspondingly high rate of post-traumatic stress disorder (PTSD) following such violence, renders women the largest single group of people affected by this disorder." "Conversely, the lifetime prevalence rate for alcohol dependence is more than twice as high in men as in women" (80).*

These gender disparities cannot be easily explained by genetic factors alone with our current level of understanding.

Yang et al. at UCLA (University of California, Los Angeles) (81) looked at patterns of gene expression in >23,000 genes in mice. The group measured the expression level in tissues from various organs, including brain, liver, fat, and muscle in men and women. There were striking and measurable differences in more than half the number of the gene's expression patterns between men and women. Although not yet studied directly in humans, because mice and humans share 99% of their genes, it is tantalizing to assume that similar gender differences occur in humans. If proved, it could explain the gender differences of the sexes to disease susceptibility and reaction to medications.

This model is complex, but likely reflects the level of intricacy associated with human mental health conditions. Fortunately the ability to store, organize, and categorize GEnES Fingerprint data can be managed through a large single computerized database. Using a sophisticated search program, elements of the database, including specific items of genetics, exogenic modification, endophenotypes, epigenetic factors, and syndromes could easily be sorted and retrieved. Computer-generated models could thereby identify potential connections between seemingly disparate data.

A growth analogy

One way to think of the production and causation of normal psychological traits and strengths as well as psychiatric disease is the analogy of growth from seeds. Seeds (both healthy and with abnormalities of plant genetic material) contain the potential blueprints for a final plant product. The seeds are a necessary, but not sufficient, condition for normal plant production. In addition to the seeds, other elements may significantly affect whether a "normal" outcome occurs, disease resiliency is present, or disease emerges. Elements such as nutrients, water, and temperature can both foster the growth of normal healthy plants and support abnormal unhealthy development (weeds, parasites, symbiotic relationships). Light, water, nutrients, and ambient temperature, too, are necessary but insufficient elements alone for the growth of plants.

There is direct analogy to the production of healthy psychological traits and psychiatric disease. Genetic material and epigenetic factors are both necessary but insufficient alone for the development of normal psychological behaviors and psychiatric illness.

If certain conditions are present (i.e., a sufficient number of abnormal genes), a psychiatric disorder may emerge spontaneously. It is possible, however, that other factors may have a significant effect either positively or negatively on the way a syndrome may emerge—either normal psychological behaviors or a psychiatric disorder. These conditions are the epigenetic factors noted earlier—gender, psychological environment, physical environment, and various treatments. In this analogy these epigenetic factors correspond to elements such as amount of sunshine, temperature, and the amount of tending or neglect given to the sown seeds. When conditions are favorable (helpful parenting and positive support for ego development) even inferior seeds can result in mild disease or potentially none at all. A toxic psychological environment (e.g., neglectful or abusive parenting or harmful physiologic environments such as the presence of acquired immunodeficiency syndrome (AIDS) or other viruses, maternal fetal alcohol, or drug usage) in an infant or young child may negatively influence a healthy genetic profile to produce illness. Treatments including psychotherapy, medication, or other physiologic treatments, are analogous to applying fertilizer, weeding the garden, or pruning so that healthy plants are encouraged and disease is neutralized.

Limitations of the model

As with all models, the GEnES Fingerprint, although innovative, has limitations. There are at least three elements that are not easily incorporated into the GEnES Fingerprint model as currently postulated. First, there is the concept of *brain plasticity*. We understand that chemical elements affect the growth and/or destruction of neurons. Brain-derived neurotrophic factor (BDNF) stimulates brain cell growth. Excess glutamate, for example, has a neurocytotoxic effect. Our understanding of how the brain repairs or regenerates damaged or otherwise faulty neurons and circuits is still in its infancy. Some epigenetic factors discussed earlier, may be partially responsible for neural plasticity, but there may be many other as yet unidentified factors in the development of neuropsychological processes.

A second modifier in this model is the concept of *critical periods* in brain development. Even if a linear model of genes to endophenotypes as modified by epigenetic factors is found to be accurate in explaining phenotypic diseases, the concept of timing of epigenetic events may be crucial to the ultimate outcome. It remains to be seen if, and how, the timing of elements such as environmental stress, non-neural hormones, infection, toxins, and other potential influences could affect the ultimate manifestation of symptoms and illness.

Third, the concept of network theory as it applies to brain neural functioning is only beginning to be explored (82). Although a linear genes–endophenotypes model may be accurate up to a point, it is possible that ultimate phenotypic syndromal expressions of mental illnesses are understood only within the concept of a *neural network*.

Briefly, a neural network is a connection of smaller processing units typically consisting of an interconnected set of nodes. The network's functioning is only understood through the interconnections of these smaller, simpler nodes or processing units. Some units are nodes of input and others are nodes of output. In a single-layer model of a neural network, there is one layer of output nodes in which the outputs of these components are given selective "weights." Depending on the "weight" given to each node, the resulting outcomes may be different. The brain is considerably more complex than a single layer and almost certainly has multiple layers of nodes in which one layer has connections to the neurons of multiple other layers.

A more precise understanding of many neural processes including learning, memory, cognitive and emotional storage, recollection and regulation, and the dysfunctions of these processes may ultimately be best viewed through the concept of a neural network (83). It is possible, and perhaps even probable, that network theory and operation are crucial to understanding brain function. Until such time as these ideas are clarified, however, elements of neural functioning can begin to be elucidated through the GEnES Fingerprint model. The elements categorized by this model may be found to provide the building blocks of any such network. If, in fact, neural networks are crucial to the development of psychiatric disease, the *GEnES* Fingerprint model would become the *GENES* Fingerprint.

Hypomania as seen through the GEnES fingerprint

As with any mental condition in GEnES Fingerprint model, the concepts of hyperthymic temperament, hypomania, mania, bipolar I and bipolar II disorders, and cyclothymia are categorized as syndromes. Targeted research should then focus on isolating and identifying critical endophenotypes of these syndromes. It has already been postulated by Akiskal, Angst, Bennazzi, and others that overactivity should be considered a behavioral endophenotype that is central to the concepts of hypomania. The Young Mania Rating Scale (YMRS), long used as a staple for measuring elevated mood, already suggests that irritability and elevated mood are central elements to our concept of hypomania. It is as yet unclear whether these will be defined as *symptomatic syndromes*, or *behavioral endophenotypes*. There is little doubt that we must further define these symptoms in ways to make them more precise. Ultimately, we will look for biologic markers and/or biochemical measures, which reliably accompany or produce such symptoms as overactivity, irritability, grandiosity, and rapidity of thought. These can then be labeled as critical endophenotypes of hypomania.

The new biology as it applies to elevated mood

Having outlined the GEnES Fingerprint system, within which genetic, neurobehavioral, and endophenotypic data can be categorized, the last part of this chapter identifies some of the significant elements of research on elevated mood that have been completed to date. As with many areas of investigation about elevated mood, there is virtually no specific research on hypomania alone. Therefore the information cited in this section relates primarily to patients with bipolar I disorder. This data is broadly divided into two sections—first, research on specific genetic localization and second, other possible endophenotypic connections between genes and our current phenotypic categorizations of elevated mood.

The genetics of elevated mood

Some of the most promising research into the genetic haplotype relationship to elevated mood is work at the University of California at San Diego, the University of British Columbia, and the University of Cincinnati, all of which participate in an eight-site consortium, sponsored by the National Institute of Mental Health (NIMH). So far, this consortium has a database of more than 700 families with bipolar disorder and has begun gene mapping, seeking areas of promising sites of potential genetic abnormality.

The region at 22q11 is of particular interest as it regulates the efficiency of all synaptic transmission by mediating the process of homologous desensitization (84). Homologous desensitization occurs when a receptor is stimulated by a neurotransmitter at high levels and/or for prolonged periods of time, resulting in that receptor becoming less sensitive to that neurotransmitter. This process is mediated in part by *G-protein receptor kinase 3 (GRK3)*. The locus for the gene coding of GRK3 shows a peak at the 22q11 region. This region was also implicated in a genome survey of 20 families with bipolar disorder and has been supported by further research using methamphetamine in rats as a model for bipolar disorder. When amphetamine is given to rats, the highest increase in expression is exactly at the GRK3 locus. Taken together, this data suggests that there may be a regulatory mutation at or near the GRK3 promoter that causes GRK3 to fail to be expressed when dopamine stimulates receptors in the brain. This results in supersensitivity to dopamine, which has been a long-held hypothesis for bipolar disorder.

A second area of susceptibility is postulated on chromosome 12q23–q24 (85). A study evaluated two families that share the pedigree of bipolar disorder and a rare skin disease, Darier's disease. Genetic samples were taken from these two families and analyzed for linkage and haplotype information from the most severely affected individuals. Several areas of interest were identified, most notably 12q23–12q24. Although a highly penetrant autosomal dominant, disease-conferring mutation was not found, the region continues to be an area of significant interest.

A large family with cosegregation of bipolar disorder and autosomal dominant medullary cystic kidney disease has been identified. It is known that there are two loci of medullary cystic kidney disease in the regions of chromosomes 1 and 16, the same chromosomes that were previously linked to bipolar disorder and schizophrenia (86). Although the exact genetics have yet to be examined in detail, this family may provide a fertile ground for further genetic study and possible identification of susceptible areas of genetic mutation leading to bipolar disorder.

Researchers have recently identified a genetic region associated not only with bipolar disorder and schizophrenia, but also one that appears to encode for a particular symptom of more severe elevated mood—namely, persecutory delusions. Schulze et al. (87), building on previous research (88,89), showed an association of the D-amino oxidase activator locus (DAOA/G30) with these delusions. Schulze evaluated genetic profiles of 300 German and 294 Polish patients with bipolar disorder with persecutory delusions. Observing four single nucleotide polymorphisms and 21 specific symptoms of psychosis, a positive association on chromosome locus 13q34 was identified. This finding has subsequently been qualified, showing congruence only between those with bipolar disorder/schizophrenia who have experienced a major mood disorder.

A final area of genetic interest is that region which codes for the protein *neuroregulin-1* (*NRG-1*). Although initial research with NRG-1 has primarily focused on schizophrenia, Green et al. (90) have begun to investigate whether the NRG-1 haplotype is more common in patients with bipolar disorder who have mood-incongruent psychotic symptoms. This haplotype was found to be significantly more common in the bipolar group (1.4:1) and especially common in those patients with bipolar disorder who had mood-incongruent psychotic symptoms (1.7:1). This suggests that NRG-1 may play a key role in the emergence of certain forms of psychosis, and may form a link between a variety of illnesses including bipolar disorder, psychotic depression, and schizophrenia.

In addition to the specific sites detailed, possible promising genetic areas of linkage for bipolar disorder have been postulated at 13q, 10p, 16p, 21q, 4q31, 6q24 (91), 4q332 and 16p12 (92), and 8q (93).

Interestingly, to date, genes that regulate the serotonin receptor, so often associated with depression and affective disorders in general, cannot consistently be associated with bipolar disorder (94–97).

Neurobiology, neurocircuits, and other biologic endophenotypes

A scattering of early and tantalizing studies of various neurocircuits and biochemical processes as they relate to elevated mood and bipolar disorder are beginning to emerge.

A variety of sources reviewed by Marchand et al. (89) suggest that *abnormalities in the frontal–subcortical circuit* are present repetitively in a variety of neuropsychiatric conditions including bipolar disorder. It is hypothesized that bipolar disorder is the result of decreased excitatory drive to the orbital frontal cortex (98) and that cortical activity is increased during manic states corresponding to changes in activation of the frontal–subcortical circuit.

The investigation of *diminished suppression of P50 auditory-evoked potential* has long been suggested as an endophenotype of schizophrenia. More recently, individuals with bipolar disorder with a longitudinal history of psychosis were evaluated for the presence of similar diminished suppression of P50 auditory-evoked potential (99). When compared with healthy subjects, patients with bipolar disorder with a lifetime history of psychosis had a significantly higher incidence of P50 suppression. This suggests then that diminished suppression of the P50 auditory-evoked potential may be a biologic endophenotype for severe bipolar disorder with psychosis.

John Port on the basis of MRI spectroscopy data from the Mayo Clinic, has suggested (100) that a long-bore magnetic resonance (MR) scanner can screen for different levels of myoinositol, N-acetylaspartate, choline, glutamate, and creatinine. By looking at *choline levels in the left caudate region and the right parietal white matter*, initial research suggests that not only could the presence of bipolar disorder be distinguished from controls, but perhaps bipolar II illness could also be distinguished from bipolar I illness. Should this process prove to be validated, it would provide a relatively simple neuroimaging technique for refinement of some phenotypic diagnosis.

Changes in the amount of *gray matter volume in the left dorsolateral prefrontal cortex* has been demonstrated in several studies of adults with bipolar I disorder (101–103) and in one study of pediatric patients with bipolar I disorder (104). Additionally, less severe reductions in gray matter were found in the left accumbens and the left amygdala.

No changes, however, were found in the hippocampus or orbital frontal cortex. McDonald et al. (105) found genetic risk for bipolar disorder specifically associated with gray matter deficits, but only in the right anterior cingulate gyrus and ventral striatum. Also, white matter volume was reduced in the left frontal and temperoparietal regions. The researchers postulate this as consistent with left frontotemporal disconnectivity, a genetically controlled brain structure abnormality common to both bipolar disorder with psychotic features and schizophrenia. Although these are gross measures of brain volume, they are potential endophenotypic screens for patients with bipolar disorder.

Neural activity in the amygdala during manic episodes was evaluated by Altshuler et al. (106). Data revealed significantly increased activation in the left amygdala and reduced bilateral activation in the lateral orbital frontal cortex relative to controls. The authors hypothesized this data to represent disruption of a specific neuroanatomic circuit during mania that may be implicated in other disorders of affect regulation.

There have been significant neuroimaging data that implicate *dopamine hyperactivity* in mania (107). PET, SPECT, and other scans have shown a variety of abnormalities including increased D_2 receptor density. Increased receptor sensitivity, increased dopamine synthesis, enhanced postsynaptic dopamine responsivity irregularities of the dopamine transporter, or inability to reabsorb dopamine presynaptically may account for this finding.

Cannon et al. have evaluated the muscarinic–cholinergic system that has been implicated by a variety of sources as indirect evidence in bipolar disorder (108). Their group specifically evaluated the type II muscarinic receptor as a possible influence in the pathogenesis of depressive symptoms. They evaluated a group of healthy controls, a group with bipolar disorder during depression, and a group with major depressive disorder. They found that the mean type II muscarinic receptor binding in subjects with bipolar disorder was reduced relative to both healthy controls and subjects with major depressive disorder to an extent that correlated with the amount of depressive symptoms. It was unclear whether this reduction in receptor density was accounted for by a reduction in receptor density or affinity, or an elevation in endogenous acetylcholine levels. This study suggests that measurement of muscarinic receptor binding would be useful in distinguishing major depression from bipolar depression and that altered muscarinic receptor function may contribute to mood regulation in bipolar disorder.

As the data begins to converge, the GEnES Fingerprint model will prove valuable in developing an evidence-based theory of causality for hypomania, bipolar disorder, and other disorders of elevated mood.

Diagnosis in the 21st century

As diagnosis is refined from a purely symptomatic, phenotypic framework into a framework with biologic underpinnings such as the GEnES Fingerprint, it will take on a multidimensional approach. It is likely that multiple aspects of neural, genetic, and psychological functioning, as well as psychopharmacologic responsiveness will be measured and recorded. This change is shown here in a hypothetical example.

Hypothetical patient with a bipolar depressive episode using phenotypic criteria of DSM-IV TR

A 32-year-old woman with a history of three earlier episodes of depression—the first at age 14. Throughout her life, the level of general functioning has been high, with greater than average energy and little tendency to become fatigued. Her typical sleep pattern is to require no more than 6 hours per night.

Depression was preceded by a lengthy period of increased productivity at work, sleeping 3 to 4 hours per night, and a subjective sense of exceptional well-being. She currently takes no medications. Six months earlier, she experienced the death of her mother. She presents with a continuous 3-week history of the following:

Self-reported depressed mood
Feeling physically "slowed down"
Excessive irritability
Insomnia
Feeling of the head being "crowded with negative thoughts."

Hypothetical patient with bipolar depressive episode described in the GEnES Fingerprint format

Genetic data
  Data from positional cloning (linkage)
    Homogeneous for short form of 5-HT serotonin transporter at SLC6A4
Exogenic mechanism data
  Gene repression/silencing
    DNA methylation at loci AA has led to silencing of gene locus BB
Endophenotypic data
  Biochemical
    Decreased density of serotonin transporter binding as measured by [^{123}I] β-CIT SPECT
    Elevated (monoamino oxidase) MAO A levels
  Endocrinologic
    Elevated resting cortisol levels
  Neuroanatomic
  Neuropsychological
  Cognitive
  Other measurements of endophenotypes
  Imaging
    Decreased density of serotonin transporter binding as measured by [^{123}I] β-CIT SPECT
  Data from pharmacologic intervention
    The first two depressive episodes remitted spontaneously without treatment. The most recent episode, 4 years ago, was treated with fluoxetine and responded dramatically within 72 hours. The patient stopped the fluoxetine within 3 weeks when she perceived that it was making her agitated and nervous.
Syndromes
  Neuropsychological activities
  Diseases/diagnoses
    Bipolar depression, type 4A1
  Temperament and personality
    Hyperthymic temperament
  Resiliency and strengths
    Elevated MAO A levels
Epigenetic influence data
  Cultural factors
    Irish/Italian descent
  Physical environment
    Drinks 3 to 4 oz of alcohol on a daily basis

Psychological environment
   Death of mother 6 months before
Medication and other treatments
   None currently
Gender
   Female

More questions

There remain many unanswered fundamental questions about elevated mood.

Of the behavioral symptoms of elevated mood, how many can be traced to distinct behavioral endophenotypes?

Does abnormal elevated mood reflect abnormal circuitry, abnormal anatomy, abnormal physiology, or all three?

Is hypomania a unified replicable syndrome as currently defined?

Is hypomania a disorder of energy regulation?

Is hypomania a disorder of thought speed?

Is hypomania a disorder of excess energy and mood, a disorder of lack of control of energy and mood, or both?

If hypomania is a disorder of energy and/or mood, what are the basic elemental building blocks of energy and mood that we seek to normalize with treatment?

If hypomania is not a disorder of energy or mood, what other underlying factors are disrupted?

Is hypomania a result of genetic errors in the same genes as mania?

If so, what other factors (genetic or epigenetic) affect severity?

Is hypomania the result of the overproduction of a gene product?

If a gene product is overproduced, is it because of a failure of a control gene (gene regulation)?

Is hypomania the result of the genetic product of one or several genes that may evolutionarily be helpful in small amounts but harmful in larger amounts?

Is there one central genetic error in elevated mood or are multiple genetic errors required for hypomania and other forms of elevated mood?

Does the permissive hypothesis apply, namely, does one genetic error only manifest itself in the presence of another genetic error resulting in the phenotypic condition of hypomania?

Are there other areas of the neuron that influence DNA (such as RNA interference) that can turn on or turn off genes and the production of their protein products in elevated mood?

How significant are epigenetic issues (such as culture, gender, physical and psychological environment) in the manifestation of hypomania?

We have many more questions than we have answers; however, we are beginning at least to ask the correct questions. These questions will lead to refined research and ultimately to answers about causation and precise treatments.

The bottom line

- Endophenotypes are more precise than phenotypic symptoms.
- Twenty-first century psychiatric research will focus on elucidating and refining critical endophenotypes in studying elevated mood.
- Neuroimaging is a helpful methodology to observe and refine critical endophenotypes of elevated mood.
- Current imaging of a variety of brain areas show mild to moderate abnormalities in bipolar disorder, but no single pathognomonic deficit has been identified as a critical endophenotype.
- The GEnES Fingerprint incorporates these elements as well as epigenetic factors such as culture, physical environment, psychological environment, and gender. It may elucidate the causal development of "normal" psychological traits, elements of personality disorders, and neuroprotective factors.
- Brain plasticity, critical periods of brain development, and neural networks could be important causative factors that may need to be incorporated into any model of the causation of elevated mood.
- The proteins G-protein receptor kinase 3 (GRK3) and NRG-1 show interesting possible connections to the pathogenesis of elevated mood.
- To date, the genetic abnormalities associated with elevated mood focus on regions 22q11, 12q23–24 and 13q34.
- Many basic questions of a genetic, neurochemical, and neurophysiological nature regarding bipolar disorder and elevated mood remain unanswered.

REFERENCES

1. Gottesman II, Gould TD. The endophenotype concept in psychiatry: Etymology and strategic intentions. *Am J Psychiatry.* 2003;160:636–645.
2. Kendler K. Psychiatric genetics: A methodological critique. *Am J Psychiatry.* 2006;162:3–11.
3. Green E, Elvidge G, Jacobsen N, et al. Localization of bipolar susceptibility locus by molecular genetic analysis of the chromosome 12q23–q24 region in two pedigrees with bipolar disorder and Darier's disease. *Am J Psychiatry.* 2005;162:35–42.

4. Shink E, Morissette J, Sherrington R, et al. A genome-wide scan points to a susceptibility locus for Bipolar disorder on chromosome 12. *Mol Psychiatry.* 2005;10:545–552.

5. Kendler KS. Reflections on the relationship between psychiatric genetics and psychiatric nosology. *Am J Psychiatry.* 2006;163:1138–1146.

6. Burian RM. Molecular epigenesist, molecular pleiotropy, and molecular gene definitions. *Hist Philos Life Sci.* 2004;26:59–80.

7. Harrington ED, Boue S, Valcarcel J, et al. Estimating rates of alternative splicing in mammals and invertebrates (reply). *Nat Genet.* 2004;36:916–917.

8. Wedekind JE, Dance GS, Sowden MP, et al. Messenger RNA editing in mammals: New members of the APOBEC family seeking roles in the family business. *Trends Genet.* 2003;19:207–216.

9. Lolle SJ, et al. Genome-wide non-mendelian inheritance of extra-genomic information in Arabidopsis. *Nature.* 2005;434:505–509.

10. Papolos DF, Veit S, Faedda GL, et al. Ultra-ultra rapid cycling bipolar disorder is associated with the low activity of catecholamine-O-methyl transferase allele. *Mol Psychiatry.* 1998;3(4):346–349.

11. Hahn CG, Han LY, Rawson NE, et al. in vitro and *in vitro* neurogenesis in human olfactory epithelium. *J Comp Neurol.* 2005;483:154–163.

12. Zhang X, Gainetdinov RR, Beaulieu JM, et al. Loss-of-function mutation in tryptophan hydroxylase-2 identified in unipolar major depression. *Neuron.* 2005;45:11–16.

13. Yehuda R, Golier JA, Halligan SL, et al. The ACTH response to dexamethasone in PTSD. *Am J Psychiatry.* 2004;161:1397–1403.

14. Allen AJ. Group A streptococcal infections and childhood neuropsychiatry disorders. *CNS Drugs.* 1997;8(4):267–275.

15. Licinio J, O' Kirwan F, Irizarry K, et al. Association of a corticotrophin-releasing hormone receptor 1 haplotype and antidepressant treatment response in Mexican Americans. *Mol Psychiatry.* 2004;9(12):1075–1082.

16. Gupta S, Aggarwal S, Heads C, et al. Brief report: Dysregulated immune system in children with autism: Beneficial effects of intravenous immune globulin on autistic characteristics. *J Autism Dev Disord.* 1996;26(4):439–452.

17. Steen E, Terry BM, Rivera EJ, et al. Impaired insulin and insulin-like growth factor expression and signaling mechanisms in Alzheimer's disease—is this type 3 diabetes? *J Alzheimer's Dis.* 2005;7(1):63–80.

18. Adler G. *Cushing syndrome.* Accessed online at http://www.emedicine.com/ PED/topic2222.html. 2006.

19. Wilson BE. *Androgen insensitivity syndrome.* Accessed online at http://www. emedicine.com/PED/topic2222.html. 2006.

20. Voderholzer U, Hohagen F, Klein T, et al. Impact of sleep deprivation and subsequent recovery sleep on cortisol in unmedicated depressed patients. *Am J Psychiatry.* 2004;161:1404–1410.

21. Plessen J, Kerstin J, Wentzel-Larsen T, et al. Altered interhemispheric connectivity in individuals with Tourette's Disorder. *Am J Psychiatry.* 2004;161:2028–2037.

22. Luby K, Joan L, Mrakotsky C, et al. Characteristics of depressed preschoolers with and without anhedonia: Evidence for a melancholic depressive subtype in young children. *Am J Psychiatry.* 2004;161:1998–2004.

23. Carlezon WJ. Antidepressant-like effects of uridine and omega-3 fatty acids are potentiated by combined treatment in rats. *Biol Psychiatry.* 2005;57(4):343–359.

24. Milak MS, Parsey RV, Keilp J, et al. Neuroanatomical correlates of psychopathological components of major depressive disorder. *Arch. Gen. Psych.* 2005;62:397–408.

25. Sawada K, Barr AM, Nakamura M, et al. Hippocampal complexin proteins and cognitive dysfunction in schizophrenia. *Arch Gen Psychiatry.* 2005;62:263–272.

26. Heckers S, Benes F. Hippocampus III. *Am J Psych.* 2005;162:450.

27. Cadenhead KS, Light GA, Geyer MA, et al. Neurobiological measures of schizotypal personality disorder: Defining an inhibitory endophenotypes? *Am J Psychiatry.* 2002;159:869–871.

28. Roiser JP, Cook LJ, Cooper JD, et al. Association of a functional polymorphism in the serotonin transporter gene with abnormal emotional processing in Ecstasy users. *Am J Psychiatry.* 2005;162:609–612.

29. Pallanti S, Quercioli L, Hollander E. Dr. Pallanti and colleague reply. *Am J Psychiatry.* 2005;162:400–401.

30. Garno JL, Goldberg JF, Ramirez PM, et al. Bipolar disorder with comorbid cluster B personality disorder features: Impact on suicidality. *J Clin Psychiatry.* 2005;66(3):339–345.

31. Oquendo MA, Galfalvy H, Russo S, et al. John Prospective study of clinical predictors of suicidal acts after a major depressive episode in patients with major depressive disorder or bipolar disorder. *Am J Psychiatry.* 2004;161:1433–1441.

32. Zimmerman M, Posternak MA, Chelminski I. Using a self-report depression scale to identify remission in depression outpatients. *Am J Psychiatry.* 2004;161:1911–1913.

33. Airaksinen E, Larsson M, Forsell Y. Neuropsychological functions in anxiety disorders in population-based samples: Evidence of episodic memory dysfunction. *J Psychiatr Res.* 2005;39(2):207–214.

34. Morey MA. Imaging frontostriatal function in ultra-high-risk early, and chronic schizophrenia during executive processing. *Arch Gen Psychiatry.* 2005;62:254–262.

35. Brewer WJ, Francey SM, Wood SJ, et al. Memory impairments identified in people at ultra-high risk for psychosis who later develop first-episode psychosis. *Am J Psychiatry.* 2005;162:71–78.

36. Jacobsen MW, Delis DC, Bondi MW, et al. Do neuropsychological tests detect preclinical Alzheimer's disease: Individual-test versus cognitive-discrepancy score and analyses. *Neuropsychology.* 2002;16(2):132–139.

37. Swedo SE, Leonard HL, Rapoport JL. The pediatric autoimmune neuropsychiatric disorders associated with streptococcal infection (PANDAS) subgroup; separating fact from fiction. *Pediatrics.* 2004;113(4):907–911.

38. Ribak CE, Roberts RC. GABAergic synapses in the brain identified with antisera to GABA and its synthesizing enzyme, glutamate decarboxylase. *J Electron Microsc Tech.* 1991;15(1):34–38.

39. Weiner HL, Selkoe DJ. Inflammation and therapeutic vaccination in CNS diseases. *Nature.* 2002;420:879–884.

40. Garvey MA, Giedd J, Swedo S. PANDAS: The search for environmental triggers of pediatric neuropsychiatric disorders. Lessons from rheumatic fever. *J Child Neurol.* 1998;13(9):413–423.

41. Plioplys AV. Intravenous immunoglobulin treatment of children with autism. *J Child Neurol.* 1998;13(2):79–82.
42. Singh VK. Plasma increase in interleukin-12 and interferon-gamma: Pathological significance in autism. *J Immunol.* 1996;66:143–145.
43. Tregellas JR, Tanabe JL, Martin LF, et al. fMRI of response to nicotine during a smooth pursuit eye movement task in schizophrenia. *Am J Psychiatry.* 2005;162:391–393.
44. Yetkin FZ, Fischer ME, Papke RA, et al. Focal hyperintensities in cerebral white matter on MR images of asymptomatic volunteers: Correlation with social and medical histories. *Am J Roentgenol* 1993;161:855–858.
45. Germain A, Nofzinger EA, Kupfer DJ, et al. Neurobiology of non-REM sleep in depression: Further evidence for hypofrontality and thalamic dysregulation. *Am J Psychiatry.* 2004;161:1856–1863.
46. van der Wee NJ, Stevens H, Hardeman JA, et al. Enhanced dopamine transporter density in psychotropic-naive patients with obsessive-compulsive disorder shown by [123I]{beta}-CIT SPECT. *Am J Psychiatry.* 2004;161:2201–2206.
47. Ashburner J, Friston KJ. Voxel-based morphometry—the methods. *Neuroimage.* 2001;11(6 pt 1):805–821.
48. Louchart-de la Chapelle S, Nkam I, Houy E, et al. A concordance study of three electrophysiological measures in schizophrenia. *Am J Psych.* 2005;162:466–474.
49. Guthrie RM, Bryant RA. Auditory startle response in firefighters before and after exposure. *Am J Psych.* 2005;162:283–290.
50. Goddard AW, Mason GF, Appel M, et al. Impaired GABA neuronal response to acute benzodiazepine administration in panic disorder. *Am J Psych* 2004;161:2186–2193.
51. Solomon DA, Leon AC, Mueller TI, et al. Tachyphylaxis in unipolar major depressive disorder. *J Clin Psychiatry.* 2005;66:283–290.
52. Vermetten E, Vythilingam M, Schmahl C, et al. Alterations in stress reactivity after long-term treatment with paroxetine in women with posttraumatic stress disorder. *Psychobiol Posttrauma Stress Disord.* 2006;1071:184–202.
53. Kirchheiner J, Nickchen K, Bauer M, et al. Pharmacogenetics of antidepressants and antipsychotics: the contribution of allelic variations to the phenotype of drug response. *Mol Psychiatry.* 2004;9:442–473.
54. Rosenblum LA, Pauly GS. Dominance and social competence in differentially reared bonnet macques. In: Ehara A, ed. *Pimatology today Xiiith congress of the International Prime Ecological Society.* Amsterdam: Elsevier Science; 1991:347–350.
55. Shively CA. Social subordination stress, behavior and central monoaminergic function in female cynomolgus monkeys. *Biol Psychiatry.* 1998;44:882–891.
56. Raleigh MJ, Brammer GL, McGuire MT. Male dominance, serotonergic systems and behavioral and physiological effects of drugs in vervet monkeys. *Prog Clin Biol Res.* 1983;131:185–197.
57. Mehlman PT, Higley JD, Faucher I, et al. Correlation of CSF 5-HIAA concentration with sociality and the timing of emigration in free-ranging primates. *Am J Psychiatry.* 1995;152:907–913.
58. Insel TR, Winslow JT. The neurobiology of social attachment. In: Charney DS, Netsler EJ, Bunney BS, eds. *Neurobiology of mental illness.* New York: Oxford University Press; 1991:880–890.

59. Pierribone VA. *Quoted in yale medicine.* at http:/yalemedicine.yale.edu, Spring 2005:18–23.
60. Gutman DA, Nemeroff CB. Neuroendocrinological research in psychiatry. In: *Psychiatry as a neuroscience.* 2002;91–124.
61. Avissar S, Matuzany-Ruban A, Tzukert K, et al. [beta]-Arrestin-1 levels: Reduced in leukocytes of patients with depression and elevated by antidepressants in rat brain. *Am J Psychiatry.* 2004;161:2066–2072.
62. http://www.medindia.net/patients/patientinfo/syndrome/home.asp. 2006.
63. Hirsch ED. *New dictionary of cultural literacy,* 3rd ed, 2002.
64. deGeus JC. Introducing genetic psychophysiology. *Biol Psychol.* 2002;61:1–10.
65. www.cogsci.princeton.edu/cgi-bin/webwn. 2006.
66. www.who.int/environmental_information/AirGuidelines/ann3.htm. 2006.
67. www.mdsupport.org/glossary/. 2006.
68. www.comtan.com/info/tools/pc_glossary_d.jsp. 2006.
69. allpsych.com/dictionary/dictionary4.html. 2006.
70. www.therubins.com/geninfo/Definit.htm. 2006.
71. Masten AS, Coatsworth JD. The development of competence in favorable and unfavorable environments. *Am Psychol.* 1998;53(2):205–220.
72. Richardson GE, Waite PJ. Mental health promotion through resilience and resiliency education. *Int J Emerg Ment Health.* 2002;4(1):65–75.
73. Bell CC, Gamm S, Vallas P. Strategies for the prevention of youth violence in Chicago public schools. In: Shafii M, Shafii SL, eds. et al, *School violence: Assessment, management, prevention.* Washington, DC: American Psychiatric Publishing; 2001:251–272.
74. Hoek HP, van Harten PN, van Hoeken D, et al. The incidence of anorexia nervosa on Curacao. *Am J Psychiatry.* 2005;162:748–752.
75. Hoek HW, van Harten PN, van Hoeken D, et al. Lack of relation between culture and anorexia nervosa—results of an incidence study on Curacao. *N Engl J Med.* 1998;338:1231–1232.
76. Estima C. Eating disorders in diverse populations. *J Pediatr Gastroenterol Nutr*2004;39(Suppl. 1):S22.
77. Humphry D. *Treat carefully when you help to die. Assisted suicide laws around the world.* Access to online at http://ww.assisted suicide.org/suicide_laws.html. 2006.
78. Goldsmith SK, Pellmar TC, Kleinman AM, et al. eds. *Reducing suicide: A National Imperative Committee on Pathophysiology and Prevention of Adolescent and Adult Suicide.* Washington, DC: Board on Neuroscience and Behavioral Health, Institute of Medicine; 2002; 193–228.
79. Woodside B, Garfinkel PE, Lin E, et al. Comparisons of men with full or partial eating disorders, men without eating disorders, and women with eating disorders in the community. *Am J Psychiatry.* 2001;158:570–574.
80. World Health Organization. Accessed on-line at http://www.who.int/mental_health/prevention/genderwomen/en/. 2006.
81. Yang X, Schadt EE, Wang S, et al. Tissue-specific expression and regulation of sexually dimorphic genes in mice. *Genome Res.* 2006;16:995–1004.
82. Jeong H, Tombor B, Albert R, et al. The large scale organization of metabolic networks. *Nature.* 2000;407:651–654.
83. Carstren E. Is mood chemistry? *Nat Rev Neurosci.* 2005;6:241–246.

84. Kelsoe JR, Spence MA, Loetscher E, et al. A genome survey indicates a possible susceptibility locus for bipolar disorder on chromosome 22. *Proc Natl Acad Sci U S A.* 2001;98(2):585–590.

85. Green E, Elvidge G, Jacobsen N, et al. Localization of bipolar susceptibility locus by molecular genetic analysis of the chromosome 12q23-q24 region in two pedigrees with bipolar disorder and Darier's disease. *Am J Psychiatry.* 2005;162:35–42.

86. Kimmel RJ, Kovacs I, Vrabel C, et al. Co-segregation of bipolar disorder and autosomal-dominant medullary cystic kidney disease in a large family. *Am J Psychiatry.* 2005;162:1972–1974.

87. Schulze TG, Ohlraum S, Czerski PM, et al. Genotype-phenotype studies in bipolar disorder showing association between the DAOA/G30 locus and persecutory delusions: A first step toward a molecular genetic classification of psychiatric phenotypes. *Am J Psychiatry.* 2005;162:2101–2108.

88. Lichter DG, Cummings JL. Introduction and overview. In: Lichter DG, Cummings JL, eds. *Frontal-subcortical circuits in psychiatric and neurological disorders.* New York: Guilford Press; 2001:1–43.

89. Marchand WR, Bennett PJ, Dilda V, et al. Evidence for frontal-subcortical circuit abnormalities in bipolar affective disorder. *Psychiatry.* 2005; 26–32.

90. Green EK, Raybould R, Macgregor S, et al. Operation of the schizophrenia susceptibility gene, neuregulin 1, across traditional diagnostic boundaries to increase risk for bipolar disorder. *Arch Gen Psychiatry.* 2005;62:642–648.

91. Schumacher J, Kaneve R, Jamra RA, et al. Genomewide scan and fine-mapping linkage studies in four European samples with bipolar affective disorder suggest a new susceptibility locus on chromosome 1p35–p36 and provides further evidence of loci on chromosome 4q31 and 6q24. *Am J Hum Genet.* 2005;77:000.

92. Gutierrez B, Arranz M, Fananas L, et al. 5HT2A receptor gene and bipolar affective disorder (letter). *Lancet.* 1995;346:969.

93. Cichon S, Schumacher J, Muller DJ, et al. A genome screen for genes predisposing to bipolar affective disorder detects a new susceptibility locus on 8q. *Hum Mol Genet.* 2001;10(25):2933–2944.

94. Gutierrez B, Fananas L, Arranz M, et al. Allelic association analysis of the 5HT2C receptor gene in bipolar affective disorder. *Neurosci Lett.* 1996;212:65–67.

95. Ogilvie AD, Battersby S, Bubb VJ, et al. Polymorphism in serotonin transporter gene associated with susceptibility to major depression. *Lancet.* 1996;347:731–733.

96. Bellivier F, Leboyer M, Courtet P, et al. Association between the tryptophan hydroxylase gene and manic-depressive illness. *Arch Gen Psychiatry.* 1998;55:33–37.

97. Vincent JB, Masellis M, Lawrence J, et al. Genetic association analysis of serotonin system genes in bipolar affective disorder. *Am J Psychiatry.* 1999;156:136–138.

98. Strakowski Sm, Sax KW. Secondary mania: A model of the pathophysiology of bipolar disorder? In: Soares JC, Gershon S, eds. *Bipolar disorders: Basic mechanisms and therapeutic implications.* New York: Mercel Dekker Inc; 2000:13–29.

99. Olincy A, Martin L. Diminished suppression of the P50 auditory evoked potential in bipolar disorder subjects with a history of psychosis. *Am J Psychiatry.* 2005;162:43–49.

100. John Port Presented at the Radiological Society of North American Annual Meetings, Chicago, IL: 2004.
101. Sax KW, Strakowski SM, Zimmerman ME, et al. Fronto-subcortical neuroanatomy and the continuous performance test in mania. *Am J Psychiatry.* 1999;156:139–141.
102. Ali SO, Denicoff KD, Altshuler LL, et al. A preliminary study of the relation of neuropsychological performance to neuroanatomic structures in bipolar disorder. *Neuropsychiatry Neuropsychol Behav Neurol.* 2000;13:20–28.
103. Ali SO, Denicoff KD, Altshuler LL, et al. Relationship between prior course of illness and neuroanatomic structures in bipolar disorder: A preliminary study. *Neuropsychiatry Neuropsychol Behav Neurol.* 2001;14:227–232.
104. Dickstein DP, Milham MP, Nugent AC, et al. Frontotemporal alterations in pediatric bipolar disorder. *Arch Gen Psychiatry.* 2005;62:734–741.
105. McDonald C, Bullmore E, Sham P, et al. Regional volume deviations of brain structure of schizophrenia and psychotic bipolar disorder. *Br J Psychiatry Suppl.* 2005;186:369–377.
106. Altshuler L, Bookheimer S, Proenza MA, et al. Increased amygdale activation during mania: A functional magnetic resonance imaging study. *Am J Psychiatry.* 2005;162:6.
107. Pollock R, Kua I. Neuroimaging in bipolar disorder. *Presented at the International Congress of Biological Psychiatry*, Sydney, Australia: Febuary 2004.
108. Cannon DM, Carson RE, Nugent AC, et al. Reduced muscarinic type 2 receptor binding in subjects with bipolar disorder. *Arch Gen Psychiatry.* 2006;63:741–747.

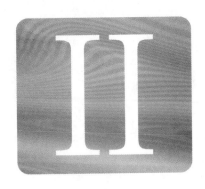

Diagnosis of Elevated Mood

3

DIAGNOSTIC ISSUES IN HYPOMANIA

As described in the previous two chapters, the detection of hypomania and elevated mood is crucial to appropriate diagnosis and management. Whether the chief complaint is elevated or (more likely) depressed mood, it is not hard to diagnose hypomania or a form of bipolar disorder when a patient acknowledges the classic symptoms of elevated mood. These classic symptoms can include lack of need to sleep, excess energy, impulsive spending, grandiose thoughts, increased talkativeness, or significantly inappropriate social and business judgments. Our diagnosis becomes much more difficult, however, when the patient presents depressed or, on direct questioning, does not clearly acknowledge hypomanic symptoms. It is most difficult, of course, if the practitioner never asks questions about elevated mood at all!

Given that hypomanic symptoms are often not the primary presenting complaints, how can we increase the odds of recognizing hypomania in the context of the myriad other psychiatric symptoms including depression, anxiety, substance abuse, and other behavioral disturbances? Until critical endophenotypic elements of elevated mood are elucidated as described in Chapter 2, we must use current phenomenologic measures to guide our

TABLE 3.1

Diagnostic omissions in evaluating elevated mood

The clinician may do the following:

• Make an incomplete assessment that fails to include collateral sources of information

• Become blinded by the chief complaint

• Misattribute hypomanic traits to other causes

• Fail to obtain a family history

• Accept a previous erroneous or incomplete diagnosis

• Fail to evaluate a longitudinal history

• Fail to reassess the diagnosis during the course of treatment

diagnosis. This chapter looks at the issue of recognition and diagnosis of elevated mood, hypomania, and bipolar disorder and provides symptom-based guidelines for the clinician.

To assist us in determining best practice techniques, it is first useful to understand the common ways that even astute clinicians may fail to diagnose hypomania. The seven most common failings of diagnosticians are listed in Table 3.1.

An *incomplete assessment* can result from many causes including a clinician in hurry or one who does not have a consistent system for assessing all aspects of a patient's condition. Good practice is facilitated by maintaining a list of symptoms and behaviors that are routinely addressed in every diagnostic assessment. Virtually all patients should be asked specific screening questions about elevated mood during an initial evaluation. These questions will be specified later in the chapter.

If the clinician doing the screening becomes narrowly *"locked on" to the chief complaint,* exploring only the patient's overt presenting problem, questioning may become unnecessarily circumscribed, and elevated mood may be left uninvestigated. This commonly occurs when depression or anxiety is the chief complaint. Under these circumstances, the clinician may perform a detailed evaluation of anxious or depressive symptoms, but fail to undertake an evaluation for the presence of elevated mood elements currently or in the past.

A corollary to becoming fixed on to the chief complaint is the failure to evaluate current complaints in the context of other symptoms and the long-term symptom pattern. For the most accurate diagnosis, it is important to *assess the patient's longitudinal history,* including his or her underlying temperament or any previous history of mood symptoms—whether diagnosed or not.

When symptoms of elevated mood are described by the patient, the clinician may mistake "feeling good" as evidence of enthusiasm, passion, or improvement from a previous depressed episode. It is critical that the period after a depression be carefully evaluated because hypomania may easily be mistaken as emergence from an episode of depressed mood.

Although not every evaluation can include information gathered from a family member or other knowledgeable person, when there is a suspicion of elevated mood, the assessment should include data from these additional sources. With every patient, inquiry should be made as to a history of psychiatric symptoms, diagnoses, or treatment in biologic relatives. Similarly, a family history of substance abuse may overlay a diagnosis of elevated mood disorder, and the clinician must be diligent in exploring this aspect of the family pedigree. Although individual patients may have limited or incomplete information about family members, an attempt should be made to obtain as much information as possible early in the process of evaluation. It may be necessary for a patient to contact relatives to obtain this information.

Routinely accepting a diagnosis made by another practitioner may point a clinician in the wrong direction, limiting his or her independent assessment of symptomatology. Many patients may present to a psychiatrist after having already been evaluated by primary care clinicians, nonpsychiatric mental health practitioners, or other mental health professionals. These clinicians may have had their own biases about diagnosis, may or may not have done a thorough evaluation, and may or may not have correctly included all symptoms in making their diagnosis. Childhood diagnoses (often made by pediatricians or non-medical therapists) can become confounding in correctly diagnosing elevated mood. Overactive or even flagrantly hypomanic symptoms may have been attributed to attention-deficit disorder (ADD)/attention-deficit hyperactivity disorder (ADHD), other developmental disorders, or "just a stage." If the clinician accepts these assessments at face value, vital clues to the presence of hypomania may be missed. Similar caution should be exercised in automatically accepting a diagnosis of bipolar disorder made earlier. There are clinicians today who see bipolar disorder "around every corner" and label almost every instance of significant functional disturbance, substance abuse, or hyperactivity as bipolar in origin.

The clinician may fail to periodically *reevaluate the initial diagnosis in light of treatment response* or lack thereof. Commonly, a patient has been diagnosed as having a major depressive disorder but has failed several antidepressant trials, or obtained some transient relief, and then rapidly lost the symptomatic response. A diagnostic reconceptualization may reveal the diagnosis of recurrent depressive mood cycling with subsyndromal hypomanic symptomatology—a disorder that mimics the course of bipolar disorder and may be more appropriately treated with mood stabilizers.

A clinician may also *fail to reassess the patient over time.* This is the long-term variation of being overly focused on an initial diagnosis. The clinician may have first diagnosed the patient with unipolar depression or an anxiety disorder, but has kept "blinders on" with regard to other possible diagnoses including that of a cycling mood disorder.

TABLE 3.2
Keys to diagnostic success with elevated mood

- Ask the appropriate questions
- Use information sources beyond the patient
- Determine family history and construct a genogram
- Use standardized screening tools
- Evaluate soft signs of elevated mood
- Use mood charting
- Review the diagnosis in light of treatment response and failure
- Reassess the diagnosis over time

The initial assessment interview

With a thought toward avoiding these errors, specific methodologies are presented in Table 3.2 and elaborated in the ensuing text. Attention to these factors can lead to improved diagnostic success.

Increasing the odds for successful diagnosis

As with any psychiatric assessment, it is best to quickly identify the patient's chief complaint and his or her reason for coming to the evaluative session. With elevated mood, two elements confound the diagnostic process.

1. Many patients present for conditions and chief complaints that do not specifically involve elevated mood; yet, elevated mood is an important component to correctly identify the ultimate diagnosis.
2. When patients with bipolar disorder or cycling moods do complain of mood problems, the complaint is most often depression, not elevated mood.

   It is, therefore, crucial for the clinician to understand bipolar disorder as a multifaceted illness that can present to the clinician with many different faces. These presentations may overtly involve mood symptoms including depression, mania, mixed states, and rapid cycling moods. There are, however, many other presentations that initially do not have mood as an obvious core element. As can be seen in Table 3.3, there is a wide variety of presenting complaints that do not readily relate to mood.

Hyperthymia and hypomania

Not all behavioral elements that are energetic, highly active, or accelerated in pace are abnormal or require treatment. Both hyperthymic temperament and hypomania can present with a constellation of these behaviors at the time of evaluation or in the history.

TABLE 3.3
Variable presentations of bipolar illness

Mania
Depression
Mixed states (agitated depression or dysphoric mania)
Anxiety or agitation
Frequent mood changes or cycling
Psychotic thoughts or behavior
Consequences of impulsive behavior (financial troubles, promiscuity, physical injury)
Aggression, violence, or legal infractions
Attention/concentration problems
Disordered intrafamily, interpersonal, or marital relationship
Substance abuse and its sequelae
Disordered sleep
Anger or rage episodes
Suicidal ideation or behavior
Repeated employment failures
No complaints at all. The patient is brought in by another person.

Although most hyperthymic individuals do not present for evaluation or treatment for accelerated and elevated mood traits, when these are seen, the clinician must differentiate the truly hypomanic individual (who may need treatment) from the hyperthymic individual (who may not). Beyond the initial complaint, the patient with minor elevated mood will likely not have problematic behaviors consistently but only a few mild ones. These will be interspersed with many desirable, beneficial, or even exceptional behaviors. In general, individuals with hyperthymic temperament but not hypomania have the characteristics in the left-hand column of Table 3.4 but few, if any, of the symptoms in the right-hand column. The hypomanic individual, however, may show some of the items in the left-hand column but will also exhibit one or more pronounced behavioral symptoms in the right-hand column. As has been depicted in Figure 1.1, a defined sharp line is not always present between what is positively perceived and what is problematic.

The four Ps of functionality

Another way to organize data so as to distinguish hyperthymia from true hypomania is to focus on the four Ps of functionality (Table 3.5).

TABLE 3.4
The range of elevated mood symptoms

May be positively regarded by the patient—mildly elevated mood	Negative behavioral consequence—significantly elevated mood
High energy	Irritability
Extroverted	Reckless
Increased plans/activities	Overtalkative
Creative	Intrusive
Self-confident	Poor judgment
Self-directed	Lack of awareness of consequences of behavior
Contagious humor	Unstable relationships
Novelty seeking	Disorderly
Consistently high output or productivity	Scattered—may start many tasks but follow through erratically
Business or financial success	Functional inconsistencies Increased substance use Rationalizing negative behavior or consequences Denial of need for help despite evidence of deficiencies

It is not only how a person *feels*, but also how they *function* on a day-to-day basis that may determine whether a psychiatric illness is present. These functional elements can be remembered as the four Ps—productivity, predictability, positivity, and people skills. Individuals with hyperthymic temperament may have appropriate functioning in each of these areas, but hypomanic persons will have exaggerated behaviors, often exhibiting deficits in one or more areas.

For example, with *productivity*, the hyperthymic individual may be consistently active in a positive way and viewed by others as more productive that the average individual. In hypomania, however, persons may feel

TABLE 3.5
The four Ps of functionality

- Productivity
- Positivity
- Predictability
- People skills

productive, but objective measurements of their activity show scattered erratic performance. At times, the hypomanic individual may be productive, but this often fluctuates and does not last. Hyperthymic persons can be consistently and predictably highly active with constant output and production. With persons with hypomania, on the other hand, *predictability* suffers and the person may have some periods of productivity, but is often erratic and unpredictable. This variability can be seen in areas such as work performance, academic success, and financial management.

With *positivity*, the hyperthymic person is found to be engaging, outgoing, and carrying a positive outlook on life. When exaggerated in hypomania, however, these criteria can yield excessive optimism, grandiosity, and poor decision making, often without regard to consequences.

Hyperthymic individuals usually have better-than-average *people skills*. They are jovial, engaging, and engender others' admiration, attention, and friendship. They mix well in social situations. They are often effective public speakers. When exaggerated in hypomania, the same skills can show social intrusiveness, increased talkativeness, and increased self-absorption, without apparent awareness about others' feelings and wishes. The hypomanic individual can be dominating and irritable, especially when his or her wishes are not met.

Depression and elevated mood

As will be seen in Chapter 4, depression is by far the most common presenting complaint in cycling mood disorders. This is not unexpected, given that for most patients, depression is much more emotionally painful and debilitating than hypomania. Patients with bipolar II disorder also spend much more of their time in the depressed phase of the illness than they do in asymptomatic or hypomanic stages.

Lish et al. (1) demonstrated that early diagnosis of elevated mood is a difficult task, given our current diagnostic acumen and patient presentation. In a survey involving members of the Depressive and Manic-Depressive Association, three fourths the number of those surveyed had given an alternative explanation for their symptoms (i.e., not a mood disorder). One fourth to one third the number of patients were misdiagnosed as having unipolar depression. More than one third of the patients took >10 years to receive an accurate diagnosis. This issue is common and sufficiently significant to merit a separate chapter on the topic.

One symptom does not a diagnosis make

There is no single symptom that is pathognomonic of hypomania. For example, isolated episodes of increased energy alone, decreased sleep alone, rapid speech, impulsivity, or any one symptom is not sufficient, in and of itself, to make a diagnosis of hypomania. To establish a diagnosis, it is important to

TABLE 3.6
Most common manifestations of hypomania

Increased activity	97%
Increased energy	96%
Increased plans and ideas	91%
Increased self-confidence	86%
Decreased sleep	84%
Increased talkativeness	72%
Decreased inhibition	71%
Increased optimism	68%

From Wicki W, Angst J. The Zurich Study. X hypomania in a 28- to 30-year-old cohort. *Eur Arch Psychiatry Clin Neurosci.* 1991;240(6):339–348, (2).

identify a constellation of symptoms that, together, point to the likelihood
of hypomania. In addition to the classic symptoms of elevated mood, the
clinician needs to be familiar with the most common symptoms of hypomania
that are shown in Table 3.6.

Another way to remember these components is the useful mnemonic
DIGFAST, which stands for the elements that, in addition to irritability, can
be used to diagnose bipolar disorder. As shown in Table 3.7, DIGFAST stands

TABLE 3.7
The elements of DIGFAST

Distractibility
Insomnia
Grandiosity
Flight of ideas/racing thought
Activities
Speech
Thoughtlessness

From Ghaemi SN. *Mood disorders.* Philadelphia: Lippincott
Williams & Wilkins; 2003:13–14,
originally developed by William
Falk, MD, (3).

TABLE 3.8
Screening questions for elevated mood

Have ever had a time when you . . .

* Were feeling so good or so "up" that people around you thought you were not your usual self?

* Were so energetic that you acted in a way to get yourself in trouble?

* Were overly active and felt like you could do much more than you are usually capable of?

* Were irritable to the point of shouting, starting fights or arguments, or yelling at inappropriate times?

* Received feedback that you were hyperactive or "manic"?

* Had periods without the need for sleep?

for Distractibility, Insomnia, Grandiosity, Flight of ideas/racing thoughts, increased Activities, rapid Speech, and Thoughtlessness.

Asking the right questions

Any patient with depression or anxiety symptoms should also be minimally asked several screening questions about elevated mood. These screening questions are listed in Table 3.8.

Follow-up questions

When one or more of the screening questions are answered affirmatively, or if there is a strong suspicion of elevated mood (e.g., because of other historical elements or a positive family history for bipolar disorder), the questions listed in Table 3.9 are useful for elucidation or elaboration. It may also be necessary to ask a question in several ways to elicit an accurate positive response; therefore, several approaches are listed for each area of inquiry.

Additional clues to diagnosis

Additional subtle signs leading to a diagnosis of bipolar II disorder and/or the presence of hypomania include instability in employment, relationships, education, body weight, or other areas of life. Cyclothymic or bipolar individuals tend to be inconsistent in work, intimate relationships, and physical parameters. While any of these areas may be erratic for reasons other than mood swings, individuals who show frequent instability in a variety of key functional areas should be evaluated carefully for bipolar disorder.

Swann et al. (4) have suggested that additional soft signs for bipolar disorder include early onset depression (prepubertal or early adolescence),

TABLE 3.9

Follow-up questions in evaluating elevated mood

Energy—Are there times when you . . .

- Have unusual excessive energy?
- Cannot slow down?
- Do not get fatigued when it would be expected?
- Can work for a very long duration without stopping?

Impulsivity—Are there times when you . . .

- Make unusual or snap decisions that are not in your best interest or may cause actual harm?
- Make decisions that are risky or where you are worried that you will be caught?
- Have ignored risks that prudent people would watch out for?
- Feel "bullet-proof" or unable to be harmed, despite risky behaviors?
- Make impulsive travel plans, especially for long distances or on short notice?

Sleep—Have there been times when you . . .

- Felt you did not need normal sleep?
- Were so energized or involved in an activity that you stayed up long hours?
- Had a period of one or more nights where you would get by on little or no sleep?
- What is that longest period of time that you have gone without sleep? How often does this happen?

Thought speed and organization—Have there been times when you . . .

- Had thoughts that race or move very quickly?
- Had too many thoughts at once so that it was difficult to focus on just one thought?
- Your mind was flooded with thoughts?
- Rapidly moved from one task to another without completing the initial task?
- Started a number of tasks simultaneously but did not finish them?

Speech—Are there times when you . . .

- Talk very rapidly?
- Receive feedback that you talk too fast, too loud, or too much?
- Receive feedback that you skip from topic to topic and others cannot follow the conversation?
- Receive feedback that you routinely interrupt other's speech, or finish other's sentences?
- Talk excessively on the phone?
- Your mind moves so fast that you cannot keep up with it?
- Telephone other individuals in the middle of the night, or call people you do not know?

Financial Issues—Do you . . .

- Spend beyond your budget? How often? By how much?
- Buy lavish, expensive items you cannot afford?

TABLE 3.9

(*continued*)

- Do you buy duplicates of items, or the same item in many colors or styles?

- Routinely buy clothes or other items that you do not use?

- Have periods of unusual generosity or give away items that you later regret?

Mood—Are there times when you . . .

- Feel the opposite of being depressed?

- Feel depressed, but are internally accelerated or speeded up (mixed states)?

- Shift from one mood state to another suddenly or unpredictably (rapid cycling)?

- Show emotion that is inappropriate to the circumstance, such as laughing at sad times or crying for no reason?

Irritability—Are there times when you . . .

- Get angry or explode over small issues?

- Get overly angry or impatient, e.g., with store clerks?

- Experience road rage?

- Have been involved in or precipitated physical altercations? How often? Was anyone hurt?

- Had levels of anger that have lead to negative consequences at your job, school, or in your family?

- Become unusually angry or dissatisfied with coworkers, bosses, or supervisors?

- Are unusually loud or demonstrative when you are angry?

- Throw objects or destroy property when you get angry?

- Have received feedback that others feel that they must "walk on eggshells" around you because of your potential short fuse?

Anxiety—Do you . . .

- Become accelerated to the point of feeling anxious or agitated?

- Have times when you cannot sit still?

- Have anxiety with physical symptoms, including rapid heart rate, shallow breathing, difficulty catching your breath?

- Frequently become anxious from rushing to perform multiple routine tasks?

Substance abuse—Do you . . .

- Use alcohol or drugs to change your mood?

- Use alcohol or drugs to make you less anxious?

- Use alcohol or drugs to slow your mind down?

- Use alcohol or drugs to curb your energy, which would otherwise be excessive?

onset of depression during the postpartum period, childhood, or adolescent psychotic symptoms accompanied by a high level of social functioning, or a family history of multiple members with mood, anxiety, and substance abuse problems. While diagnostically helpful, it is unreasonable to diagnose bipolar mood swings or cyclothymia on the basis of soft signs alone. Rather, these data are additive elements that supplement more classical bipolar symptoms. Having said this, as the concept of bipolar spectrum disorder becomes more defined and accepted, soft signs alone may guide the clinician to make a diagnosis of bipolar disorder in a patient who might be diagnosed to have some other disorder.

Akiskal reviewed >1,000 depressed patients he had personally examined with the initial diagnosis of unipolar depression. Subsequently, these patients were confirmed to have periods of hypomania, cyclothymia, or revealed additional soft signs that made it more likely that the patient should be diagnostically categorized in the bipolar rather than the unipolar domain (5). Traits seen in these patients and their blood relations included periods of creative achievement, professional instability, substance/alcohol use/abuse, multiple axes I and II comorbidity, multiple marriages, a broad repertoire of sexual behavior (including brief interludes of homosexuality), impulse control disorders, increased ornamentation, and flamboyance. Often these individuals showed an ability to thrive on hyperscheduling that has been labeled as being "an activity junkie."

The value of family history

The evaluation of any patient with a mood disorder would be incomplete without assessing psychiatric disorder in biologic family members. While it is not always possible to ascertain the exact psychiatric status in a relative, the clinician should ask about family members who

• have carried a formal psychiatric diagnosis;
• have been psychiatrically treated or hospitalized;
• have significant substance abuse;
• have displayed traits characteristic of a psychiatric disorder, even if formal evaluation and treatment have never been completed.

In cases where a diagnosis may be equivocal between a unipolar and a bipolar diagnosis, for example, the presence and nature of a positive family history for a specific psychiatric disease can often point the clinician toward the most appropriate diagnostic sector.

Creating a genogram

With information gleaned from the patient, it can be very helpful for the clinician and patient to collaboratively create a genogram detailing blood relatives with various psychiatric conditions. Examples of these genograms are shown in Figures 3.1, 3.2, and 3.3. Figure 3.1 is reproduced in Appendix 1

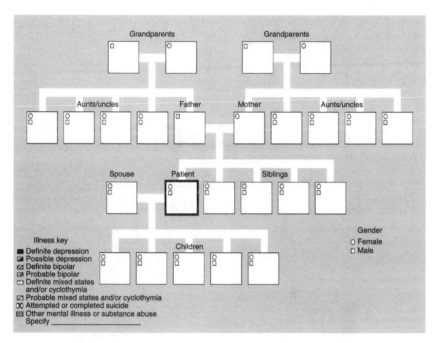

Figure 3.1 Genogram template.

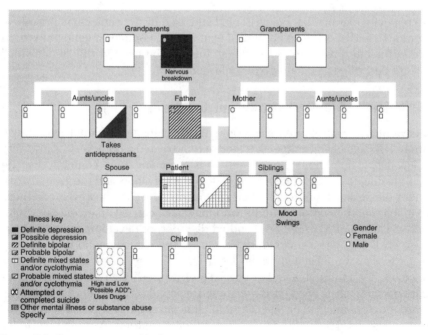

Figure 3.2 Genogram example 1.

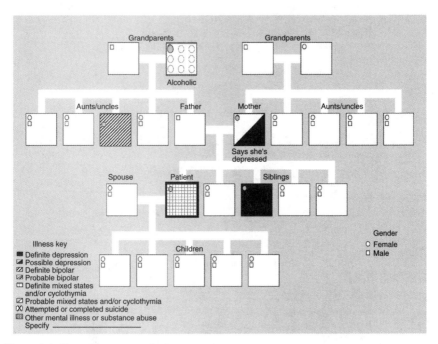

Figure 3.3 Genogram example 2.

as a blank genogram that can be copied and used by the clinician in the office. Figures 3.2 and 3.3 show hypothetical examples of completed genograms with a code for interpretation. Such genograms can be used in the "re-viewing" process described in Chapter 6 on treatment.

The patient's childhood history and diagnoses

In current psychiatric care, it is common for teenage and adult psychiatric patients to have been evaluated, tested and/or treated as children for a variety of psychiatric conditions. Fortunately, it is becoming more common that the accurate diagnosis of childhood mood disorders is made, and the groundwork laid for future adult treatment. This is not always the case, however, and there are many mood-disordered adults who may have carried an erroneous childhood diagnosis of ADD/ADHD, conduct disorder, or developmental disorder. These earlier diagnoses should not dissuade the clinician who is evaluating the patient as a teenager or as an adult from making a new mood disorder diagnosis if a careful evaluation suggests otherwise. Such ADD/ADHD diagnoses or other labels of cognitive dysfunction, conduct disorder or personality disorder can be misleading and the adult clinician should reevaluate (de novo) as much as possible for the presence of mood symptoms. As noted by Geller et al. (6,7), if as a child, the person has experienced the presence of elated mood, grandiosity, hypersexuality, decreased need for sleep, racing thoughts, and any other manic symptoms (with the exception of excess energy and distractibility), these individuals are much more likely to have had bipolar disorder rather than ADD/ADHD. Likewise, the report of multiple failures of psychostimulants to adequately treat "hyperactivity" may indicate a misdiagnosis. A history of the need to stop a stimulant because it produced excessive nervousness, psychotic symptoms, or behavioral overactivity may also lead the clinician in the direction of making a diagnosis of bipolar disorder rather than an ADD/ADHD diagnosis.

Axelson et al. (8) suggest that children and adolescents who have elevated mood symptoms will often show symptom duration that is less than the necessary criteria to meet DSM-IV (*Diagnostic and Statistical Manual of Mental Disorders-IV*) requirements for a diagnosis of bipolar I disorder. From their data on 438 youths, they found that those with bipolar NOS diagnoses differed from those with a diagnosis of bipolar I disorder, primarily on duration and severity of manic symptoms, not on the fundamental phenomenology. They opined that their study underscores the likelihood that children and adolescents with bipolar I, bipolar II and bipolar NOS diagnoses exist on a continuum and support the concept of a bipolar spectrum disorder. What remains to be discovered in a more longitudinal study is if those with subsyndromal elevated mood (at least by DSM-IV criteria) will remain so into adulthood or will morph into a bipolar I clinical picture.

Making a longitudinal diagnosis

The investigating clinician should always attempt to discern the pattern of mood episodes that may have preceded the current index episode. Either by life cycle charting or through careful history taking, the clinician should establish the presence of any earlier depressed, hypomanic, or mixed episodes, their duration, and the circumstances that led to their resolution. The treatment regimen for the presenting episode may be influenced considerably by the presence of hypomanic or elevated mood symptoms in the past. Such elevated mood episodes in the past should also alert the clinician to the possibility of a dysphoric mania or a mixed episode, even if the presenting chief complaint is a very severe depression.

Assessment of temperament

In addition to current mood symptoms, past mood episodes, and family history, the clinician should inquire about elements of temperament. What is the patient's usual state of optimism or pessimism? What is his or her usual state of energy and enthusiasm? Is the current episode an intensification of usual temperament or is it considerably out of character? It is often useful to assign a temperamental category to the patient on the basis of the delineation of various personality types as defined in Chapter 1. The presence of a dysthymic temperament, a hyperthymic temperament, or a temperament characterized by significant mood fluctuations (cyclothymic temperament) may guide both diagnosis and treatment with medication. This is discussed more fully in Chapter 7 on treatment with medication.

Identification of a mood pattern

The clinician's goal is to understand the context and pattern of the patient's moods. It is this pattern that forms the backdrop against which the clinician will identify current symptomatology and the chief complaint. Patients with a down dominated mood, who are currently depressed, may be treated differently than a patient who has an up dominated mood pattern and who similarly presents with depression (see Chapter 7).

It is also important to establish whether there is a cycling pattern to the patient's mood. Some patients will have regular mood cycling patterns with depression followed by hypomanias; others will have hypomanias followed by depressions. Some patients will have periods of mood cycling that last for several weeks or months, and then are not present for months or years. Still others have no discernible pattern. The process of establishing the presence of patterns has several uses. Mood patterns may provide clarification of the nature of the current index episode, and also provide a context of understanding for breakthrough episodes that may occur during treatment.

Additional history sources

Accurate mood diagnosis cannot be determined based solely on the identified patient's perception of his or her mood state. As has been noted, patients may have an inaccurate perception of their own mood state or have a bias against seeing hypomania as part of a pathologic condition. At other times, current depression may impair cognition, rendering patients unable to remember accurately how he or she felt several months or years ago. It is important, therefore, to use sources of information in addition to the identified patient. This means interviewing the patient's spouse, children, parents, guardians, or other individuals who have knowledge of the patient's behavior on a day-to-day basis. If necessary, a phone call to an out-of-town source may also be useful. When mood charting is utilized as discussed subsequently, it may also be helpful to give a copy of the mood chart to a spouse or other family member to complete. The family member's perceptions of the patient's behavior may shed a different perspective on the intensity and stability of the patient's condition. Behaviors that are "usual" or "normal" for the patient may only come to be identified as "symptoms" when seen through the eyes of the family.

Using standardized screening tools

Although detailed history taking may be the most effective way to evaluate the presence of hypomanic symptoms, many practitioners do not have the time or expertise to do so. This is particularly the case with primary care clinicians who suspect many bipolar patients "hidden" in their practice, but may have limited time for a confirmatory evaluation. For these practitioners, the use of standardized screening tools can be a timesaving measure and lead to more accurate diagnosis. Two of the most commonly used screening questionnaires are the Mood Disorders Questionnaire (MDQ) and the Bipolar Spectrum Disorder Scale (BSDS).

The MDQ was developed by Robert Hirschfeld et al. and is a 13-item, self-administered screening tool that has been psychometrically validated (9). It has a high sensitivity and specificity and has been in use for >5 years. The questions on MDQ and the scoring system are shown in Tables 3.10 and 3.11.

The BSDS, developed at Harvard Medical School by Ronald Pies and Nassir Ghaemi (10), is a short story consisting of 19 elements that can be endorsed or denied by the patient. Another question is about how well the story "fits" this individual. The patient's total score is indicative of the probability of having a bipolar spectrum disorder. The BSDS and its scoring system are shown in Tables 3.12 and 3.13.

Although somewhat less precise and not validated for large clinical populations, simple daily and monthly screening done by the patient between sessions can sometimes alert the clinician to mood swings and mild hypomanic symptoms if the patient is educated as to what constitutes evidence of elevated mood. An example of such a chart and a discussion of its use are contained in Chapter 6.

Reaction to medication trials

Additional clues to the presence of bipolar spectrum disorder and hypomania may be revealed in the patient's reaction to specific psychotropic medications. By inquiring about response to previous psychotropic medication trials during the initial history, important clues to a bipolar diagnosis can be uncovered. Although patients may not remember each particular medication, an effort should be made to identify previous response, lack of response, or the production of any new symptoms for each psychotropic trial. Particular attention should be paid to the patient's reaction to previous antidepressant medication trials, whether they are tricyclic antidepressants, selective serotonin reuptake inhibitors (SSRIs), serotonin–norepinephrine reuptake inhibitors (SNRIs), or other antidepressants. The clinician should ask about the extent and the speed with which an antidepressant response was obtained. Unusually rapid response to an antidepressant (e.g., marked or full response within a period of 1 to 3 days) may be a factor suggesting a possible bipolar diagnosis.

It has been frequently debated whether a manic or hypomanic response to an antidepressant constitutes a true form of bipolar disorder. It is the opinion of the author and other writers (see Chapter 4) that elevated mood symptoms, as a response to an antidepressant, does in fact reflect a bipolar diathesis and places the patient along the bipolar spectrum. That is to say, a

TABLE 3.10

The mood disorder questionnaire (MDQ)

INSTRUCTIONS: Please answer each question as best you can.	YES	NO
Has there ever been a period of time when you were not your usual self and . . .	—	—
. . .you felt so good or so hyper that other people thought you were not your normal self or you were so hyper that you got into trouble?	—	—
. . .you were so irritable that you shouted at people or started fights or arguments?	—	—
. . .you felt much more self-confident than usual?	—	—
. . .you got much less sleep than usual and found that you did not really miss it?	—	—
. . .you were more talkative or spoke much faster than usual?	—	—
. . .thoughts raced through your head or you could not slow your mind down?	—	—
. . .you were so easily distracted by things around you that you had trouble concentrating or staying on track?	—	—
. . .you had more energy than usual?	—	—
. . .you were much more active or did many more things than usual?	—	—
. . .you were much more social or outgoing than usual, for example, you telephoned friends in the middle of the night?	—	—
. . .you were much more interested in sex than usual?	—	—
. . .you did things that were unusual for you or that other people might have thought were excessive, foolish, or risky?	—	—
. . .spending money got you or your family in trouble?	—	—
If you checked YES to more than one of the above, have several of these ever happened during the same period of time?	—	—
How much of a problem did any of these cause you—like being able to work; having family, money, or legal troubles; getting into arguments or fights?		
_____No problem_____Minor problem_____Moderate problem_____ Serious problem		
Have any of your blood relatives (i.e. children, siblings, parents, grandparents, aunts, uncles) had manic-depressive illness or bipolar disorder?	—	—
Has a health professional ever told you that you have manic-depressive illness or bipolar disorder?	—	—

TABLE 3.11

The mood disorder questionnaire (MDQ)—scoring algorithm

Positive screen

All three of the following criteria must be met:

Scoring:	Question 1: 7/13 positive (yes) responses
	+
	Question 2: Positive (yes) response
	+
	Question 3: "moderate" or "serious" response

bipolar disorder is "uncovered" or "unmasked" by the use of an unopposed antidepressant. The bipolar condition has not been "created" by the use of an antidepressant.

Regardless of this debate, there are significant clinical implications when a manic/hypomanic reaction occurs in response to an antidepressant. Such a response indicates a vulnerability to an antidepressant as monotherapy. With such a history and a presentation of depression, the patient should not be placed on antidepressant monotherapy. Initial therapy should consist of a mood stabilizer, an atypical antipsychotic, or potentially a combination of one of these drugs with an antidepressant, as discussed in Chapter 7.

Frankly manic and hypomanic responses, even when they have been unrecognized by the patient are, by definition, indicators of the presence of a bipolar spectrum disorder. Less dramatic subsyndromal responses should also be noted and serve as a warning to the clinician that bipolar spectrum condition is a possibility. These softer responses include the following:

• A marked sleep disorder as a side effect to the antidepressant, especially if there is no fatigue with the loss of sleep
• Markedly anxious responses to an antidepressant, including frank panic attacks

In other cases, patients who have had multiple trials of antidepressants with virtually no antidepressant response may indicate a missed bipolar diagnosis. Also, within this group are patients who are placed on an antidepressant and respond to the antidepressant medication, but lose the response within a few weeks to several months. These patients may periodically "cycle down" into depression rather than "lose" the medication response. A useful therapeutic strategy in such patients would be to use a mood stabilizer, alone or in combination with an antidepressant.

Lack of response to potential mood stabilizers, such as lithium, valproic acid, or carbamazepine, generally does not, unfortunately, give the clinician significant diagnostic information. The lack of response to monotherapy with a

TABLE 3.12
The bipolar spectrum diagnostic scale

Description	Response (tick)
1. Some individuals notice that their mood and/or energy levels shift drastically from time to time	
2. These individuals notice that, at times, their mood and/or energy level is very low, and at other times, very high	
3. During their "low" phases, these individuals often feel a lack of energy; a need to stay in bed or get extra sleep; and little or no motivation to do things they need to do	
4. They often put on weight during these periods	
5. During their low phases, these individuals often feel "blue," sad all the time, or depressed	
6. Sometimes during these low phases, they feel hopeless or even suicidal	
7. Their ability to function at work or socially is impaired	
8. Typically, these low phases last for a few weeks, but sometimes they last only a few days	
9. Individuals with this type of pattern may experience a period of 'normal' mood in between mood swings, during which their mood and energy levels feel "right" and their ability to function is not disturbed	
10. They may then notice a marked shift or "switch" in the way they feel	
11. Their energy increases above what is normal for them, and they often get many things done that they would not ordinarily be able to do	
12. Sometimes, during these "high" periods, these individuals feel as if they have too much of energy or feel "hyper"	
13. Some individuals, during these high periods, may feel irritable, "on edge," or aggressive	
14. Some individuals, during these high periods, take on too many activities at once	
15. During these high periods, some individuals may append money in ways that cause them trouble	
16. They may be more talkative, outgoing, or sexual during these periods	
17. Sometimes, their behavior during these high periods seems strange or annoying to others	
18. Sometimes, these individuals have difficulty with coworkers or the police, during these high periods	
19. Sometimes they increase the alcohol or nonprescription drug use during these periods	

TABLE 3.13
Scoring the Bipolar Spectrum Disorders Scale (BSDS)

Add the check marks from the first 19 sentences. To that total, add the number in parentheses below for the line you selected:

• This story fits me very well, or almost perfectly **(6)**
• This story fits me fairly well **(4)**
• This story fits me to some degree, but not in most respects **(2)**
• This story does not really describe me at all **(0)**
The maximum is 19 plus 6, for 25 points
Here is how to interpret your score:
19 or higher = bipolar spectrum disorder highly likely
11–18 = moderate probability of bipolar spectrum disorder
6–10 = low probability of bipolar spectrum disorder
<6 = bipolar spectrum disorder very unlikely

mood stabilizer says little about whether bipolar disorder is present, but could simply indicate that this particular medication is ineffective for this patient. With bipolar patients in the depressed phase, insufficient antidepressant response from mood stabilizer monotherapy is not unusual and says little about the underlying diagnosis.

Another clinical situation with diagnostic significance is when patients present with symptoms of an affective mixed state. When placed on a mood stabilizer, these patients quickly note feeling "much worse," and significantly more depressed. In these cases, the response to the mood stabilizer may be a confirmation of the presence of mixed states with depressive and hypomanic symptoms (see Chapter 8).

The bottom line

- For a variety of reasons, elevated mood symptoms are often missed or discounted by clinicians.
- The clinician should ask questions about elevated mood of every patient with depression, anxiety, or substance abuse as a chief complaint.
- The most important elements for success in diagnosing elevated mood include the following:
  1. Asking appropriate questions
  2. Using sources of information beyond the identified patient
  3. Determining family history
  4. Looking for soft signs of elevated mood

5. Documenting response to previous medication trials and
6. Reassessing the diagnosis over time in light of treatment response and failure
- Bipolar disorder may present to the clinician with a wide variety of chief complaints.
- In milder forms, elevated mood symptoms may be initially viewed as positive, productive, and helpful. When exaggerated or intense, however, they create significant negative behavioral consequences.
- The most common manifestations of hypomania are increased activity and plans, increased energy and self-confidence, decreased amount of sleep, increased talkativeness, and decreased inhibition.
- When distinguishing hyperthymic traits from hypomanic dysfunction, utilize an assessment of the four Ps—productivity, positivity, people skills and predictability.
- Always reevaluate the validity of a diagnosis made by other clinicians in light of current diagnostic criteria for elevated mood.

REFERENCES

1. Lish JD, Dime-Meenan S, Whybrow PC, et al. The National Depressive and Manic Depressive Association survey of bipolar members. *J Affect Disord.* 1994;31:281–294.
2. Wicki W, Angst J. The Zurich Study. X hypomania in a 28- to 30-year-old cohort. *Eur Arch Psychiatry Clin Neurosci.* 1991;240(6):339–348.
3. Ghaemi SN. *Mood disorders.* Philadelphia: Lippincott Williams & Wilkins; 2003: 13–14, originally developed by William Falk, MD.
4. Swann AC, Geller B, Post RM, et al. Practical clues to early recognition of bipolar disorder: A primary care approach. Prim care companion. *J Clin Psychiatry.* 2005;7(1):15–21.
5. Akiskal Hagop S. Bipolar depression: Focus on phenomenology. *J Affect Disord.* 2005;84:279–290.
6. Geller B, Williams M, Zimerman B, et al. Pre-pubertal and early adolescent bipolarity differentiate from ADHD by manic symptoms, grandiose delusions, ultrarapid and ultradian cycling. *J Affect Disord.* 1998;51:81.
7. Geller B, Zimerman B, Williams M, et al. DSM-IV mania symptoms in a prepubertal and early adolescent bipolar disorder phenotype compared to attention deficit hyperactive and normal controls. *J Child Adolesc Psychopharmacol.* 2002;12:11.
8. Axelson D, Birmaher B, Strober M, et al. Phenomenology of children and adolescents with bipolar spectrum disorders. *Arch Gen Psychiatry.* 2006;63:1139–1148.
9. Hirschfeld RM, Williams JB, Spitzer RL, et al. The mood disorder questionnaire (MDQ). *Am J Psychiatry.* 2000;157(11):1873–1875.
10. Nassir Ghaemi N, Miller CJ, Berv DA, et al. Sensitivity and specificity of a new bipolar spectrum diagnostic scale. *J Affect Disord.* 2005;84(2–3):273–277.

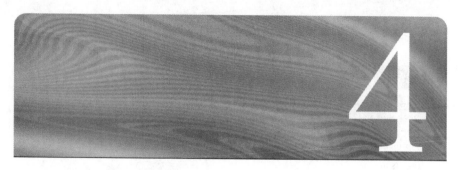

UPSIDE DOWN—
DEPRESSION AND HYPOMANIA

- Differentiating a major depressive episode from the depression of bipolar disorder
- Searching for historic periods of elevated mood
- Temperament as the context for depression
- Suicidality and antidepressants

- Treating depressed mood in patients with elevated mood symptoms
- Light therapy in depressed mood
- Omega-3 fatty acids
- The bottom line

  References

Although the focus of this book is elevated mood, any discussion of hypomania must include its interface with depression. Whether the appearance of depressed symptoms is discrete or concurrent with episodes of elevated mood, the diagnosis and treatment of elevated mood must take into account its relationship to depression. The prevalence of depression in patients with elevated mood occurs so frequently that this topic deserves special attention here. Depressive symptoms occurring simultaneously with elevated mood are covered both in this chapter and under mixed affective states in Chapter 8.

If one were to construct a "Top Ten List" of the reasons that patients with elevated mood present for mental health treatment, it might appear like the list in Table 4.1.

Because the presenting complaints of elevated mood, patients have not been systematically researched or quantified, experts might disagree on the exact order of this "top ten list," but few would dispute that depression is, by far, the most common reason for presentation. Because evidence of elevated mood may be only commingled with symptoms of depression in patients with mixed states, or may only be historically evident but not present at the time of evaluation, careful diagnostic exploration is crucial.

Data gathered in several large-scale studies has shown that depression is extraordinarily common in patients with elevated mood. Judd, Akiskal et al. demonstrated that patients with bipolar I disorder spent an average

TABLE 4.1

Top 10 reasons for persons with elevated mood to present for treatment

- Depression
- Depression
- Depression
- Depression
- Depression
- Sleeplessness
- Anxiety
- Alcohol/drug use and abuse
- Irritability and explosiveness
- Problems with relationships

of one third of their time in a depressed state (1). Another study by this same group (2) showed that patients with bipolar II disorder spent at least half of their time in a clinically depressed state. In a naturalistic perspective, 7-year follow-up study of 908 patients with bipolar disorder, Suppes et al. looked for subtle signs of hypomania and depression as scored on the Young Mania Rating Scale and the Inventory of Depressive Symptomatology (3). Hypomania was present in 392 (43%) of these patients. In those patients with hypomania, 71% presented with depression mixed with hypomania during at least one visit. Overall, in 57% of the visits in which hypomania was present, depressive symptoms also occurred.

Bauer et al. (4) performed a cross-sectional analysis of 441 individuals with bipolar disorder treated at an American health maintenance organization and investigated the distribution of manic and depressive symptoms in that population. They found that clinically significant depressive symptoms occurred in 94.1% of those with mania or hypomania whereas 70.1% of those in a depressive episode had clinically significant manic symptoms.

Beyond the frequency of depression in patients with bipolar disorder, as documented by the studies mentioned in the preceding text, there is now evidence that depressed episodes incur a significant level of psychosocial impairment. Judd et al. (5) followed 158 patients with bipolar I disorder and 133 patients with bipolar II disorder for 20 years. Their findings suggest that any level of depression in patients with bipolar disorder is more disabling than any form of mania, further highlighting the necessity of identifying depression as well as elevated mood.

Perlis et al. (6) followed a subset of 1,469 patients who had been symptomatic for bipolar disorder with 58% achieved recovery. During a 2-year follow-up period, 49% of those who had recovered subsequently experienced recurrences with twice as many patients developing depressive episodes as manic/hypomanic/mixed episodes combined. These episodes of depression also occurred significantly earlier than manic or hypomanic recurrences. Their data suggests that residual mood symptoms at the time of recovery are a "powerful predictor" of recurrence. The risk of a depressive relapse increased by 14% for every *Diagnostic and Statistical Manual of Mental Disorders-IV* (DSM-IV) depressive symptom still present at the time of recovery. This led the researchers to conclude "Overall, these results suggest that despite modern evidence-based treatment, bipolar disorder remains a highly recurrent, predominantly depressive illness." Therefore, the principle of treating depression to full remission, the clinical goal for major depressive episodes, also appears to apply to depressive episodes within the context of a bipolar disorder.

Differentiating a major depressive episode from the depression of bipolar disorder

It is helpful to think of depression not as a *diagnosis* but rather as a *constellation of symptoms* that can be present in multiple psychiatric disorders. Just as sepsis is a constellation of symptoms that requires further diagnostic assessment to determine etiology, "depression" should not be considered an end point. Once a depressive constellation of symptoms is identified, further clinical assessment is necessary to fully solve the diagnostic puzzle. A constellation of depressive symptoms could (in our current nomenclature) reflect unipolar depression, dysthymic disorder, bipolar I disorder, bipolar II disorder, a mixed affective state, a side effect to medications such as interferon or corticosteroids, or a response to certain viral illnesses such as mononucleosis or hepatitis. As this text focuses on elevated mood, we will concentrate our discussion on the interface between depressive symptoms and elevated mood in primary mood disorders.

Until there is solid endophenotypic and/or genotypic data to assist in more precisely diagnosing various types of depressed mood as described in Chapter 2, we must depend on clinical signs and symptoms and solid diagnostic skills to differentiate bipolar depression from unipolar depression. Even with potentially useful phenotypic signs and symptoms, it is important to realize that these are still only broad generalizations.

Some of the other signs that may assist clinicians in distinguishing unipolar depression from bipolar depression include differences in the course of the depressive symptoms as well as which symptoms are present. These are shown in Tables 4.2, 4.3, and 4.4 adapted from (7–9).

Searching for historic periods of elevated mood

When a patient presents with depression, it is important not to limit diagnostic queries to symptoms and time courses of depressive episodes alone. In

TABLE 4.2

Time considerations more common in bipolar depression when compared with unipolar depression

- Earlier age of onset
- Higher frequency of episodes
- Shorter duration of episodes
- Longer total duration of illness
- Quick onset and/or more rapid improvement of symptoms

TABLE 4.3

Symptom presentation in bipolar and unipolar depression

Symptoms more common in bipolar depression	Symptoms more common in unipolar depression
Family history of bipolar disorder	Agitation
Higher incidence of psychosis	Insomnia
Atypical features such as psychomotor retardation	Weight loss
Hypersomnia	—
Weight gain	—
Extroversion	—
Mood liability	—
Novelty seeking	—

TABLE 4.4

Symptoms that occur with equal frequency in unipolar and bipolar depression

- Guilt
- Low self-esteem
- Decreased energy
- Poor concentration
- Increased suicide risk

addition to the diagnostic principles discussed in Chapter 3, each depressed patient should be asked specifically about the presence of mood shifts including the frequency, intensity, rapidity, and the character of the changing moods.

Akiskal and Benazzi (10), in their review of 563 consecutive, private outpatients, have emphasized the presence of *overactive behavior* rather than mood change as the crucial and sentinel event of hypomania. These researchers suggest that episodes of behavioral activation should be the primary field of inquiry, followed by questions about euphoria and irritability. They further suggest that there is an increased diagnostic sensitivity if the following questions are asked:

- Do you feel better in the summer?
- Do you feel much better right before depression or soon after it?
- Do you have periods of excess energy?
- Do you not become tired when other people do?
- Do you have periods of crowded thoughts (your head is so continuously full of ideas that you are unable to stop thinking)?
- Do you have episodes of high activity that depart significantly from your usual routine?
- Do you have frequent mood changes from happiness to sadness without apparent cause or reason?
- Do you have any of the issues mentioned earlier that occur while feeling depressed?

Temperament as the context for depression

Akiskal and Angst, as well as others, emphasize the longitudinal context of a patient's personality against which the emergence of depressive episodes should be understood. They particularly focus on the depressive temperament, the cyclothymic temperament, and the hyperthymic temperament as defined in Chapter 1. Depressive episodes, presenting as a chief complaint, should be viewed against the backdrop of an individual who is subsyndromally depressed, has subsyndromal affective cycling or, conversely, has high energy and is hyperthymic. Not only is this information of theoretic and causative importance, but temperament factors can also affect the clinician's choice of medications (see Chapter 7). Individuals with a depressive or dysthymic temperament may be at low risk for elevation into mania when antidepressants are prescribed, whereas cyclothymic or hyperthymic individuals may be at a greater risk for this complication. Cyclothymic or hyperthymic individuals may benefit substantially from mood stabilizer monotherapy or a therapy using a combination of mood stabilizers. Antidepressants would be used less frequently in this group. Depression in patients with a dysthymic temperament may be at less risk for the induction of cycling or a switch into hypomania if antidepressants are used.

Suicidality and antidepressants

In addition to the intense mental pain and significant dysfunction, in social role associated with depression, a great clinical concern is the incidence of suicidality in bipolar patients with depression. It has long been known that patients with bipolar disorder comprise a population who are at high risk for suicide (11–14). Prompt recognition, treatment, and prophylaxis of depressive episodes in a bipolar disorder have a marked beneficial effect on diminishing suicide rates in this group.

Warnings by the United States Food and Drug Administration suggest that the use of antidepressants may be associated with increased suicidality. While the exact incidence of such suicidality has been debated and is generally thought by most clinicians to be relatively small, there is little additional information to date that elucidates the nature of suicidal ideation and behavior in patients with a bipolar disorder. A recent large-scale study, however, as part of the Systematic Treatment Enhancement Program for Bipolar Disorder (STEP-BD) gives some relatively reassuring data (15). In this study, the first 2,000 participants were observed and evaluated for a new-onset major depressive episode. The study participants were given standardized rating scales for suicidality and monitored for antidepressant exposure. The study found no association between new-onset suicidality with the initiation of antidepressant treatment, increased exposure to antidepressants, or change in antidepressant exposure. This study suggests that there is no increased suicidality when antidepressants are used in a bipolar population. Although reassuring, the clinician must continue to carefully monitor and assess for suicidal ideation and intent. The incidence of suicidality in patients with bipolar disorder remains high secondary to the underlying illness itself, particularly with patients with bipolar II disorder and those with mixed affective episodes.

Treating depressed mood in patients with elevated mood symptoms

The issue of the use of antidepressants in treating depressed mood in patients with bipolar disorder is discussed in Chapter 7. However, it is important to note other treatment modalities that are helpful in the treatment of depression that do not include prescription medication. Many of the strategies described in Chapter 6, which are useful in the elevated mood states, are also useful for the depressed phase of the illness. Cognitive Behavioral Therapy (CBT) has long been a staple of treatment of depression and can be effectively used in the depressed phase of bipolar illness as well as with major depressive episodes. CBT has neither noted incidence of bipolar exacerbation nor any increased incidence of hypomania with its use. Likewise, it is easily adaptable for use on its own or in combination with medication.

Light therapy in depressed mood

Patients and clinicians have known that a period of early morning awakening may provide a transient boost in mood, usually lasting several hours or part of a day. Recently, Benedetti et al. (16) extended this concept by treating 60 inpatients with drug-resistant bipolar depression with one week of repeated total sleep deprivation and light therapy combined with ongoing antidepressants and lithium. Their chronotherapy consisted of a series of three consecutive cycles of total sleep deprivation for a period of 36 hours (days 1, 3, and 5). Patients/subjects were then allowed to sleep during the nights of days 2, 4, and 6. In addition, patients/subjects were exposed to an artificial light source (400 Lux of green light) for a 30-minute period during sleep deprivation and in the morning after recovery sleep. With this protocol, 70% of patients with non–medication-resistant bipolar disorder and 44% of medication-resistant patients achieved at least a 50% reduction in Hamilton Rating Scale for depression. This response was significant, particularly for drug-resistant patients. When these patients were followed for a 9-month period, 57% of the non-resistant responders and 17% of the drug-resistant responders were euthymic at 9 months. Although unrealistic over an extended period, light and chronotherapeutic interventions do merit further investigation for bipolar depression, particularly when medicines have failed.

Omega-3 fatty acids

Over the past decade there have been a number of reports, albeit with small patient populations, that suggest that the use of cold water fish oils containing omega-3 fatty acids have been useful in prophylaxis of unipolar depression (17–20).

Parker et al. (21) have also hypothesized that deficits in dietary fatty acids may play a partial causal role in the development of mood disorders. Two recent studies, one by Osher et al. (22) and a second by Frangou et al. (23), suggest that 1 to 2 grams per day of eicosapentaenoic acid (EPA) have favorable results in the treatment of bipolar depression. This treatment has been supported by a variety of biochemical studies that suggest that fatty acids may modulate neurotransmitter metabolism and cell signal transduction. Although the numbers in the studies are small (12 in the Osher study and 75 in the Frangou study), both studies showed a significant improvement on the Hamilton Depression Rating Scale over a 6-month period for a significant number of participants. No patients experienced precipitation of a manic episode and, in general, the therapy was well tolerated. This adds then to the growing evidence for omega-3 fatty acids being useful acutely or prophylactically for bipolar depression.

The bottom line

- Depression is frequently present in patients with elevated mood and is often the presenting complaint in patients with bipolar disorder and mixed states.

- Soft signs may help differentiate a unipolar depression from a bipolar depressive episode; however, the distinction is not easy to make on symptoms alone.
- Family history of bipolar disorder, early onset, shorter and more frequent episodes, and atypical features may point to a bipolar depression.
- Patients with bipolar disorder are at high risk for suicide.
- CBT, omega-3 fatty acids, chronotherapy, and phototherapy can be useful treatment modalities for bipolar depression.

REFERENCES

1. Judd LL, Akiskal HS, Schettler PJ, et al. The long-term natural history of the weekly symptomatic status of bipolar I disorder. *Arch Gen Psychiatry.* 2002;59:530–537.
2. Judd LL, Akiskal HS, Schettler PJ, et al. A prospective investigation of the natural history of the long-term weekly symptomatic status of bipolar II disorder. *Arch Gen Psychiatry.* 2003;60:261–269.
3. Suppes T, Mintz J, McElroy SL, et al. Mixed hypomania in 908 patients with Bipolar disorder evaluated prospectively in the Stanley Foundation Bipolar Treatment Network. *Arch Gen Psychiatry.* 2005;62:1089–1096.
4. Bauer MS, Simon GE, Ludman E, et al. Bipolarity in bipolar disorder: A distribution of manic and depressive symptoms in a treated population. *Br J Psychiatry.* 2005;187:87–88.
5. Judd LL, Akiskal HS, Schettler PJ, et al. Psychosocial disability in the course of bipolar I and II disorders: A perspective comparative longitudinal study. *Arch Gen Psychiatry.* 2005;62:1322–1330.
6. Perlis RH, Ostacher MJ, Patel JK, et al. Predictors of recurrence in bipolar disorder: Primary outcomes from the Systematic Treatment Enhancement Program for Bipolar Disorder [STEP-BD]. *Am J Psychiatry.* 2006;163:217–224.
7. Bowden CL. Strategies to reduce misdiagnosis of bipolar depression. *Psychiatr Serv.* 2001;52:51–55.
8. Akiskal HS, Walker P, Puzantian VR, et al. Bipolar outcome in the course of depressive illness: Phenomenologic, familial, and pharmacologic predictors. *J Affect Disord.* 1983;5:115–128.
9. Akiskal HS, Maser JD, Zeller PJ, et al. Switching from "unipolar" to bipolar II: An 11-year prospective study of clinical and temperamental predictors in 559 patients. *Arch Gen Psychiatry.* 1995;52:114–123.
10. Akiskal HS, Benazzi F. Optimizing the detection of bipolar II disorder in outpatient private practice: Toward a systematization of clinical diagnostic wisdom. *J Clin Psychiatry.* 2005;66(7):914–921.
11. Chen YW, Dilsaver SC. Lifetime rates of suicide attempts among subjects with bipolar and unipolar disorders relative to subjects with other Axis I disorders. *Biol Psychiatry.* 1996;39(1):896–899.
12. Tondo L, Isacsson G, Baldessarini R. Suicidal behavior in bipolar disorder: Risk and prevention. *CNS Drugs.* 2003;17(7):491–511.
13. Goodwin FK, Jamison KR. *Manic-depressive illness.* New York: Oxford University Press; 1990:227–244.
14. Slama F, Bellivier F, Henry C, et al. Bipolar patients with suicidal behavior: Toward the identification of a clinical subgroup. *J Clin Psychiatry.* 2004;65(8):1035–1039.

15. Bauer MS, Wisniewski SR, Marangell LB, et al. Are antidepressants associated with new-onset suicidality in bipolar disorder? A prospective study of the participants in the STEP-BD. *J Clin Psychiatry.* 2006;67:48–55.

16. Benedetti F, Barbini B, Fulgosi MC, et al. Combined total sleep deprivation and light therapy in the treatment of drug-resistant bipolar depression: Acute response and long-term remission rates. *J Clin Psychiatry.* 2005;66:1535–1540.

17. Su KP, Huang SY, Chiu CC, et al. Omega-3 fatty acids in major depressive disorder. A preliminary double-blind, placebo-controlled trial. *Eur Neuropscyhopharmacol.* 2003;13(4):267–271.

18. Peet M, Stokes C. Omega-3 fatty acids in the treatment of psychiatry disorders. *Drugs.* 2005;65(8):1051–1059.

19. Nemets B, Stahl Z, Belmaker RH. Addition of omega-3 fatty acid to maintenance medication treatment for recurrent unipolar depressive disorder. *Am J Psychiatry.* 2002;159(3):477–479.

20. Silvers KM, Woolley CC, Hamilton FC, et al. Randomized double-blind placebo-controlled trial of fish oil in the treatment of depression. *Prostaglandins Leukot Essent Fatty Acids.* 2005;72(3):211–218.

21. Parker G, Gibson NA, Brotchie H, et al. Omega-3 fatty acids and mood disorders. *Am J Psychiatry.* 2006;163:969–978.

22. Osher Y, Bersudsky Y, Belmaker RH. Omega-3 eicosapentaenoic acid in bipolar depression: Report of a small open-label study. *J Clin Psychiatry.* 2005;66(6): 726–729.

23. Frangou S, Lewis M, McCrone P. Efficacy of ethyl-eicosapentaenoic acid in bipolar depression: Randomized double-blind placebo-controlled study. *Br J Psychiatry.* 2006;188:46–50.

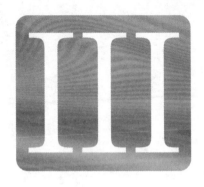

Treatment of Elevated Mood

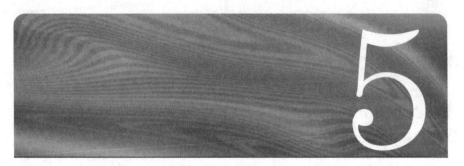

TREATING ELEVATED MOOD—
PRINCIPLES AND THE CHALLENGES

T he first several chapters of this text describe the evolution in understanding hypomania and elevated mood starting from a purely phenomenologic perspective and moving to a more biologic and genetic perspective. As the understanding of causality and the underlying biologic parameters that lead to hypomania become elucidated, more precise treatments will emerge. Meanwhile, we must continue to treat hypomanic individuals with the information we have. This chapter, as well as those that follow, is devoted to elements of treatment that we can utilize now. We will focus first on management principles of mildly elevated mood and activity, before discussing treatment of more severe conditions. In addition to identifying the elements of treatment that facilitate improvement, we will also look at potential therapeutic pitfalls and how to avoid or remedy them.

What is normal?

Many factors play into the assessment of what, on the surface, appears to be a simple question, "What is normal?" The clinician's response to this query is essential in devising a treatment strategy that has been mutually agreed upon for elevated mood. Many clinicians are afraid of a potential "wildfire" of mania and may become overly concerned about even minimal elevations of mood or energized behavior. If the clinician assumes a suppressive monolithic approach toward this condition, the patient will rebel, become noncompliant, or drop out of treatment altogether. Therefore, the more appropriate question is not *"What is normal?"* but *"What is normal for this patient?"* In many cases, reestablishing a previous, but not necessarily optimal, level of functioning will be adequate treatment that is agreeable to the patient. On occasion, there may be the patient who wants to remain hypomanic, however, the clinician is aware that such a mood state is inappropriate, dysfunctional, or likely to result in increased mood swings. In these cases, the therapist must educate the patient about the dangers of flagrant hypomania. In circumstances where a reasonable treatment plan cannot be reached between the therapist and the patient, the therapist will need to withdraw from treatment. Further exploration of the topic, patients wanting to remain hypomanic, is presented later in the chapter.

Stability is in the eye of the beholder

Even with considerable mood instability, a patient may not necessarily see this as a problem. Stability is in the eye of the beholder. Some patients are remarkably willing to accept an unstable mood if the alternative is seen as becoming "flat" or "boring." They may view stabilizing treatment as modifying essential elements of their individuality or personality, which they do not wish to relinquish. Many patients with elevated mood tolerate mood instability if their functional deficits and/or depressive episodes are infrequent or mild. In such cases, the patient may be unlikely to seek treatment unless symptoms markedly impair functioning. Other patients decide "This is the way I am," tolerate the cycling, and reject psychotherapeutic or medication interventions. This may be in spite of clinical recommendations, family, or workplace pressure.

The pain of dealing with hypomania/depression cycling prompts the patient to seek and maintain treatment. If patients feel minimal or no psychic pain/discomfort, or have no family, financial, or work consequences to their cycling disorder, they are less likely to see a need for treatment. Medical analogies to the situation include the treatment of blood pressure or arteriosclerotic cardiovascular disease. An asymptomatic hypertensive patient may be erratic or resistant to treatment, whereas a patient experiencing a transient ischemic attack (TIA) from elevated blood pressure is likely frightened and therefore more amenable to treatment. Likewise, when patient's poor diet and exercise habits result in weight and cholesterol abnormalities, changes may be made only when an episode of angina occurs. And so, hypomanic patients become more amenable to treatment when the pain or consequences of impulsive elevated mood or depression interfere significantly in their lives.

"Just a little off the top"

This instruction, often given to a barber, also provides us with a way of thinking about hypomania treatment. Even as patients with significant symptomatology wish to minimize their cycles of hypomania, they do not wish to lose the positive attributes that are inherent in hyperthymic temperament and/or mild hypomania. Few of these patients desire or require a "buzz cut." Just "a little off, here and there" is the desired approach. In the collaborative patient-centered approach discussed in this text, moderation and modulation of the most severe and frequent symptoms of elevated mood is an appropriate goal of treatment and may be the only one acceptable to the patient. Totally eliminating elevated mood, although sometimes possible, is seldom desirable or acceptable to the patient.

When is treatment needed?

As with any mental health condition, even when hypomania is diagnosed, it may or may not require treatment. This section describes collaboration with patients in deciding whether treatment is necessary and appropriate.

Patients with relatively mild symptomatology of elevated mood may never present for treatment. Those with hyperthymic temperament may function adequately, or even at a superior level without any psychiatric intervention. As has been discussed in Chapter 4, by far the most common problem that brings a person with hypomania to mental health practitioners is the presence of depression. In these cases, hypomania is diagnosed using the principles described in Chapters 3 and 4 to elucidate a history of hypomania in the patient presenting with depression. At times, hypomanic or hyperthymic individuals present in the mental health setting not because of depression but because one or more symptoms of elevated mood have become bothersome, intense, exaggerated, or intrusive in the patient's life. Such symptoms can include excessive irritability, agitation, or a sleep disorder resistant to typical treatment modalities. Other patients request treatment for conditions that are ancillary to hypomania itself such as alcohol, or drug abuse, or marital dysfunction. In most cases, however, hypomanic individuals tend not to seek treatment solely for hypomania unless their hypomania is spiraling up toward mania, contains significant elements of anxiety or panic, or when they have previously experienced a hypomanic prelude to mania. This latter group has often had a hospitalization or outpatient treatment with medication to bring down the symptoms of mania but may have residual symptoms of a mild, moderate, or severe nature that require follow-up treatment.

Treatment by functional severity

Arriving at a diagnosis of elevated mood may not be sufficient enough to undertake treatment. Although the therapist may feel that treatment is appropriate, the patient must see the benefits of treatment. In general, rather than commenting about one symptom, the therapist's approach should focus on a more general assessment of the patient's life and how this hypomanic and/or depressive mood pattern fits in. It is within this broader picture that the current presenting symptoms are viewed. Two separate but equally useful techniques to accomplish this can be summarized in the phrase "use both a telescope and a microscope."

First use a "telescope" to look at the whole of the patient's life to determine if treatment is necessary at all. How does this episode fit in the overall functionality of the patient's life? Is this a distinct aberration? How often have such aberrations occurred? What is the level of severity of this particular episode? Who else is affected by the patient's behavior other than the patient himself? What risks may be taken by *not* treating the identified episode? As was discussed in Chapter 3, the use of lifetime charting can be a useful tool to visually and graphically view the patient's functionality over time. It is only in the context of unpredictability, irregularity, and periods of functional disability that some patients can see the impact of their condition on the overall fabric of their lives.

The converse is also a useful technique. Here, the therapist attempts to use a "microscope" to tease apart the various phenomenologic and symptom elements of the patient's condition. The practitioner identifies those elements of the patient's life that work well and those that are functionally problematic and need attention. Examine separately symptoms such as irritability, sleep pattern and fatigue, work productivity, marital and family relationships, income production, and the presence or absence of depression. This way, the patient and the practitioner attempt to recognize strengths and useful behaviors, as well as potentially problematic symptoms and behaviors. A patient is much more likely to participate in treatment for specific problem areas when the entirety of their mood and behavior is not challenged. Once individual strengths and weaknesses are assessed, a "bottom line analysis" can be made, from which a treatment plan can be forged.

Presenting the diagnosis

After completing diagnostic questions using the techniques previously outlined, the manner in which the diagnosis and prognosis are presented to the patient is crucial to patient acceptance. Receiving any psychiatric diagnosis may be "bad news" for some patients and the therapist will need to carefully determine the best way to proceed with each individual.

For example, it is not always necessary to use a formal psychiatric diagnosis when first presenting an assessment. If the therapist feels that this patient would be distinctly upset about receiving a diagnosis of hypomania or bipolar disorder, it may be preferable to present the assessment in a less formal way. Although it may be necessary to make a formal diagnosis for insurance or paperwork purposes, the therapist's conclusions can be stated in a less alarming way with phrases such as

- "mood swings,"
- "a problem with irritability,"
- "being unable to slow down,"
- "being in overdrive," or
- "cycling."

It may be much easier for a patient to accept a specific symptom assessment rather than deal with being labeled as "bipolar" or "hypomanic." The evaluator simply discusses those symptoms that are most problematic and identifies treatment options. At a later date, the concept of bipolarity or hypomania may be made clearer, once the patient has stabilized and the therapeutic alliance is firmly set. In some cases, the "official" diagnosis is never used except for insurance purposes and discussed only if patients ask. This request for a diagnosis usually signifies that the patient is now ready to hear the answer.

For other patients, breaking the "bad news" is actually "good news," in the sense that the patient may now have an explanation for behaviors that previously they attributed to personal weakness, a seemingly senseless series of adverse consequences, or "bad luck." With this group, receiving a diagnosis is a great relief and will provide considerable understanding and clarity. As noted in Chapter 6 on the nonmedication treatments of elevated mood, making a diagnosis followed by a "re-view" of the patient's life in the context of the diagnosis may provide significant illumination. The understanding of previously mysterious elements of the fabric of a person's life can provide significant benefit even before any other treatment is undertaken. Broad generalizations such as "you have unstable mood that we need to stabilize," "You are too high and we need to help you come down" are likely to be rejected out of hand by the patient.

The patient must see the advantage of treatment

The therapeutic alliance with the hypomanic patient can be fragile, particularly at the beginning of treatment. With elevated mood, the therapist must go to significant lengths to outline the nature and course of treatment and the expected benefits. Be prepared to answer questions about how treatment might negatively affect the patient, how medications might have side effects, or how creativity, energy, and productivity may be impacted. Clear transparency as to the potential advantages and disadvantages of treatment is critical. Forthrightness will cement the relationship for those patients who are willing to undertake treatment. Forging a therapeutic alliance and a contract to work may not be accomplished in the initial session. For some patients, particularly those with significant anxiety about treatment, developing and agreeing on a treatment contract may take several sessions.

In some situations, the sum total of an initial agreement may consist of a plan to conduct a more extended evaluation. If symptom intensity is mild and the risk of dangerous behavior is low, it is helpful and appropriate for the therapist to take a "wait-and-see" approach while monitoring symptoms and behaviors. Some patients may take weeks or months to agree to fully participate in therapy. Initially, a patient may be only willing to fill out mood and behavior charts, or have their spouse come in for further input about their condition. Some therapists, especially inexperienced ones, might feel that they will "lose" the patient if they do not solidify a therapeutic agreement at the first or second session. Although this is possible, particularly with some grandiose hypomanic patients, there is simply no viable alternative. A larger percentage of hypomanic patients will be engaged in therapy if the slower, more patient approach is taken.

For example, when patients present at the insistence of another person (e.g., a spouse, a parent, an adult child, or a supervisor), they are often wary, angry, and less amenable to problem recognition. These individuals will often label the problem as originating and residing in the person who insisted on the evaluation and be unable to see any deficits within themselves. In such situations phrases such as *"Let's put ourselves in his/her shoes and see what they see,"* can be a useful way to gain perspective. It is also useful to ask the patient *"Do you respect him/her?" (the person who insisted on an evaluation) "Would there be any reason for this person to exaggerate or insist on an evaluation other than for your own good?"*

Despite a clinician's therapeutic technique, a certain number of individuals with elevated mood may be simply unwilling to enter a treatment contract. Even when identifying potential risks, we cannot, as practitioners, always protect individuals from themselves. Some patients need to "hit bottom" before they are more willing to accept their diagnosis, engage in therapy, or take medication. An approach by the therapist such as, *"I think you would benefit by being in treatment, but if you need time to think about this, I remain open to seeing you at some point in the future,"* may sometimes be all that is possible during an initial evaluation.

Principles of clinical treatment

Basic supportive or psychodynamically oriented technique often falls short with the hypomanic patient. Likewise, typical psychoanalytic therapy using primarily free association and intermittent interpretation is also not likely to be the best method in treating hypomania. Although listening is important, hypomanic patients require an active therapist who is willing to intervene with limit setting, psychoeducation, and suggestions for behavioral change. As with any patient, the therapist must listen carefully and attentively but intervene with limits if necessary. Additionally, the therapist may need to interrupt the patient in order to make appropriate verbal or behavioral interventions.

Broad-brush maxims or assessments rarely work. To tell patients that they are "high," "too speeded up," or hypomanic" may well produce an angry and resistant patient. It is far more therapeutic to precisely identify target symptoms necessitating treatment or intervention.

The hypomanic patient is often skeptical that there is need for therapy at all and may be openly doubtful of any therapeutic process. Grandiose, hypomanic patients often feel superior in their self-knowledge and feel free to say so! Interpretations or advice are, in their view, unneeded and unwanted. Hypomanic individuals may directly challenge the therapist's knowledge and/or expertise. The clinician should ignore or minimize any such challenges unless they directly threaten continuation of the evaluation or therapy. Participating in a challenge of egos with a hypomanic patient is not only unproductive, but may also result in creating emotional distance between therapist and patient. Although patients indeed know their own story best, they may be unwilling or unable to see any problems resulting from their moods or behaviors. If the patient berates or minimizes the treater's ability, this can serve as an opportunity to not only gain more information but also to defuse and calm an upset patient. One possible approach is *"You are right. You do know yourself better than I do. Can you help me get to know you better?"*

Additional challenges to the therapist may present when the patient's history involves some indiscretions or embarrassing behaviors. In such cases, the patient may attempt to minimize the therapist's skills as a defense against feeling belittled or humiliated. Here, a helpful technique would be to recognize value in the patient's positive traits, but to point out that when not controlled, even positive traits may result in negative consequences. One way to help the patient recognize both these positive and negative outcomes could be phrased in this way:

> *"Your level of energy is of obvious benefit in certain situations such as at work. It allows you to be in the upper echelon of productivity. As long as your drive to produce does not alienate or irritate other coworkers, I suspect that your supervisor values your efforts. This same energy and activity may work against you at home. Your wife has indicated that your wish to be constantly active and always "on the go," leaves her feeling fatigued and she becomes irritated with you. It may be useful for us to look at how you utilize your energy in family and social situations. As you become better able to recognize when others may not wish to operate at the same speed that you do, you may have increased*

control and increased ability to have others respect you rather than be irritated with you."

Or,

"I know that you expect much of yourself and have perfectionistic traits. With your schoolwork, this has been helpful in obtaining good grades. When you feel that you are "tuned in" and that your mind is "really clicking" you have the energy to make your essays and term papers of consistently high quality. Your boyfriend however gets angry when you apply this same level of scrutiny and drive for perfection to his behavior and appearance. Rapid-fire comments about his hair, his dress, or his interactions with others when you are together are driving you apart."

The soft, slow, and persistent approach

Therapists who treat patients with elevated mood must earn the patient's respect, not expect it. Such respect is earned through gentle persistence rather than abrupt pronouncements. Often when patients are speeded up, clinicians may themselves feel accelerated. Additionally, there may be a tendency for the therapist to insert too much material into a session. It is generally better to make a single comment or interpretation on which you both can agree. Similarly, the therapist must take a cooperative and gentle approach to interpretations and interventions. When dealing with a patient who may be brusque, accelerated in thought and speech, grandiose, or even openly antagonistic, there is a temptation to respond in kind or to be intense in order to be heard. Without realizing it, therapists may feel they need to "hit patients over the head" in order to get them to "see the problem." These approaches are not only unhelpful, but also counterproductive. The therapist may also feel that unless significant interventions are made rapidly with a hypomanic patient, the patient might leave therapy before help can be given. Some patients may terminate treatment, but it is very unlikely that strong or rapid-fire interpretations will save a therapy. As with any psychiatric condition, a strong bond between treater and patient is essential for productive treatment. If patients see the therapist as knowledgeable, balanced, and with the patient's best interests at heart, they are much more likely to be willing to participate in therapy for hypomania.

Although the quality of the relationship between therapist and patient is always important, nowhere is it more important than when treating the patient with elevated mood. Patients with irritable, self-inflated and, at times, frankly grandiose personality elements must have adequate confidence in the therapist to maintain satisfactory compliance. In addition to such elements as professional office milieu, helpful and friendly office staff, an open and direct manner with patients, and an ability to speak in plain language, the therapist needs to take special note of how the patient is responding to interventions and attempt to provide therapy "with the patient" rather than "to the patient." When the treatment relationship is strong, the patient is more likely to comply with recommendations and the overall response to treatment is likely to be enhanced. A strong therapeutic relationship also helps overcome "errors" that the therapist will inevitably make. These "errors" can be psychotherapeutic—lack of understanding or lack of recognition of the patient's feeling of specialness, or with medication, prescriptions that are intolerable because of side effects or lack effectiveness. These mistakes are often overlooked or tolerated in the context of a strong therapeutic alliance.

Life stressors and elevated mood

Although elevated mood and mood disorders have strong biologic underpinnings that usually require biologic treatment, their ultimate course and outcome are substantially affected by life stressors and the patient's ability to successfully manage those stressors (1,2). Such stressors may include divorce, deaths, job change, and family dysfunction, to name a few.

Stressful life events can significantly complicate the course of bipolar disorder (3). It has been shown that negative life events are linked with a threefold increase in time to recover from a bipolar episode and also increase rates of relapse into another episode (4). It is critical that psychotherapeutic interventions in modulating, adjusting to, or eliminating sources of stress be employed to lessen the likelihood of a manic or depressive relapse.

In general, for persons with more significant hypomania, the initial focus should be on moderating elevated mood with medication. However, the therapist cannot settle for lowered mood as a sole end point. Following mood stabilization, the therapist can be exceptionally helpful in clarifying complex interpersonal situations, assisting the patient to simplify and "detoxify" their lifestyle, and advising on the management of specific behavioral crises. By working in partnership to identify and solve life stressors, patient and therapist can often ameliorate situations that might otherwise destabilize a balanced state.

When patients want to take on additional tasks, a useful question is "*What are you going to eliminate in order to make room for this new activity?*" A common patient response is "nothing" as they can "shoehorn" this new activity into an already busy schedule. In such cases, it is useful to make an hourly assessment of the patient's daily activities over the course of a week, determining how much time is required for current tasks and how much can be allotted to additional activity. Often without realizing it, the patient has minimized the impact of the time necessary for the new activity. Alternatively, the patients may assume they will shorten sleep time to accommodate the new activity. In both the long and short run, such sleep loss is not healthy and should be advised against.

The wish to remain hypomanic

It is sometimes assumed that patients "like to be manic" or cannot give up "being high." Depressed patients *can* yearn for a return to a hypomanic state to remedy the pain of depression. When patients are feeling depressed, many miss "that old spark" or wish to return to the "quick pace" that they felt when hypomanic. Managing this wish to return to hypomania is one of the central challenges to the therapist. A treatment approach that advocates that the patient can "never be hypomanic again" or "must remain level" may well alienate the patient. A more helpful technique is to identify with the patient the pros and cons of their hypomanic behavior, particularly in its extremes. By identifying hypomanic symptoms, behaviors, and their consequences, the therapist and patient can arrive at reasonable goals for therapy. For example, using a combination of medication and sleep hygiene to achieve a minimum of 6 hours of sleep per night may be a reasonable compromise for the patient who insists on working a 14-hour day.

Another useful technique is helping the patient understand the trade-offs in allowing full hypomania to recur. The most distressing of these trade-offs is an almost certain depression that will follow the high. Although being seemingly attractive, hypomanic episodes are often followed by deep depression in an ongoing repeated pattern, the occurrence of depression, with loss of productivity, intense mental pain, and damage to work, social, and family relationships can be a powerful disincentive to the wish for elevated mood. When a cycling pattern is present, it is important for the therapist to underscore the temporal connection between hypomania and depression. Even with great therapeutic encouragement, patients may need to endure several episodes of hypomania/depression before the cycle is identified and accepted. Once understood, patient and therapist can use this cycle to form the basis for a solid and mutually accepted treatment contract.

Down from the high—necessary grieving

Some cycling patients find that when a diagnosis of their symptoms is made, they are relieved that someone (the therapist) can make sense out of the chaos in their lives. For these patients, diagnosis is a great relief. As the patient's mood and energy level therapeutically decrease to more normal levels, there is an inevitable sense of loss. It is extremely important for the therapist to be aware of this feeling and to help the patient grieve the losses that occur over the ensuing weeks or months. Even if euthymic, the patient may continue to idealize their previous level of hypomanic functioning. The therapist needs to help the patient be realistic in assessing his or her current and past clinical state. Many patients have the perception of great positive benefits and increased levels of functioning when in an elevated state. The chaos created by the hypomania is often diminished or forgotten. The therapist should recognize with the patient any positive value of hypomania that may be missing in the euthymic states.

When true hypomania is present, however, patients usually feel that they functioned much better than they actually did in reality. Levels of productivity or the ease of sociability tend to be exaggerated. Patients may have functioned rapidly and completed more tasks, but not necessarily as effectively as they thought. More work may have been produced, but it may have been less organized than remembered. The patient may have stayed up late at night and arisen early; however, the commotion that it created in the house may have been totally overlooked. By working with the patient on the effects of hypomanic behavior, elements of truly increased productivity and interactivity can be separated from those that just appeared to be improved, or were improved at a price.

Usually the traditional stages of grief resolution include denial, anger, sadness, bargaining, and acceptance. Successful treatment of elevated mood requires that each of these elements be dealt with as they emerge. Some patients will handle grief satisfactorily on their own. Most patients, however, will require therapeutic help to recognize and resolve the loss, and move from one stage to another.

Three elements of loss commonly emerge in a stabilized hypomanic patient. They are

- loss of the perfect self,
- loss of the "the way I used to be," and
- loss of missed opportunities.

The *loss of the perfect self* is a principle that can be generalized to most individuals when diagnosed with any illness. Patients' view of themselves as whole and healthy persons without imperfection is punctured when a medical condition is uncovered. When a cycling diagnosis becomes a reality, patients often realize they need to make compromises in their lifestyle and, more importantly, adjust their view of themselves. Although this adjustment occurs naturally as part of maturation, the process is hastened and intensified when a major mental illness is diagnosed.

This leads to the second element of loss—*the loss of the way I used to be*. In grieving this loss, it is helpful for the therapist and patient together to identify personality elements that might be lost from those that may have been exaggerated or imagined. Some areas may be particularly problematic. For example, as patients become more stable in mood and energy level, they realize they can no longer work with the intensity and long hours that they had without suffering significant mood or functional consequences. For example, patients who procrastinated in assignments and pulled "all nighters" to complete tasks, find that they are no longer able to do this. Even when it is possible, the sleep loss creates significant aftereffects such as increased irritability, fatigue, or depression. Other patients perceive that they had a "photographic memory" or other mental abilities that far exceeded those of the average individual. The patient may find that the speed of mental processing or memory recall feels significantly less accurate and their mind sluggish. The therapist's task is to realistically assess the patient's current mental functioning. Often, the patient's mental abilities are well within the normal range even if they are perceived by the patient to be less than they used to be. When there is a genuine decrease in mental speed, the therapist can point out the rewards of mental stability and the many gains that are achieved by treatment. This may be a "tough sell," especially initially, as the patient grieves the lost self.

In the assessment process, a therapist should be careful to search for areas of impaired mental functioning that do have possible remedies. Overmedication with mood stabilizers can often leave the patient mildly depressed and less cognitively sharp. Simply reducing the amount of medication could remedy this situation. In other cases, certain medications may cause specific mental impairments. For example, lithium and topiramate are well-known causes of short-term memory impairment. If this memory impairment is significant, it is important to decide if lithium and/or topiramate are crucial elements of the patient's medication regimen. If not, a substitute medication may be chosen. In some cases, one or both must be continued for safety and mood stability. In these cases, the therapist helps the patient deal with minor memory interference by using written notes, clock alarms for time reminders, and an appointment book for scheduling. When this approach is taken, it is useful to identify for the patient that the cognitive impairments of lithium and topiramate are not cumulative and will disappear when and if medication is stopped. It is often very reassuring to the patient that "permanent brain damage" is not occurring.

A third area of grief and loss experienced by patients when diagnosed with an elevated mood disorder is the *loss of missed opportunities*. Undiagnosed patients with a lifelong history of mood disorder have often had significant life reversals, social or occupational impairment, or interpersonal relationships that have "failed" because of their unstable behavior or judgment. Although simultaneously being pleased with their new state of mood stability, patients may be quite sad for relationships that ended, jobs that were lost, achievements unfulfilled, or other life events that may have been hampered or caused by illness-related behavior. It is important that the therapist help sort out illness-related losses from those areas that might have been grandiose, unreachable goals.

Reinforcement and repetition

Although many hypomanic individuals are bright and intellectually gifted, an important therapeutic principle is it that this cognitive ability does not necessarily lead to treatment compliance. These patients require repeated interventions to incorporate behavioral change. Reviewing unhealthy behavior and reinforcing positive action must often be repeated to help the patient accept difficult recommendations or lifestyle changes. Written materials that the patient can take from the office and read at home will reinforce ideas discussed in the office. A written prescription can be a helpful tool for emphasizing and underscoring the need for therapeutic lifestyle change recommendations. Using a prescription pad, the therapist can write a "behavioral prescription" for a specific activity. Such prescriptions can be given for sleep hygiene recommendations, taking restorative short walks during work activities, getting distance from sources of overstimulation, or getting "prescribed" exercise.

A treatment plan for elevated mood

When the clinician is with presented a patient who has elevated mood, there are a variety of factors to be considered when developing a treatment plan. These are shown in Table 5.1. If the elevated mood is severe, with the presence of full mania (with or without psychosis), treatment is initiated at level 1. With hypomania only, treatment is begun at level 2.

For many, if not most, patients, bipolar II disorder, which includes periods of hypomania, is a chronic, lifetime diagnosis with frequent exacerbations and remissions. The reality of this chronicity may take time for the patient to accept. In order to build a therapeutic alliance, this issue should not be mentioned unless the patient brings it up. Clinicians should recall that a diagnosis of a long-term condition does not automatically mean long-term treatment. Even if long-term treatment is ultimately proven to be necessary, long-term maintenance may only occur after an initial shorter period of treatment, one or more treatment-free intervals, and re-occurrence. In some cases, this may need to occur several times before the patient is willing to consider maintenance therapy.

Strategies for full-blown mania

As this text focuses on hypomania, it is not intended to provide extensive details of the management of the acutely manic patient. However, elaboration of treatment approaches in the manic patient is helpful. As is well known, verbal interventions with a significantly manic patient are seldom useful. Manic patients are so preoccupied with racing internal thoughts and overwhelmed with ideas that they literally cannot hear or digest psychotherapeutic interventions with any degree of success.

With full-blown mania, the initial interventions should be physiologic, with an aim toward decreasing manic symptoms. Most often, this involves the use of medication or electroconvulsive therapy (ECT). Rapid tranquilization, intramuscular medication, and combinations of medication may be necessary to lessen the severity of hypomanic symptoms.

In the course of diminishing manic symptoms (this usually occur in an inpatient setting), there should also be a focus on regularizing the patient's physiologic patterns including sleeping, eating, and activity levels. In the most serious situations, involuntary hospitalization, seclusion, and/or restraint may be necessary while medication takes effect. Limit setting on

TABLE 5.1

Treatment stages of elevated mood

Level 1—interventions—acute phase stabilization with severely elevated mood
- Assessment, with input of family or social support network
- Establish whether a previous treatment plan has been in place and the level of the patient's compliance
- When necessary, take the patient out of their environment (often involving inpatient care)
- Behavioral control, restraint, or seclusion, if necessary
- Regularization of physiologic process (sleeping, eating, physical activity)
- Stabilize any withdrawal symptoms from alcohol or drugs, when indicated
- Eliminate the presence of and access to intoxicating substances
- Implement biologic treatments (medication, ECT). If a previous regimen has been satisfactory, re-establish the biologic regimen. If relapse has occurred despite apparent compliance, reformulate the biologic regimen.
- Verbal limit setting
- Minimal psychotherapeutic interpretation
- Maintain and gradually reduce behavioral controls
- When appropriate, transition to the home environment

Level 2—Initial interventions: mild to moderate elevated mood
- Assess primary patient complaint (this may be an element of mood disorder or a psychosocial stressor). First, focus on this problem initially to engage the patient
- Establish or solidify a biologic treatment regimen
- Monitor for regularity of physiologic patterns
- Assist to discontinue or minimize use of intoxicating substances
- Assess need for financial constraints or controls
- Monitor compliance with medication
- Begin investigation of precipitants to current mood episode
- Obtain a history of previous mood episodes
- Obtain a history of previous treatments and outcomes
- Obtain detailed history of previous psychotropic medication use, dose, duration, and outcome
- Identify patient's support systems
- Establish consensus on issues to be treated psychotherapeutically
- Illness education
- Assess the extent of elements of elevated mood and make a mood diagnosis
- Establish a mechanism for follow-up care

Level 3—Interventions during follow-up and maintenance care
- Begin or adjust physiologic treatments to modulate mood
- Utilize specific psychotherapeutic strategies from Chapter 7
- Monitor compliance with medication

TABLE 5.1
(continued)

- ○ Illness education
- ○ Discuss chronic intermittent nature of elevated mood disorders
- ○ Engage family/support systems in recovery
- ○ Monitor for relapse, and intervene when necessary
- ○ Monitor for substance abuse
- ○ Concur on a "psychotherapy only," "medication only," or combined treatment approach for short- and medium-term care

Level 4—Long-term maintenance
- ○ Regular or intermittent therapeutic contact
- ○ Support healthy initiatives and maintenance strategies
- ○ Observe for medical issues including new medication prescriptions by other providers or medical illness that might disrupt a stable treatment regimen
- ○ Assess age-related changes that could disrupt a stable treatment regimen
- ○ Reinforce need for long-term treatment for a chronic disease
- ○ Incorporate new treatments into regimen when appropriate
- ○ Eliminate treatments no longer needed
- ○ Maintain flexibility in the treatment plan
- ○ Identify and aggressively treat relapse

amounts of activity and moderation of verbal outbursts are essential parts of a therapeutic milieu for actively manic patients. The treatment team should be cognizant that substance withdrawal can often complicate manic behaviors and, therefore, carefully watch for withdrawal symptoms. It is only when the flood of manic symptoms has been diminished that the other treatment principles listed in this chapter and in Chapter 6 can be successfully utilized. Research supports this graduated sequential treatment approach as successful for a variety of mood disorders, especially bipolar disorder (1,2).

Mild to moderate elevated mood

As outlined in the treatment stages mentioned in the preceding text, the therapist's approach will be significantly determined by the current chief complaint and presenting symptoms. The initial treatment approach will differ significantly, depending on whether the patient is depressed (the most common presentation) or displays symptoms primarily of elevated mood. Early in treatment, it is useful to discern how many active mood episodes have occurred prior to the index episode for which the patient presents. As discussed in Chapter 3, this can be documented through life charting and careful history taking. In any case, it is important to note how many discreet mood episodes have occurred and whether they were depressed, hypomanic manic or mixed. It is likewise important to assess the patient's baseline temperament—hyperthymic, cyclothymic, or dysthymic—as a background to full mood episodes because these elements may affect the optimal selection of the medication (see Chapter 7).

Another important consideration in devising a treatment plan is to assess the patient's level of social support. Patients who live alone and do not have other reliable observers of their behavior are more at risk. Patients who are not good self-observers are less likely to recognize the onset of mood swings and behaviors that can carry negative consequences. Patients with a rapid cycling condition, whose moods fluctuate quickly and unpredictably, need much more careful monitoring, more frequent consultation, and often a higher level of medication dosage. On the other hand, if a patient has a supportive, informed spouse, family members or other caretakers who are in regular contact with the patient they can serve as valuable assistants to the therapist in both assessing the effects of treatment and noting the warning signs of clinical deterioration.

Research suggests that in hypomania, as in other psychiatric conditions, the most effective treatment is a combination of psychotherapy and medication. However, the treatment that will most likely succeed for any given individual is one with which the patient concurs. Therefore, treatment approaches need to be modulated depending on the patient's wishes and attitudes. Some patients are clearly oriented toward talking therapy, but may be resistant to medication. Unless the patient's elevated mood is causing urgent or intense dysfunction, it is quite appropriate to use psychoeducation and other psychotherapeutic techniques before medication usage is urged. It is useful to mention the possibility of medication during an initial visit as part of a thorough treatment plan. Medication-avoidant patients, however, will see this as a last resort, which will only be tried if and when other methodologies fail. Other patients are not only in favor of medication, but come to treatment with the expectation that taking medication will help them considerably. These patients often see the sole role of the treater as prescribing an appropriate "pill for their ill." They may be skeptical about psychotherapy and meetings beyond what is needed to monitor their medications. Although the therapist may require several initial sessions for appropriate illness education and to assess the effectiveness of the medication regimen, these patients will often lobby for infrequent medication checkups with minimal psychotherapeutic intervention.

Paralysis by analysis—useful analogies

It is normal and expectable that in the early phases of treatment, the patient will become much more focused on his or her mental state. Depending on the patient, this can be a positive or a negative factor. For those patients who have never been self-reflective, awareness of one's mental state can lead to both better compliance and refinement of treatment. Other patients however become overly self-reflective and experience "paralysis by analysis." They are so focused on their mood state that they may experience difficulty in day-to-day functioning. When such a state exists, a useful analogy for the therapist is to compare the patient's mood to walking. When people walk they have an integrated "swing" to their step, such that they do not have to think about each individual motion. The movement of arms, legs, and torso is automatic and not directed by the patient in individual elements. When the patient becomes overanalytical, he or she focuses extensively on each individual element and "loses his/her swing." It can be useful to have patients stand up and attempt to walk, focusing on each individual element of walking: setting the heel down, rotating to the ball of the foot, setting the other heel down rotating to the ball of that foot, and turning their attention to their arms, raising and lowering them individually. As patients walk awkwardly and with hesitancy, the therapist can use this as a model for what the patient is doing to himself emotionally. Although it may take some time, the therapist encourages the patient to avoid focusing on individual details of mood, but take a broader view of how they are functioning to "regain their swing."

Another analogy in the treatment of hypomania is hitting a golf ball. Anyone who has played golf or has taken golf lessons knows how complicated it can be to "fix" a swing. When many suggestions are given at once, the golfer becomes overwhelmed and unable to focus on any one element satisfactorily. "Paralysis by analysis" is the golfing result. Similar thinking applies to treatment of hypomania. If the therapist attempts to address all symptoms at once, whether it is through psychotherapy, medication, or a combination of both, frustration and probable failure are in store. The patient must be helped to limit attention to a hierarchy of symptoms, and address only one or two at a time. Even if patients are willing to consider multiple personal changes, they seldom succeed. Faced with this frustration, the patient may well discontinue treatment, with or without notice to the therapist.

Resistance

Some hypomanic patients are considerably resistant to evaluation or any form of treatment. It is a skill that requires considerable practice, to be able to see the "holes in the Swiss cheese" i.e., those areas of the patient's life that, in fact, are not functioning well despite his or her verbalizations to the contrary. As noted earlier, it is well for the therapist to remember that even if there are multiple areas of patient dysfunction, it is best to limit the area of treatment focus.

Especially at the beginning of treatment, therapists should view their role as less "in charge" of the therapy with the hypomanic patient, and more an intelligent companion, sharing treatment decisions, goals, and outcomes.

Pitfalls for the therapist

Whether serving as a psychotherapist, a prescriber, or both, there are therapeutic pitfalls in treating hypomanic patients. This section will describe those pitfalls and provide practical advice to avoid these problems.

Diagnostic oversight

The most common of all pitfalls is the diagnosis ignoring the signs and symptoms or history of hypomania. For all the reasons listed earlier in Chapter 1, hypomanic symptoms are simply not identified by some therapists, the patient, or the patient's family. The possibility of elevated mood may be missed by exclusively focusing on a patient's presenting complaint such as depression or anxiety.

Another common mistake is to make a diagnosis (e.g., depression or an anxiety disorder) and become so focused on the treatment of that condition that hypomanic symptoms that may have been minimally present or present only by history are ignored. Diagnosis is further complicated by the fact that patients themselves may be either unaware of their symptoms or do not feel the need to describe them to the therapist.

Assuming a diagnosis of elevated mood is made, there are still traps into which the therapist can fall that will slow down or prevent adequate treatment. Unwittingly, some therapists may be drawn into psychotherapeutic relationships with hypomanic patients which are not healthy. Hypomanic individuals are engaging and can be at times alluring in their style; at other times, they can be annoying, intrusive, and challenging. Countertransference feelings are easily stirred up that result in "responses in kind," which are not therapeutic and may even serve to perpetuate the hypomania. Therapists need to be sensitive to reacting overly positively or negatively to hypomanic patients.

Joking and awe

Hypomanic patients are often humorous, charming, and charismatic, and can spend entire sessions telling jokes, describing exploits, travels, or adventures, or otherwise "entertaining" the therapist. A patient's ability to be funny, particularly when combined with efforts to get the therapist to "loosen up" can sometimes engender a relationship that is unhealthy. When the therapist likewise becomes engaged in telling jokes and/or funny stories rather than focusing on the real needs of the patient, the treatment dangerously loses focus on the patient's issues. Under the guise of matching the patient's style or gaining his trust, inappropriate comments may be made or funny personal stories can be revealed by the therapist that have little therapeutic purpose.

As many hyperthymic and hypomanic patients are accomplished, skilled, and successful persons, the novice therapist may be awed with the patient's success and fail to differentiate between dangerous/risky and successful behaviors. There are several indicators that therapists are being drawn into nontherapeutic treatment stances. These include finding themselves describing their own exploits, travels, writings, academic accomplishments, and possessions, or bragging about the fame or notoriety of certain patients that they are treating.

Riding the stagecoach

In general, a passive, nondirective style is less effective in working with hypomanic patients than a more active therapeutic stance. Therapists who take a therapeutic approach of listening with minimal verbal interventions can find themselves spending long periods of a single or many sessions on the "outside" of a therapy, not actively engaged. Although listening is important, merely "watching" the patient reduces the therapist to a spectator rather than being an active participant in therapy. This is a warning sign that active therapy is not occurring.

Verbose patients who talk rapidly may "bulldoze" the therapist so that it is difficult to make interventions at all. It is incumbent on the therapist to periodically interrupt a rapid-fire monologue in order to therapeutically direct the person. This can be challenging. Therapy with a hypomanic patient can feel like attempting to chase down a runaway stagecoach in a vintage Western movie. As a therapeutic rule, it is not necessary to stop the stagecoach but only to slow it down sufficiently for directional adjustments. The pace of interaction with a severely hypomanic patient, can feel more like a speeding bullet train rather than with a stagecoach. Attempting to intervene with such a patient without medication to help moderate the patient's hyperactivity is generally an exercise in frustration. The patient must be helped to slow down before other interventions will be effective.

Angry challenges

Hypomanic patients who are confrontive, irritable, or aggressive present a different challenge to the clinician. They may actively disagree with, and openly defy the therapist's position or interventions. They can be dismissive of potentially accurate and helpful comments. Such patients may attempt to dominate a therapist, engendering competition. It is not only unhelpful for the therapist to be louder, faster, or more intense in response to this behavior, but also serves to drive the patient away. Rather than respond directly, it is often more helpful to tolerate such emotions at least for a time and interpreting them later when the therapeutic alliance is strengthened. At a later date, such behaviors can be interpreted as both part of the hypomania and a defense against therapeutic change.

A useful analogy for this latter technique is swimming in heavy ocean surf. To attempt to stand up in large waves usually results in the swimmer being knocked over and gasping for air. When swimmers learn to duck under a wave and come up on the other side, they can swim safely and have fun mastering the waves. Similarly with the hypomanic patient, it is neither necessary nor desirable to confront strong waves of emotion and intensity. It is better to listen, "duck under the wave," and come up later on the other side to make interventions or observations.

Crossing the line

The most serious concern for a therapist working with hypomanic patients is being lured into a boundary violation of the therapeutic process. These violations can be minor such as inappropriately revealing personal information, or entering into a joke-telling contest. However, violations can be more serious. Energetic, intrusive hypomanic patients, especially those with poor impulse control, may attempt to engage the therapist in improper behaviors both during and outside the therapy session. Such behaviors may include suggesting financial transactions, such as loans or gifts, both from the therapist or to the therapist. Some hypomanic individuals will offer the clinician extra compensation or expensive gifts for what the patient describes as "being the best therapist I have ever had." It is unfortunately easy to become flattered by such comments, perhaps accepting inappropriate remuneration or gifts. At times, the patient may make recommendations about financial matters, engaging the therapist in business advice, joint business activities, or stock tips. Even when such information appears accurate, it is inappropriate for the therapist to utilize or engage in business decisions based on patient encouragement or advice.

Seductive hypomanic patients may attempt to engage the therapist in social engagements or frank sexual encounters. Unless interpreted and steadfastly avoided, some hypomanic patients, especially those with borderline tendencies, can be doggedly persistent in subtle and not-so-subtle ways to engage the therapist in a relationship that would lead to a nontherapeutic and potentially injurious form of personal or sexual relationship.

A major analogy—the diabetes management model as it applies to elevated mood

It has been common to apply a chronic medical disease model to mental illnesses such as schizophrenia, depression, and bipolar disorder Diagnosis and treatment principles of hypomania will now be addressed similarly. The chronic medical condition of diabetes mellitus will serve as a comparison. Specifically, we will look at the continuum between prediabetes, type 2 diabetes and type 1 diabetes as it has parallels, and some differences with the continuum from hyperthymic temperament to hypomania to mania.

Understanding the medical model of the diagnosis and treatment of diabetes can clarify our approach to elevated mood diagnosis and treatment and may point the way to future therapeutic directions. This analogy also

TABLE 5.2

Parallels between diabetes mellitus (DM) and elevated mood (EM)

Stage of the illness	Intervention with DM	Intervention with EM
Level A—Positive family history with minimal or no symptoms	Disease education and watchful waiting	Disease education and watchful waiting
Level B—Mild symptoms and/or multiple risk factors	Use level A interventions plus more frequent screening Intermittent treatment may suffice	Use level A interventions plus more frequent screening Intermittent treatment may suffice
Level C—Moderate symptoms	Ongoing treatment with periodic reevaluation and adjustment	Ongoing medication treatment with or without ongoing psychotherapy
Level D—Severe symptoms	Hospitalization and emergency care	Hospitalization and emergency care

provides a conceptual bridge in understanding milder mood states through hypomania to full mania and is summarized in Table 5.2.

Common diagnostic issues

In both diabetes and elevated mood, many patients with mild symptoms are not diagnosed or are never present for medical evaluation. There are a large number of patients who have mild to moderate symptoms, but who view these symptoms as "normal" or bothersome annoyances, and not as diagnosable illness.

For many patients, a first diagnosis may be made while investigating another problem. For example, a patient might present for a urinary problem, which, in fact, is the polyuria of diabetes. Other patients may be seen for fatigue, changes in appetite and/or weight, or erectile dysfunction without any idea that underlying diabetes may be the cause of their symptoms. With elevated mood, patients may present for evaluation of depression, alcohol or drug abuse, irritability, anxiety, or marital dysfunction caused by elevated mood. They, too, may be quite oblivious to the underlying nature of their mood disorder until it is identified.

With diabetes, there may be warning signs and specific laboratory tests that can confirm the diagnosis. Elevated fasting blood sugar or a mildly impaired glucose tolerance test may precede the diagnosis of diabetes. This patient is often labeled as "prediabetic." There are other warning signs and symptoms that, from the patient's point of view, may seem to have little to do with diabetes. To a trained clinician, however, a constellation of symptoms including increased thirst, increased urination, and hyperphagia may point toward the diagnosis of diabetes and be directly correlated with dysregulation of blood sugar.

At this time, we have no specific laboratory tests, which can be measured before the onset of elevated mood. A constellation of symptoms including frequent mood swings, particularly without obvious cause, unexplained increased energy, lack of need for sleep, irritability, and rapid speech and thought, however, will direct the experienced clinician to a diagnosis of hypomania or bipolar disorder.

Another parallel is that type 2 diabetes was once considered primarily an "adult onset" illness. However, it is now increasingly common in children and teenagers. Ignored or misdiagnosed, the illness is particularly dangerous when it strikes early in life, because later complications can include microvascular retinopathy and nephropathy, cardiovascular complications including ischemic heart disease, stroke, and peripheral vascular disease.

Similarly, elevated mood and hypomania were, in the past, thought to exist primarily in adults. It is now clear that elevated mood can be exhibited even in very young children and early adolescents. If not diagnosed early, these disorders may lead to significant complications including future episodes of depression, severe mood swings, academic underachievement, family dysfunction, lack of success in relationships and, most alarmingly, suicide.

Further comparison between diabetes and mood disorders finds both illnesses complex to treat, requiring a multifactorial approach. In diabetes, lifestyle adjustments are often essential to successful treatment. However, many patients, even when given appropriate diagnosis, treatment, and education, do not comply with recommended therapies. Repeated patient education about the course of the illness can help with compliance.

In elevated mood, treatment can be complex and also requires a multifactorial approach. In addition to physiologic treatments such as medication, lifestyle modification is likewise critical to maintaining satisfactory treatment outcomes. Illness education often helps with compliance.

In each condition, complications of the primary illness may require additional therapy. For diabetic patients, this may include increased lipids, high blood pressure, and coagulopathies. Elevated mood patients may show increased anxiety, vocational difficulties, marital and social deficits, and psychosis.

Another useful comparison between diabetes and mood disorder is the need to follow up the illness over time. With diabetes, an acute "snapshot" view of blood sugar level may not provide the most valuable information. Hemoglobin A1C, which measures an average blood sugar over time, is a more valuable measure of the amount of control and/or the progress of the illness than a single measure of fasting glucose. However, even with this measurement, the clinician must remain alert. Hemoglobin A1C can be affected by pregnancy, uremia, hemolytic anemia, blood transfusion, and other medical conditions. Therefore, a clinician cannot base an assessment and treatment recommendations solely on one laboratory test.

Similarly, with elevated mood, an isolated one-time view of the patient's condition may not tell the whole story. It is helpful and more accurate to see a patient over time, view patient mood charts over time, or have input from other family members in order to see the mood patterns that signify the presence of disease. External situational life stressors or medical conditions can also affect mood. In making a diagnosis, the informed clinician can assess a mood chart, but must also take into account such factors as marital dysfunction, parent/child stressors, job changes, and relocation. Other medical conditions and certain medications can have a profound effect on mood. Such illnesses include mononucleosis, hepatitis, and hyper- or hypothyroidism. Over-the-counter or prescription stimulants or oral steroids may create significant changes in mood, resulting in hypomania or depression. There are as yet no replicable endophenotypic traits of elevated mood. Laboratory and biologic assessment of mood disorders is in its infancy.

With both illnesses, one serious episode of life-threatening symptomatology may indicate the need for chronic treatment. With diabetes, this could be one episode of diabetic ketoacidosis. With elevated mood or bipolar disorder, it could be one serious suicide attempt or a major manic episode resulting in loss of job and/or breakup of a marital relationship.

Further parallels

Both conditions appear *on the surface* to be diseases of "too much" and "too little" of a crucial entity. For diabetes, this is the level of blood sugar as mediated by insulin production. For mood disorders, this appears to be mood that is "elevated or activated" versus mood that is "underactive and depressed." For both entities, there are changing criteria and changing definitions of health and pathology. Even nationally respected experts and agencies such as the American Diabetes Association (ADA) and the World Health Organization (WHO) differ as to what constitutes adequate control and what constitutes risk. According to the ADA, normal fasting plasma glucose is now defined as <100 mg per dL, where it had previously been allowed up to 126 mg per dL. Impaired fasting glucose is now defined by a fasting glucose level between 100 and 125 mg per dL. There is also controversy as to what is the best and most cost-effective screening test for diabetes—impaired glucose tolerance or impaired fasting glucose. With mood, we are still struggling with what is the best indicator to evaluate elevated mood, elevated activity and energy, or both.

An initial screening and baseline treatment for both conditions can be performed by primary care physicians, but as a condition worsens or a patient's symptoms become more severe, specialty care may be required.

Medications used in both diabetes and elevated moods are two-edged swords. They can be extraordinarily helpful but also create significant side effects. High doses of medication alone can create an exacerbation of the central condition. Overprescription of insulin or oral antidiabetic agents (e.g., sulfanylureas) can cause hypoglycemia, which can be life-threatening. Other serious side effects such as lactic acidosis (metformin) and cardiovascular disease (congestive heart failure with glitazones) are potential complications of therapeutic treatments.

In mood treatment, overprescription of mood stabilizers or antipsychotic medication can initially create excessive flattening or blunting of the patient's affect. When used at higher doses, they can lead to depression with all its complications including suicidal behavior. Valproic acid can lead to elevated liver functions, pancreatitis, and weight gain. Carbamazepine can cause Stevens-Johnson syndrome, blood dyscrasia, elevated liver functions and agranulocytosis. Lithium can cause hypothyroidism, weight gain, diabetes insipidus, psoriasis flare-ups, and lithium toxicity. Atypical antipsychotics can cause hyperglycemia, weight gain, increased mortality in the elderly and, rarely, neuroleptic malignant syndrome.

Important differences in this analogy

Analogies clearly abound between the assessment and treatment of diabetes and those of mood disorders. There are, however, some important differences, particularly when it comes to understanding underlying causality. Type 2 diabetes, which superficially appears to be a lesser form of type 1 diabetes, has a totally different physiologic cause and mechanism. In type 2 diabetes the patient develops insulin resistance, that is, cells in the body become resistant to the effects of insulin. Depending on islet cell functioning in the patient's pancreas, the patient may initially stay normoglycemic when mild insulin resistance is present. With lessened β cell functioning, however, there is relative insulin deficiency. Hyperglycemia and type 2 diabetes occur. This insulin resistance can come from inherited genetic transmission including mutations that result in changes in the insulin receptor, glucose transporter, or signaling proteins, but these are rare. The other genetic causes are largely unidentified at this time. We also know that insulin resistance may be acquired from lifestyle factors including overeating, obesity, inactivity, and repeated episodes of hyperglycemia and glucose toxicity. Type 1 diabetes, on the other hand, comes from underproduction of insulin by the pancreas. This is often caused by an autoimmune disorder in which the body's immune system destroys, or attempts to destroy, the cells in the pancreas that produce insulin. Immune-mediated diabetes is the most common form of type 1 diabetes but in some other cases the cause is idiopathic. Therefore, what appears to be phenotypically similar but milder illness, type 2 diabetes, has a totally different underlying causal mechanism than type 1.

We do not yet know if the relationship between hyperthymic temperament, hypomania, and mania is one of severity or results from fundamentally different causes. It is only as we develop endopenotypic and genetic underpinnings of these disorders that we will discover if these conditions have similar or different causality as discussed in Chapter 2.

The role for primary care clinicians

In the past, bipolar disorder treatment was solely the realm of mental health professionals. This is changing. It is already known that only one third of mental illness patients are treated in the mental health sector, whereas primary care clinicians see approximately one half of all patients with mental illness (3). Anxious patients, who form one fourth to one third of patients with depression presenting in primary care practices, may have a bipolar illness (5).

Therefore, the chief complaint to the primary care practitioner may be depression, anxiety, or other conditions that do not immediately alert the clinician to the presence of elevated mood. Clinicians may see patients complaining of a sleep disorder, fatigue, headaches, or weight loss that may ultimately be shown to be related to elevated or depressed mood. As Judd et al. have shown, bipolar II disorder patients experience symptoms in only 54% of their lives, and of this segment, the patient is purely hypomanic only 1.5% of the time. Mixed states contribute 2.5% of the symptomatic episodes, but depression occurs a full 50% of the time. Because depression is much more commonly seen in primary care offices initially, primary care clinicians must be vigilant for signs of hypomania in the assessment or during treatment response. As primary care clinicians become more comfortable with the concept of elevated mood, they will become more expert at recognizing the condition. This is not to say however that consultation with specialists (psychiatrists and advanced practice psychiatric nurses) will not be necessary and useful. Collaborative efforts between specialists and primary care clinicians will appropriately utilize mental health resources in the treatment of mood disorders.

Kai MacDonald (6) has given labels that are easy to remember for primary care clinicians when considering referral to a specialist. These are shown in Table 5.3.

In the following scenarios, therefore, a primary care clinician should seek specialist referral.

- ***Perilous Presentations.*** Patients who present with serious suicidal risk, full-fledged mania and/or psychotic mania should be immediately referred to a psychiatrist and considered for inpatient hospitalization because the combination of impulsive behavior, hyperactivity, and delusional grandiose beliefs can lead to significant behavioral risk.
- ***Diagnostic Dilemmas.*** Although primary care clinicians may use some of the screening tools mentioned in Chapter 3, such as the Mood Disorder Questionnaire and the Bipolar Spectrum Disorder Questionnaire from Ghaemi et al., there may be significant confusion or uncertainty as to the presence of a bipolar diagnosis. Primary care clinicians may also not have

TABLE 5.3

MacDonald's criteria for specialist referral in bipolar disorders

- Perilous Presentations
- Diagnostic Dilemmas
- Medical Maladies
- Comorbid Conundrums
- Arduous Ages
- Cruise Control

From MacDonald K. Optimizing outcomes: Bipolar disorder and specialist referral. *Prim Psychiatry*. 2006;13(6):52–59.

sufficient time for the other elements necessary to diagnosis, such as extensive history taking and obtaining information from collateral sources. A referral to a specialist may clarify diagnosis for possible follow-up with the specialist or possible referral back to the primary care clinician once a regimen is stabilized.

- *Medical Maladies.* When medical comorbidity exists simultaneously with the bipolar diagnosis, a psychiatrist referral may help clarify the most appropriate medication treatment that will not exacerbate the medical condition. Similarly, if medical comorbidity emerges during the course of initial care by the primary care physician, a specialist referral may be useful in outlining the next best mood treatments. This could occur, for example, when hypothyroidism secondary to lithium, weight gain and hyperlipidemia secondary to atypical antipsychotics, or any significant side effect emerges secondary to a mood medication.
- *Comorbid Conundrums.* As has been noted throughout this text, bipolar disorder is comorbid with a variety of psychiatric conditions. In the complicated comorbid individual who presents with bipolar symptoms in addition to substance abuse, anxiety disorder, attention deficit/hyperactivity disorder, a personality disorder, or pregnancy, the expertise of a specialist is desirable both in sorting out diagnostic elements and in planning and implementing a treatment regimen.
- *Arduous Ages.* Bipolar disorder that presents in children and adolescents or in the geriatric patient can present special challenges that would benefit from a specialist referral. When available, a child and adolescent psychiatrist is desirable for youth who demonstrate bipolar symptoms. In the elderly patient, as will be discussed in the section on secondary mania, a thorough neurologic and medical work-up should be performed by the primary care doctor to rule out possible medical causes of mania or bipolar disorder that emerges for the first time late in life.

- *Cruise Control.* Some primary care clinicians are uncomfortable with managing psychiatric treatment in general or with bipolar disorder in particular. They may refer the patient to a mental health specialist for ongoing psychiatric care even when the patient is relatively stable. Likewise, a stable patient who develops an episode of elevated or depressed mood may also benefit from consultation and/or ongoing follow-up.

There are a number of factors that make bipolar disorder, even in its milder forms, a candidate for a disease management approach. These include the following:

- Frequent medical and behavioral morbidities.
- Early diagnosis and treatment can prevent more costly interventions later.
- A small number of persons with the illness account for most treatment costs.

It is, therefore, incumbent on large group practices or managed-care organizations to insist on appropriate collaboration between primary care and mental health speciality components to ensure that bipolar disorder is adequately managed both for the benefit of patient care and for cost containment.

The bottom line

- A decision to treat elevated mood should be determined by the functional severity of the symptoms, and not merely by the presence of a diagnosis.
- The patient must concur with the necessity for treatment. Individuals may only agree to treat one or two dysfunctional target symptoms.
- The strength of the treatment relationship is crucial not only to initiating therapy, but also to maintaining it for as long as the patient needs it.
- Many patients wish to maintain traits they associate with their hypomania and may be resistant to giving them up unless a good rational reason or trade-off is identified.
- In treatment, relinquishing hypomania is a significant loss for the patient and will require grieving for
  - the loss of their perfect self,
  - the loss of "the way I used to be,"
  - the loss of missed opportunities.
- In the manic patient, behavior control, regulation of physiologic processes such as sleep and activity, removal of intoxicating substances, and establishing a medication regimen are crucial first steps before any psychotherapeutic regimen can be undertaken.
- Common therapeutic pitfalls when clinicians treat hypomania include the following:
  - Diagnostic oversight
  - Joking and awe
  - Angry challenges
  - Boundary violations

- There are many parallels between the treatment of diabetes mellitus in its full spectrum and the treatment of elevated mood in its entire spectrum.
- With increasing frequency, primary care clinicians will now be required to participate in the treatment of elevated mood and bipolar disorder with the consultation and assistance of mental health specialists.

REFERENCES

1. Giovanni A. Fava and chiara ruin. What is the optimal treatment of mood and anxiety disorders? *Clin Psychol: Sci Pract.* 2005;12(1):92–96.
2. Miklowitz DJ. Psyhcological treatment and medication for the mood and anxiety disorders: Moderators, mediators, and domains of outcome. *Clin Psychol: Sci Pract.* 2005;12(1):97–99.
3. Regier DA, Narrow WE, Rae DS, et al. The de facto US mental and addictive disorders service system. Epidemiologic catchment area prospective 1-year prevalence rates of disorders and services. *Arch Gen Psychiatry.* 1993;50:85–94.
4. Otto MW, Miklowitz DJ. The role and impact of psychotherapy in the management of bipolar disorder. *CNS Spectr.* 2004;9(11 Suppl 12):27–32.
5. Manning JS, Haykal RF, Connor PD, et al. On the nature of depressive and anxious states in a family practice setting: the high prevalence of bipolar II and related disorders in a cohort followed longitudinally. *Compr Psychiatry.* 1997;38:102–108.
6. MacDonald K. Optimizing outcomes: Bipolar disorder and specialist referral. *Prim Psychiatry.* 2006;13(6):52–59.

6

TREATING ELEVATED MOOD WITHOUT MEDICATION

- Schools of psychotherapy effective in elevated mood states
- Other useful psychotherapeutic strategies
- Analogies
- "Re-viewing" history
- "Re-viewing" family history
- "Re-viewing" from a new perspective
- Mood recognition and charting
- The internet and bibliotherapy
- Recognizing the warning signs of hypomania
- Identifying triggers
- Speed does not equate to efficiency
- Too much of a good thing is a bad thing
- Decreasing stimulation in an elevated state
- Pauses in thought and Activity
- Feedback from others—whom do you trust?
- Taking on new tasks

- Advisors—both well-meaning and self-serving
- Saying "No"
- Making decisions
- The value of routine
- Financial controls
- "The high goeth before the fall"
- You are not alone—identification with others
- The myth of making up for lost time
- Self-soothing techniques
- Treating depressed mood in patients with elevated mood symptoms
- Light therapy in depressed mood
- Can light (or lack of it) help elevated mood?
- The bottom line

References

Treating elevated mood and upside symptomatology with medication is commonplace and is expected in most treatment settings. However, this does not negate the therapeutic advantages of a psychotherapeutic approach. Many mental health practitioners have not learned this, having been given the overt or covert message that therapy for patients with grandiose or elevated symptoms was either not possible or at best, minimally helpful. As with so many issues involving elevated mood mentioned previously, this message was based on full-blown manic symptoms in elevated mood. Manic patients, whether psychotic or not, *are* minimally accessible to verbal interventions. The practitioner rapidly recognizes that such patients cannot or will not attend to instructions, education, limit setting, or interpretation. Although one needs to be mindful of the pitfalls listed in Chapter 5, specifically targeted verbal interventions can greatly help hypomanic patients (1). Psychotherapeutic interventions, either alone or in combination with medication, are useful in both the short and long terms and can be accomplished for individual patients or in a group setting.

An additional consideration is that direct treatment of elevated mood may also, in the long run, protect against the emergence of depressive episodes. Therefore, modalities that treat elevated mood may indirectly decrease the emergence of depressed symptoms. Hypomanic and manic patients are frequently overactive and attempt to function on little or no sleep. This combination of excessive activity and little restorative rest can lead to periods of physical exhaustion that may also predispose the patient to slipping or "crashing" into depression. Therefore both medication and nonmedication treatments of hypomania listed in this chapter and the next should be vigorously advocated by the clinician.

This chapter is divided into two sections. The first covers various schools of psychotherapy applied in treating elevated mood and a brief review of the literature supporting their effectiveness. This is followed by sections devoted to specific elements of hypomania education and other psychotherapeutic techniques that can be employed by virtually any practitioner regardless of his/her therapeutic orientation.

Schools of psychotherapy effective in elevated mood states

There are five forms of research-based psychotherapy found useful in conditions, which include elevated mood. These are listed in Table 6.1.

Each of these techniques is somewhat different than traditional psychoanalytic methodology but each focuses on a constellation of treatment elements, which is shown in Table 6.2. As with most of the research on elevated mood disorders, subjects included a mixture of patients with a diagnosis of both

TABLE 6.1

Forms of psychotherapy useful in treating hypomania

Cognitive behavioral therapy
Psychoeducation
Family-focused therapy
Interpersonal/social rhythm therapy
Prodrome detection

TABLE 6.2
Common elements of psychotherapeutic techniques used in elevated mood

- Identify signs of relapse and make plans for early detection and response
- Use education to increase treatment consensus between doctor, patient, and family
- Emphasize the need to continue medication even when euthymic
- Problem solving, stress management, and focus on improving relationships
- Monitor regular daily "rhythms" of sleep, exercise, eating, and activities of daily living

From http://www.psycheducation.org/depression/Psychotherapy.htm, (2).

bipolar I and bipolar II disorders. There is virtually no specific research on psychotherapy in hypomania alone. It is therefore by extrapolation and clinical experience that we assume this research demonstrates that these modalities would be helpful in treating hypomania as well.

Cognitive behavioral therapy (CBT) is a well-known and effective treatment for depression. There is also some evidence (3–5) of its usefulness in bipolar disorder. This evidence focuses particularly on early detection and intervention, medication adherence, stress management, and treatment of co-morbid conditions and bipolar depression (6). As with all psychotherapeutic techniques mentioned in this section, CBT has the advantage of not inducing or precipitating mania and has essentially no side effects (7).

A study that specifically looked at the use of CBT in bipolar disorder and focused on the amount of long-term change was conducted by Ball et al. (8). In this study, 52 patients with bipolar I or bipolar II disorder were randomly allocated to a 6-month trial of CBT or treatment as usual. Both treatment groups were also receiving mood stabilizers. At post-treatment analysis, patients allocated to CBT had less severe Beck Depression and Montgomery-Asberg Depression scores and lower Young Mania Rating Scales scores when compared with controls. The differences were less strong with time but did persist for the succeeding 12 months.

Psychoeducation is useful in a wide variety of psychiatric conditions, including virtually all mood disorders. Although not often studied directly, Colom et al. researched a group of mixed bipolar I and bipolar II patients, adding 21 sessions of structured psychoeducation about bipolar disorder to their management. This was provided in a small group setting of approximately 10 patients, and then compared to a control group of unstructured meetings with the same therapists, which included minimal teaching about bipolar disorder. When compared to controls over a 2-year period, those patients given psychoeducation had a 67% decrease in psychiatric hospitalization (9).

Family-focused therapy. Miklowitz et al. applied a family management strategy in treating patients with bipolar I and bipolar II disorders that had been previously successful in the treatment of schizophrenics (10). In addition to psychoeducation, patients and their families also learned communication techniques in anticipation of relapse. Therapists helped patients and their families develop a plan of action and communication techniques if symptoms of relapse occurred. Using 21 therapy sessions over 9 months, there was a significant reduction of relapse rate in patients who had been previously hospitalized for mania.

Interpersonal and social rhythm therapy (IPSRT) was developed specifically for bipolar disorder. It had been noted that disruption of sleep and circadian rhythms often exacerbated or instigated affective symptoms. Using interpersonal principles, Frank et al. taught patients self-monitoring techniques as well as regular routines for daily activities, such as sleeping and eating. When used in conjunction with medication, this form of therapy was shown to increase lifestyle regularity and decrease manic episodes (6). When IPSRT was withdrawn, higher relapse rates occurred (10,11). IPSRT could not, however, be correlated with faster recovery from mania (12)

Prodrome detection is a strategy in which a therapist meets with an individual patient and discusses the signs and symptoms of manic and depressive relapse for this specific patient. In concert with the therapist, the patient rehearses a plan of action should relapse occur. Perry, et al. (13) devised an individualized plan written on a laminated card, which was to be carried by the patient. A symptom diary kept on a daily or weekly basis helped the patient to monitor symptoms. Studying a group of primarily bipolar I patients, those using prodrome detection treatment suffered a 20% relapse rate after 1 year, whereas the control group not using prodrome detection suffered a 50% relapse rate.

Other useful psychotherapeutic strategies

Although not associated with any one school of thought or treatment, the strategies and approaches outlined throughout the rest of this chapter can be utilized by any therapist, regardless of training. Some of these incorporate the same essential elements listed in Table 6.1.

Analogies

Analogies, especially ones using non–mental health subject matter that are easily recognizable by the patient, can be helpful in explaining diagnostic concepts, treatment goals, and the expectations of response. For the hypomanic patient with bipolar or cyclothymic disorder, analogizing their condition to sitting on a raft in the middle of an ocean storm is particularly illustrative.

THE OCEAN STORM

> *Your life has been a marked series of ups and downs as if you were sitting on a raft in the middle of an ocean gale. When the wind whips up, you are tossed from the peak of high waves to their trough. The strength of the weather, the length of the storm, and the turbulence of the waves can feel quite unpredictable. Although the ride may be exhilarating at times, it can*

also be very frightening. At times, it may feel as if the raft will capsize, and you are hanging on for your very life. While at the bottom of the trough a large wave may splash over you and engulf the raft to the point that you may feel suffocated or as if you are going to drown. As terrifying as this situation may feel, without warning you may be taken back up to the peak of a wave and feel as if you are again riding the crest, on top of the wave, only to crash again.

Our treatment will attempt to smooth out the waves to a gentle swell, such that you will remain comfortable sitting on the raft without fear of being tossed overboard or drowning. By working together, we will minimize the likelihood that you will be unpredictably taken to heights, which you cannot control, only to fall again. As you adjust to calmer seas, you will be better able to clearly view your surroundings and assess what course of action and direction you wish to take. Do you wish to paddle toward a ship in the distance? Paddle to a nearby island? Or rest comfortably in the sun? In any case, it will feel much more under your control. No one's life is ever a totally calm sea; however, an increased sense of control will feel empowering.

Another analogy, which can be useful when using mood stabilizers and antidepressant medication as well as explaining the risks of administering antidepressants alone, is that of a seesaw or a teeter-totter.

THE TEETER-TOTTER

Using medication in elevated mood or mood swings is like balancing a teeter-totter. When in a depression, the left end of the seesaw is down. When in the midst of unstable mood episodes, the teeter-totter often moves up and down with seeming unpredictability. When the seesaw is in the down position and an antidepressant alone is added, the lower end may rise. It may help transiently, making you feel better but often this positive effect is unpredictable. Either the seesaw falls again (you revert to the depressed state), balances briefly (your mood is transiently even) or can zoom up off the ground in the high position (spiral into a hypomania or mania). In this latter state, you may feel elated for a period of time, but this is not likely to last, as you crash to the ground again. At other times, the frequency of the oscillations increases. Therefore we use medications to stabilize mood and keep the seesaw level. When mood stabilizers alone are insufficient to eliminate or reduce depressed periods, a specific mood elevating medication may also be carefully added.

"Re-viewing" history

Many patients with elevated mood have lived with their condition for years, even a lifetime, without a diagnosis. Some may have the sense that they have a condition, which could never be positively affected by treatment. When periods of depression and low functioning are intermingled with periods of hypomania, patients (and those around them) may develop inaccurate explanations for their erratic behavior and lack of consistency. Impulsive business and social decisions, overspending, and other money mismanagement and poor judgment may be attributed to lack of discipline, personality weakness, or simply "not caring." These evaluations may be made by the patient himself or by the patient's family, and invariably lead to decreased self-esteem and negative assessments by others.

When the diagnosis of hypomania or cycling is made and mood is sufficiently stable, it can be extraordinarily helpful to "re-view," that is, *view the patient's history again in light of the new diagnosis*. In doing so, it may be clearer to patients that some of their erratic and excessive behaviors—personally, financially, sexually, or otherwise—are symptoms of their illness. It can be quite relieving to understand that such behavior does not automatically mean the patient is a "bad person" or has a fundamentally flawed personality. They have had the behavioral symptoms of an illness that can be treated. This is not to say that all negative behaviors can be ascribed to hypomania or illness. On a person-by-person basis, it is necessary to sort out what may be illness-related behavior and what may be referable to other personality characteristics and/or other causes. It may be similarly helpful to invite the spouse, children, parents, or other family members for a session and explain directly the relationship between hypomania and problematic behaviors. A meeting such as this may provide a useful context for the patient's family to understand their loved one and assess these problematic activities in a less negative way.

"Re-viewing" family history

It is not uncommon when identifying a patient's cycling mood disorder to find other close biologic relatives who have been similarly diagnosed or have a presumptive diagnosis based on their behavior. Therefore, a similar analysis of the patient's close blood relatives may be useful in helping the patient understand negative behaviors as part of an illness instead of viewing the relatives as being "mean", "weird" or "thoughtless". It would be an advantage to evaluate a patient's relative in person to establish a cycling mood diagnosis. Even when this is not possible however, patterns of family behavior may be sufficiently classic or similar to the patient's own behavior to classify them as symptomatic of manic/hypomanic episodes. Excessive anger and irritability, sexual acting out, poor financial decisions, or inability to hold a job in the context of major mood swings may be interpreted for the patient as relating to that relative's own cycling mood episodes. Even abusive behavior may be partially "re-viewed" and reinterpreted in light of an absence of anger control that can often occur in the context of hypomania or mania. Although not removing the necessity of psychotherapy for the patient, it may be quite helpful to understand that an abusive parent, for example, was ill and not just "mean."

"Re-viewing" from a new perspective

A third way of "re-viewing" is to help the patient see his/her own mood state and actions from "the outside" rather than from his own internal perspective.

Patients may see the world solely from their own perspective, unable to absorb feedback from others and act "with blinders on." Helping patients to get a more balanced view of themselves can be helpful in changing this view and modulating behavior. When hypomanic, patients with elevated mood often believe that their ideas are "meant to be," "perfect," "sharply focused," or ideal. Although valid at times, the more hypomanic an individual becomes, the higher the likelihood that such notions are unique to the hypomanic person but viewed differently by others. When re-viewed later, behaviors or ideas that "seemed right at the time" are often viewed as overly impulsive, or frankly impossible.

Although it would be optimal if such perspective could be achieved when the patient is most hypomanic and therefore most at risk, this may be difficult. Obtaining a more accurate perspective may only occur after the lowering of mood with medication. One psychotherapeutic technique useful in obtaining perspective is drawn from the field of psychodrama. A "two-chair technique" involves having the patient sit in a second chair, not the usual chair where the patient sits. The patient and the therapist together then view the patient's behavior as if he or she was a third person in the room sitting in the empty chair. Comments and dialogue are conducted in the third person; for example, *"How would you characterize his (patient's name) behavior?" "What risks is Jill taking?" "Let's compare the benefits of how Frank is acting with the risks he is taking." "What would Jennifer's husband think of what she's doing?" "How would you advise Matthew if you were his best friend?" "Let's assume that you were Anna's supervisor. What if any corrective action is necessary and how would you tell that to her?"*

After such a series of questions, the patient then reverts to his usual chair and the therapist and the patient discuss possible changes in perspective as a result of this exercise. With new insights, a specific behavioral plan can be put in place with a higher potential for success.

Mood recognition and charting

One might assume from all that has been written about elevated and depressed mood in this book that patients are acutely aware of their mood state. This is hardly the case. Some individuals may be aware of their behavior, energy level, and mood, whereas many are oblivious to these parameters. Although unrecognized mood/behavior states are more prevalent at the elevated end of the spectrum, they can also apply to depression, particularly dysthymia. During a hypomanic episode, patients often do not recognize marked changes in activities, moods, and routines that are readily apparent to others. One goal of therapy is to help individuals recognize specific mood-related behavioral cues, especially those that serve as "red flag" warnings of incipient mania or depression. A particularly effective technique in this recognition is the use of graphic charting.

Lifetime mood charting in patients with a cycling disorder is extremely useful. These charts can be self-completed or constructed during a therapy session by therapist and patient together. Such charts depict a long-term picture of the patient's mood history, focusing on significant mood episodes, whether depressed or elevated. Periods of psychiatric treatment or hospitalizations are noted. In addition to significant dysfunctional moods, it is useful to indicate milder deviations including periods of euthymia, temperamental hyperthymia, dysthymia, or subsyndromal traits. This graphic information is helpful in diagnosis and treatment planning, especially in determining a medication regimen (see Chapter 7). Lifetime charting can illustrate long patterns of mood swings and, therefore, is useful in the "re-viewing" of the patient's life as noted earlier in this chapter.

Shorter-term graphic charts, completed by the patient between therapy and medication management appointments, can be organized by the day, week, or month. Although many formats have been used for graphic charting, the most typical chart will be completed for a 1-month period during which the patient rates his mood on both a graphic and numeric scale, the number of hours of sleep, and the presence of any life events which might affect mood (see Figure 6.1). Women will include menstrual cycle data and observe for any correlation with mood changes. All medications taken are noted down, along with dosage and any side effects. Charts may be customized to track other target symptoms including irritability, binge/purge episodes, anxiety and panic attacks, headaches, or other specific physical pain. These too are rated on a numeric scale.

Yearly charting is helpful in highlighting any seasonal changes in elevated or depressed mood. Even with significant mood stabilization, when followed over time, seasonal changes may clearly emerge. A very common seasonal pattern is a progressive elevation of mood in the spring, reaching an apex in the summer, and then falling in autumn to a depression in winter. Other seasonally related patterns show depressions regularly appearing in the summer or mood elevations each spring and fall.

Most patients find the opportunity to self-chart as a way of becoming actively involved in their own care. Charting can be an especially helpful graphic tool for patients who are not particularly sensitive to their mood and activity changes. Additionally, medication management and compliance can be enhanced by these graphic and objective reports of changes in the patient's mood state and activity.

Occasionally, there may be resistance to mood charting. Patients may worry that they do not know what constitutes "normal" and are concerned that they will give a false impression of their condition. Reinforcing that learning and recognizing one's moods is a gradually learned skill, and the fact that there is no "right or wrong" to charting can be reassuring. Other patients, especially those newly diagnosed, may decide that attempting to recognize, analyze, and rate their feelings is a waste of time. Such patients would not complete their charts or would have "forgotten" to bring them. Gentle persuasion and the therapist's skill in utilizing these charts will help most patients to eventually comply.

YOUR PRESCRIPTION		1	2	3	4	5	6	7	8	9	10	11	12	13	14	15	16	17	18	19	20	21	22	23	24	25	26	27	28	29	30	31
Medication Name	Dose Pills																															

TOTAL NUMBER OF PILLS TAKEN PER DAY

	1	2	3	4	5	6	7	8	9	10	11	12	13	14	15	16	17	18	19	20	21	22	23	24	25	26	27	28	29	30	31
Record Hours of Sleep / Night																															

Dysphoric Mania: check if yes

		1	2	3	4	5	6	7	8	9	10	11	12	13	14	15	16	17	18	19	20	21	22	23	24	25	26	27	28	29	30	31
SEV	Essentially incapacitated or HOSPITALIZED																															
HIGH	GREAT difficulty with goal-oriented activity																															
LOW	SOME difficulty with goal oriented activity																															
MILD	More energized & productive; usual routine not affected much																															
STABLE																																
MILD	Usual routine not affected much																															
LOW	Functioning with SOME effort																															
HIGH	Functioning with GREAT effort																															
SEV	Essentially incapacitated or HOSPITALIZED																															
MOOD (1-100)																																
Number of Mood Changes/Day																																
Menstrual Cycle																																

Figure 6.1 Daily mood chart

DATE	LIFE EVENT	IMPACT	SIDE EFFECTS	MILD	MOD	SEV	COEXISTING SYMPTOMS
1							
2							
3							
4							
5							
6							
7							
8							
9							
10							
11							
12							
13							
14							
15							
16							
17							
18							
19							
20							
21							
22							
23							
24							
25							
26							
27							
28							
29							
30							
31							

Figure 6.1 (continued)

Another useful technique in helping the hypomanic patient is the therapist routinely asking the patient at the end of a therapy session *"Where do you think you fall on a minus 10 to plus 10 scale in rating your mood today?"* (+10 being the most manic and −10 being the most depressed). On the basis of knowledge of the patient and the tenor of the session, the therapist can then provide his or her own assessment. Comparing the assessments helps the patient become more accurate in his understanding of normal, accelerated, or depressed mood.

The internet and bibliotherapy

Internet searches for reference materials as well as bibliotherapy, the use of educational reading materials, can be extremely helpful to some patients, but not all. At the outset of treatment, many patients will find references, textbooks, and informational books written by patients and professionals as useful adjuncts to the information provided by the therapist. Many hypomanic individuals are voracious readers. It is worth asking patients if they wish to read about their illness when the diagnosis is made. One should not assume that all patients prefer to read about their condition. Some individuals find that reading only confuses them, raises anxiety, or describes symptoms that they do not have. Some patients will find themselves to be suggestible, "developing" symptoms only after reading about them.

There are few, if any, sites on the Internet specifically related to hypomania. Most search engine results for the term *hypomania* will result in articles or other references related to elevated mood in general and often describing symptoms and disease states of full mania rather than hypomania. Such Internet access is constantly changing and, therefore, rather than trying to recommend specific sites to patients, it is preferable to have patients do their own search and bring in copies of materials that they think may be applicable to their own treatment.

A bigger problem is that although the Internet is a rich source of information for patients, individuals are unfortunately not able to adequately differentiate factual sites from sites with a particular bias, which may make their information irrelevant or suspect. Particularly when it comes to specific treatments or medications, many patients assume that any material "in print" (or published on the Internet) is valid and applies to their particular condition. It is important, therefore, to provide guidelines to help patients use the Internet wisely but effectively and selectively.

A handout left in the waiting room or distributed to patients as needed, such as the one here, can be quite helpful.

The Internet and your treatment (14)
There are ever-increasing numbers of sites on the Internet that purport to give information about mental health problems, general health issues, medications, and possible side effects. In general, I am supportive of your having information about your treatment and any medications that you may be

taking. Some of these sites are quite helpful and informative, whereas others contain merely opinions without adequate factual backup, biased information disguised as "fact" and, occasionally, information that is simply inaccurate. Even solid, authoritative sites may present data or mention side effects that are highly unlikely, or will not apply to you.

Here are some tips on assessing the possible usefulness of Internet sites:

- Your "search engine" results do not guarantee quality.
- Information that is "in print" on a web site says nothing about its accuracy, or relevance to you, even if it is colorful and appealing to the eye.
- Even sites allegedly "sponsored" by official-sounding organizations may not be unbiased.
- Who sponsors the site? More reliable sites are sponsored by those with credible medical credentials including medical and nursing associations, hospitals, medical centers, and accredited schools of medicine and nursing.
- Is the information factual or an opinion?
- Does the site have a vested interest? Does it attempt to get you to buy any product or service? This is usually a sign of possible bias.
- How up-to-date is the information? Has it been updated recently? The date of the most recent revision should be clearly evident on the site. Sites that are the most accurate and medically valid are updated regularly, but recent updates do not necessarily guarantee quality content.
- What is the privacy policy? How does the site treat any personal information given?

Even if you see something on one of these sites, I would suggest not making any changes in your regimen or the medicines that I prescribe for you without discussing the issue with me first.

A list of web sites that have information on mood disorder and that are sponsored by not-for-profit organizations can be found in the Appendix.

In addition to the general treatment approaches and overarching treatment modalities useful in the treatment of hypomania, there are many more specific interventions, interpretations or specific behavioral advice that are useful. These more specific treatment interventions are covered in the subsequent subheadings.

Recognizing the warning signs of hypomania

Identifying specific warning signs labeled as "danger signals" or "red flags" of hypomania with patients is useful. When these occur, the patient is advised to seek more intense consultation from the therapist.

Changes in patterns of speech or interpersonal communication are particularly valuable clues to emerging or worsening hypomania. When patients begin to interrupt or "talk over" individuals, it is often a sign that the patient is speeding up mentally. Talking fast, loud, or in excited tones are other cues to hypomania. It is often useful for therapists to advise that persons with elevated mood consciously attempt to tune in to the responses of their listeners in conversation. Hypomanic individuals all too often become self-absorbed or believe that the value of their comments is so significant that they lose sight of whether a conversation partner is staying up with them, understanding the concepts, or paying attention at all! Suggest to hypomanic patients that when they find themselves with listeners who appear bored, uninterested, or puzzled, they take it as a sign that they may be talking too rapidly or making connections in a way that the listener is not following. It can also be mentioned that if this practice of becoming tuned in to the listener is not followed with regularity, the patient may find that friends and acquaintances begin to avoid him or her rather than deal with someone who talks too rapidly or in a mildly disorganized manner. The therapist may also suggest that the patient will want to tune in to his or her own feelings and thoughts during conversation. If the patient finds that he or she is racing ahead, thinking of other subjects, and finishing their partner's sentences, suggest that the patient consciously attempts to slow down and tune in to what the partner is saying. Although hypomanic individuals may initially feel that they are becoming "bored" with their partner's comments or "know what they are going to say before they say it," suggest that this is not likely true and that they attempt to digest as fully as possible what their partner is attempting to say before thinking of responses or rebuttals.

As will be discussed in more detail later in the chapter, another signal is *ineffective multitasking*. The patient starts several tasks, but finishes none or feels that he or she can attempt multiple tasks simultaneously, but is ineffective in each. Multitasking often involves forgetting important details, or missing important appointments or dates.

Increased irritability and aggression can develop in interpersonal relationships with family, colleagues, or strangers. Spouses, coworkers, store clerks, or others might be the objects of explosive anger and rage. More severe aggravation can result in interpersonal explosions and intense rage briefly or over an extended period. Driving the behavior might be denial of instant gratification, approval, or attention. Hypomanic individuals may be very quick to show displeasure, becoming argumentative, hostile, or aggressive when not getting what they want. Such self-absorbed behavior often results in the alienation of others.

Mildly hypomanic individuals can often identify their own irritability or proneness to anger and make a voluntary effort to suppress it. As hypomania becomes more intense and progresses toward full mania, the expression of anger may be less under voluntary control and emerge spontaneously, unpredictably. Even when trying to do so, patients may find themselves unable to voluntarily control expressions of anger and irritation. Such uncontrolled anger, which shows up as excessive reaction to small events, explosions of anger (the "Vesuvius eruption"), or frequent or almost constant irritability with people in the patient's life, can often be strong indicators that the patient's hypomania is getting out of control and that additional treatment and/or medication may be needed.

Increased activity can also signal hypomania. As noted earlier, overactivity is one of the most consistent and predictable signals of hypomania. In contrast to the hyperthymic individual who is often purposely and productively active, hypomanic individuals are hyperactive without a clear purpose or direction. Increased activity is often accompanied by nocturnal activity and reduced need for sleep.

Other warning signs of hypomania include the following:

Wearing excessively bright colors
Spending money or being overly generous
Increased contact with people through letters, e-mails, and phone calls
Increased travel, particularly on the spur of the moment
Taking risks, often without regard to the consequences
Hypersexuality or risky sexual behavior

Identifying triggers

There are both biologic and behavioral events, which, with a high degree of predictability, can trigger episodes of unstable mood. In addition to knowing these triggers and being on the lookout for them, the therapist can educate the patient about their possible effects. These triggers are listed in Tables 6.3 and 6.4.

The most toxic triggers from Tables 6.3 and 6.4 are *sleep disruption* and the *use and abuse of substances*. These two elements are potent and frequent triggers to destabilization of mood. Any behavior including shift work, long-distance travel, "burning the candle at both ends," or simply staying up too long can cause significant and dangerous disruptions in sleep. It is well known that even one or two nights of shortened sleep can disrupt an otherwise stable patient. It is critical to impress upon patients that regular and sufficient sleep hours are essential for mood stabilization. Although sleep will be discussed in more detail later, it is important to emphasize here that every therapist must be keenly aware of the importance of sleep in the stabilization of hypomania

TABLE 6.3
Biologic triggers to unstable affect

Sleep loss	Substance abuse—alcohol or recreational drugs
Hypothyroidism	Subclinical or clinical seizures
Migraine headache	Oral steroids
Nicotine withdrawal	Stimulants
Stopping or starting reproductive hormones	Bronchodilators

TABLE 6.4
Behavioral/interpersonal triggers to unstable mood

Interpersonal conflict and stress

Emotional trauma

Grief

Loss of support systems

Long-distance travel

Shift work

Failure or success!

and elevated mood states. Liberal use of hypnotic or sedative medications for sleep stabilization can be an important part of the biologic management of elevated mood.

Use of alcohol, cocaine, marijuana, amphetamines, barbiturates, and opioids is common in the hypomanic population. Many patients with elevated mood will use alcohol and other drugs, either consciously or without conscious intent, as a method of self-medication. Heavy infrequent use (binges) or frequent regular use of any of these substances makes mood stabilization difficult. Any episode of heavy alcohol or recreational drug use can destabilize an otherwise calm, controlled patient.

Speed does not equate to efficiency

Many hypomanic patients have learned to approach tasks speedily and may be pleased with their ability to do so. Although there is a positive cultural value assigned to efficiency and quantity of activities accomplished, it is also true that *faster* may not equate to *better*. When patients become overzealous and speeded to the point of being scattered, or move beyond the ability of family members, coworkers, or teammates to work together, speed can create decreased accuracy, decreased effective work output, and increased friction in interpersonal functioning or chaos.

In 21st century Western culture, multitasking—accomplishing several tasks simultaneously—is highly valued. Hypomanic persons may be seen by themselves or others as having an exceptional ability to multitask. If the level of energy and activity falls into the range of hyperthymic temperament or mild hypomania, this may, in fact, prove true. The hyperthymic patient *is* more productive and functions at a faster pace as compared with others. Truly hypomanic individuals, however, go beyond efficient speed. Many hypomanic individuals assume "If 60 miles per hour is good, 100 mph is better, and 120 mph is better still." It is often necessary to emphasize that multitasking and/or speed may come at a price in efficiency and emotional connectedness.

This price can also include lack of attention to detail, lack of memory recall, and a propensity to become scattered, having several tasks that are started but not finished. On an individual basis the patient should be evaluated for his or her ability to be able to function effectively, or when increased speed leads simply to carelessness, irritation, and inefficiency.

Although obvious, it may be necessary to impress upon the patient that *the rest of the world does not move at a hypomanic pace.* The source of much frustration in hypomania can result from a perception of life moving too slowly.

> *Charlie, your speed can be helpful when used in a controlled and directed way. Faster is not always better though. Your wife and children do not think or act as rapidly as you do. This is not a good/bad situation. Speed is a two-edged sword. You may get more accomplished but don't assume that to be a given. By going faster, you may just become scattered and irritate those who love you. Sitting in the car honking the horn for them to come out will likely set the stage for an unhappy picnic. It might be more helpful to have a mutually agreed upon plan for when you all will leave.*

Clinical intervention may include the need to direct patients to "do less" when feeling like they are capable of "doing more."

Consequences of hyperactivity are listed in Table 6.5.

Too much of a good thing is a bad thing

In the throes of hypomania, patients often lose perspective on the speed of their thinking, the quantity and quality of activity, and the effects of their behavior. When mildly increased, productivity is useful and often rewarded. As hypomania progresses, however, the patient can be seen as being overzealous, annoyingly persistent, racing, or expressly demanding. Although difficult to accomplish when the patient is in the midst of a hypomanic episode, it is nonetheless incumbent on the therapist to be direct and forthright. Inappropriate behaviors and other hypomanic sequelae may come to the therapist's attention directly in face-to-face patient contact, through input from the family or caretakers, or through extrapolation based on the patient's activity report.

TABLE 6.5
Consequences of hyperactivity

1. Precipitation of a subsequent depression
2. Excess fatigue following a hypomanic burst of activity
3. Difficulty in maintaining a constant level of productivity
4. Decreased accuracy when hypomanic
5. Increased irritability and friction with family or coworkers
6. Need for increased medication

Attempts by the therapist to point out hypomania, redirect behavior, or alter medication may meet with resistance from the patient. If patients are engaged solidly in a psychotherapeutic relationship, they come to trust the therapist's judgment and may attempt to view their behavior as hypomanic and to limit their level of activity. A way to phrase this for the patient is, often, "less is more."

For example, the ability to work long hours whether at the office or at home is often one by-product of hypomania. This behavior may be viewed with pride, and often incentivized with increased financial remuneration, worker recognition, or increased productivity. Inflated self-esteem and admiration of superiors or colleagues may further reinforce that more activity achieves more results. This behavior may be especially difficult to change if financial indiscretions, also secondary to hypomania, make working long hours essential to offset obligations. The therapist should evaluate the number of hours worked by patients and, when excessive, encourage patients to moderate their activity even when it may be encouraged or, at times, mandated by the patient's employer. A signed medical letter to the employer limiting the hours of overtime or the frequency of travel "for the patient's health" may be necessary.

Decreasing stimulation in an elevated state

One of the most useful behavioral interventions with a moderately hypomanic patient with elevated energy and mood state is to encourage strategies for decreasing stimulation. Hypomanic individuals often generate positive responses from other people, and exhibit increased social interaction. Hypercommunication face-to-face, on the telephone, or through the Internet can stimulate others to respond in kind. Helping the patient obtain space in terms of time and distance from others can help settle the patient and prevent further acceleration. At a social gathering, for example, the patient can be encouraged to take a "time out" and go for a brief walk interrupting accelerated interactions. Similarly, in busy or intense family interactions, the patient can be encouraged to take breaks in activity and conversations. Sound is often overstimulating and the patient should be encouraged to turn down or mute television volume and turn off radios or sound systems in the car or at home. Encourage finding a quiet place for a "time out" when the patient feels overstimulated.

Pauses in thought and Activity

Individuals with mild hypomania may have the ability to hyperfocus and the energy to remain at tasks or thought patterns for sustained periods. Within this context, they may actually "lose track" of time, spending hours on a particular activity with sustained productivity. However, the patient may also engage in nonproductive activities to the exclusion of other necessary tasks. These can include playing video games, spending time with a handicraft or hobby, talking on the telephone, watching television, writing, cleaning, organizing the household, and Internet e-mailing or "surfing." The therapist should identify these activities and, if counterproductive, suggest a strategy for setting appropriate timing mechanisms. This can be accomplished by setting a kitchen timer, a wristwatch alarm, or a computer alarm to alert the person to the need to take a restful and restorative break. The patient may also ask a spouse, parent, or roommate to help. When the alarm sounds or they are notified by the other person, the patient is instructed to take a significant break. Walking, stretching, light exercise, performing relaxation activities, or having a healthy snack can refresh and allow the person to evaluate subsequent time usage decisions.

This same principle holds in work situations. The patient should be encouraged to take regular breaks from work including, as a minimum, a 15-minute break during the morning, a lunchtime break, and a 15-minute afternoon break. During these times, the patient should be instructed not to work, take phone calls, or engage in business conversation. Additionally, the activities mentioned in the previous paragraph can also be undertaken in the workplace.

Feedback from others—whom do you trust?

Hypomania, especially when it encompasses grandiosity, can result in over-reliance on internal judgment and assessment of situations. In these cases, reliance on oneself may supersede appropriate attention to others' concerns. A useful strategy early in treatment is to have the patient identify one or more persons who he or she feels can be trusted for feedback about his or her behavior. If the patient has any question about the extent of possible hypomanic behaviors, he or she should be encouraged to ask this person for direct assessment. Likewise, these identified persons should be encouraged to provide ongoing feedback about behaviors they feel are excessive or counterproductive.

Overactive hypomanic patients may engender anxiety in relatives or friends. Impulsive, reckless and/or aggressive behaviors often worry those around the patient. In an effort to be helpful, family members who become anxious may overscrutinize the patient, commenting on behaviors, remarks, or activities which they see as "spiraling up" signals and precursors to more serious problems. It is incumbent on the therapist to help the family strike a balance in this process. If the family seems overzealous in efforts to monitor and/or control, the minimally hypomanic individual may feel criticized and watched like a "bird in a cage" or as if they are "walking on tiptoes." When patients express frustration at being excessively scrutinized, the therapist needs to intervene both with the family and the patient. This is especially important because excessive or unwarranted criticism worsens bipolar prognosis (15). Reassure the family about the "red flag" warning signs that need comment, and those that may be of minimal significance. Outline specific activities, intensity, and time-lengths, which may signal justified concern. Indicate appropriate times to intervene with the patient or, if episodes are more severe, when to call the therapist. In these cases, unfortunately, patients may find that no matter how gently the family gives feedback they may still feel watched, judged, or criticized. This feeling cannot be avoided entirely and should be identified as part of normal recovery, especially early in the course of treatment.

Taking on new tasks

During periods of excess energy and overactivity, there may be, for the patient, a tendency to take on new tasks: responsibilities at home, new work assignments, volunteer activities, or new hobbies. The therapist and patient together may need to construct an hour-by-hour schedule of current activities, assessing if such additional time is realistic when considering a new activity.

Because individuals with hypomania often have very busy baseline activity levels, a useful question to ask the patient is *"What are you going to give up in order to make room for this new activity?"* If the patient cannot come up with a valid response or implies "I'll just fit it in somewhere," the therapist should be skeptical and openly question whether this is healthy. Hypomanic individuals also often have the tendency to take on new responsibilities at the cost of decreasing sleep, which itself is counterproductive.

Even when a patient is satisfactorily able to find time to perform a new activity, task, or assignment, the therapist should be on the lookout for activities, which may be demanding. It can be pointed out to the patient "Just because you *can*, doesn't mean you *should*." Activities, which overstimulate or have the potential to mushroom into increasing responsibilities, are particularly problematic for the hypomanic individual. Similarly, optional experiences or relationships with a high emotional content or the potential for significantly turbulent interactions should be questioned closely. Activities involving public appearances or high-risk decision making should be monitored carefully.

Advisors—both well-meaning and self-serving

There are some family members, relatives, friends, bosses, or coworkers who may unknowingly support or encourage hypomanic manic behavior. They may encourage the patient to be talkative, make more money, take on onerous tasks, or volunteer for difficult assignments at work. Most times, this encouragement is offered without intending harm to the patient. At other times, the encouragement seems deliberate, come what may for the patient. Families or partners may encourage hypomania in order to avoid having to do the work themselves. Coworkers or bosses may relish the patient's increased productivity. Not all people are well meaning. Some may take advantage of the patient for selfish motives.

Examples include quiet individuals who encourage hypermanic talkativeness to keep themselves in the background. A substance abuser invites hypomanic individuals to drink or use drugs, thereby having a partner for drinking or drug-using. Free-spending spouses may encourage or even demand more income at any price from their hypomanic partner. Likewise, family members who like to stay up late and feel lonely if left alone may encourage those with hypomania to avoid a reasonable bedtime. Sexual partners may encourage promiscuous or unhealthy sexual practices to serve their own sexual needs. Intervention is necessary to discuss and rectify these situations.

Saying "No"

Although not necessarily an integral part of the hypomanic syndrome *per se*, an inability to refuse a request for fear of disappointing or angering others can be dangerous for a patient. When the patient is unable to say "No," it may be necessary to diagnose and specifically treat this lack of assertiveness. Marital or family therapy may also be useful in relationships where others "over ask" or refuse to take the patient's "No" for an answer. The therapist needs to advocate for the patient, protecting him/her from behaviors that may foster hypomanic elevation or mood swings.

Making decisions

A corollary of helping the patient say "No" when necessary and decreasing simulation is helping the patient suspend acting on feelings at times of significant symptoms. Whether it is during a hypomanic or manic episode or in the throes of depression, patients should be encouraged to minimize decision making, particularly in situations that may be relatively irreversible or have long-term consequences. Buying or selling a house, changing jobs, getting married, separated or divorced, buying or selling items that involve a large financial commitment are some examples of behaviors that should be limited or postponed until the patient feels that his or her mood is stable. Significant mood states can profoundly color or distort the person's judgment even when he or she is normally level-headed and logically thinking. It is often important for the therapist to at least try to "save the patient from his own clouded thinking." This principle of management of elevated (and depressed) mood often appears contrary to recommendations made by some nonmedical psychotherapists. It is not uncommon for therapists to encourage a patient to change jobs, begin or end a relationship, or other significant life endeavor as part of the treatment to "bring them out of" the mood episode. Although some patients do benefit from these recommendations, in general there is no urgency to make such decisions and it is significantly safer in the long run to advise the patient to wait until they are mood stable before making such decisions.

The value of routine

Hypomania may result in erratic and unpredictable sleep habits and dysregulation of physical or work activity. It is useful to support the concept of routine with these activities. In addition to taking time outs, the extent of activity should be monitored. "Moderation in all things" is a good maxim for hypomanic individuals. The therapist may find repeating this maxim useful at many stages of treatment.

One issue that is universally detrimental to all patients with mood disorders, particularly so in hypomania, is shift work. In rotating schedules or intermittent night shifts, sleep is invariably disrupted and mood flare-ups are more likely. It is ironic that persons with elevated mood often function with little sleep and in fact may be drawn to shift work or night work hours because they *can* get by with little sleep. Patients should be strongly cautioned that this is a potential danger, which may exacerbate their mood disorder. When necessary, the therapist may intercede with an employer to limit patient erratic work schedules or excessive overtime.

Financial controls

In severe hypomania, there may be little control over impulsive buying and excessive spending. The therapist and sometimes the patient's family may need to intervene in this costly symptom. Therapeutic strategies may include a "cash only" system of purchase, limiting the number and amount of checks that may be written, giving up the use of credit cards, and approval by a spouse or family member before purchases over a set amount of money can be made. In the most extreme cases, strict financial oversight must be instituted. A spouse may need to manage bank accounts and credit cards or in severe cases when a friend or family member is not available, a financial custodian may be hired at a bank or law office.

"The high goeth before the fall"

One of the most helpful verbal techniques with cycling hypomanic patients is "Everything has a price" including hypomania. For most patients the "high" of increased activity, the "rush" of success, and generally feeling "great" are often followed by a period of debilitating depression that lasts days, weeks, or months. In cyclothymia, the depression may be relatively brief or mild, but patients with bipolar I or II disorder have major depressive episodes accompanied by a substantial impairment of functioning. For hypomanics, the "high" is gone, replaced by the "hell" of despair. Grasping this concept when a serious depression has yet to occur might be difficult. However, once depressions have occurred, the patient often becomes more amenable to intervention, having now experienced the dreadful pain of depression—the "fall" after the "high." This depression, with its pain, immobility, lack of energy, sleep disruption, lack of productivity, and possible suicidal ideation, is excruciating for the patient accustomed to functioning at an accelerated, high-energy, productive level. Even if they intellectually understand that "The High goeth before the Fall," the best compliance often occurs after patients experience one or more depressive episodes and their devastating aftermath.

You are not alone—identification with others

When given a new diagnosis of hypomania, many patients are understandably frightened. It may be useful to hear about successful persons in the entertainment world, the literary world, the sports arena, politicians, or business leaders who have identified themselves as having elevated mood disorder. There is now a long list of public figures who have identified their own ongoing struggles with bipolar disorder (see Table 6.6). From such a list, it is simple for the therapist to highlight individuals who have struggled and succeeded with their illness.

The myth of making up for lost time

Following a depressive episode, hypomanic individuals frequently fear they have "fallen behind" in their work or social obligations. When feeling better, they may accelerate to make up for time lost to depression. When depression causes a deceleration even to a pace considered normal for most individuals, hypomanic patients may feel nonproductive and guilty for what they perceive as "sloughing off." Therapists can be enormously helpful in offering perspective on appropriate production—what is overproduction, normal, and underproduction. Additionally, accelerating to "make up" for time lost may actually precipitate mania.

Because dysfunctionality in hypomania can be worsened through excessive speed both mentally and behaviorally, teaching the patients techniques to slow thought and actions can lead to a significantly better control of their illness.

Self-soothing techniques

There are a variety of techniques (see Table 6.7) that can help hypomanic individuals soothe and calm themselves. Any of these, used alone or in combination, can be therapeutically useful in managing accelerated thoughts, feelings, and actions. These techniques also help maintain a psychological equilibrium. Such methods should be part of the therapist's treatment options, even if referral to another practitioner for consultation is necessary.

Progressive deep muscle relaxation is simple to learn. Although methodologies vary slightly, the central technique involves the contraction and relaxation of each major muscle group in sequence. Some practitioners will start with the feet and work upwards, whereas others go in reverse. One by one, the muscle groups are contracted and then allowed to relax with ease and smoothness. As patients move from one muscle group to another they periodically check that previous muscle groups remain relaxed. Once the sequence is completed, patients are instructed to stay in this state for a period of 5 to 10 minutes, consolidating the relaxation gains.

Often associated with Hinduism, *yoga*'s original purpose of assuming specific postures and breathing exercises was designed to bring mental stability

TABLE 6.6

Some individuals with bipolar disorder

Rosemary Clooney, singer	Ernest Hemingway, author
Dick Cavett, writer and media personality	Samuel Clemens (Mark Twain), author
Kitty Dukakis, former First Lady of Massachusetts	Tennessee Williams, author/playwright
Patty Duke, actor and writer	Jane Pauley, TV personality
Connie Francis, actor and musician	Robert Louis Stevenson, author
Peter Gabriel, musician	Robert Burns, poet
Charley Pride, musician	Virginia Woolf, author
Abraham Lincoln, United States President	Wolfgang Amadeus Mozart, composer
Kay Redfield Jamison, physician and writer	Cole Porter, composer
Margot Kidder, actress	Kurt Cobain, musician
Jimmy Pearsall, Red Sox baseball player	Emily Dickinson, poet
Robin Williams, actor and comedian	Walt Whitman, poet
Axl Rose, musician	Georgia O'Keefe, artist
Ted Turner, entrepreneur and media mogul	William Blake, author
Napoleon Bonaparte, General	Robert Schumann, composer
Art Buchwald, writer and humorist	Charles Dickens, author
Tim Burton, artist and movie director	Jackson Pollock, artist
Ilie Nastase, tennis champion	Vincent Van Gogh, artist
Edgar Allan Poe, author	Kristy McNichol, actress
Winston Churchill, British Prime Minister	Kate Millett, writer
Muffin Spencer-Devlin, pro golfer	Sylvia Plath, author
William Faulkner, author	Paul Gauguin, artist
Ralph Waldo Emerson, author	—
Herman Melville, author	—
Leo Tolstoy, author	—
Peter Tchaikovsky, composer	—
Irving Berlin, composer	—
Noel Coward, composer	—

TABLE 6.7

Self-soothing techniques useful in hypomania treatment

Deep muscle relaxation
Yoga
Meditation
Abdominal breathing

and physical relaxation as preparing for meditation. Current readers might assume yoga to be solely connected to balance, stretching, and physical stability. However, practitioners of yoga see body and breath as intimately connected with the mind. Yoga utilizes movement, breath, posture, and relaxation to integrate and harmonize body, mind, and emotions. Control is a key aspect of yoga—control of the body, breath, and mind—and one who practices yoga seeks balanced moderation in every area of life. Hatha yoga, one of the most popular types of yoga in the Western hemisphere, consists of asanas or postures that embody controlled movement, concentration, flexibility, and conscious breathing. The practice of yoga and its combination of physical and mental relaxation generally benefits individuals with hypomania.

Meditation can be combined with the physical techniques of yoga or practiced independently. The simplest form of meditation involves breathing in a deep, slow, relaxed manner. Beyond this basic meditation, more advanced practice demands the brain not to focus on any single thought or entity, thereby attempting to relax the mind and allow less conscious thoughts to emerge. There are a wide variety of techniques used in meditation including various mental foci, physical positions, mantra repetition, and visualization techniques. Although the exact mechanism of action is not known, many therapists have found that encouraging daily meditation can be a useful technique to help hypomanic individuals.

Abdominal breathing, the technique of abdominal versus chest breathing, is useful in the treatment of many anxiety disorders including panic attacks. This same utility and its ability to prevent hyperventilation and provide for deep relaxation can be useful in hypomanic mental or physical "raciness." Abdominal breathing technique asks the patient to slowly breathe by pushing the stomach outward and inhaling deeply through the nose to a count of four. Exhalation is slow and gradual through pursed lips to the count of four. It is impossible to hyperventilate or remain tense when appropriately applying this breathing technique.

Treating depressed mood in patients with elevated mood symptoms

Before beginning the discussion on the use of medications in treating depressed mood in bipolar patients in Chapter 7, it is important to mention the treatment modalities that are helpful in the treatment of depression that do not include prescription medication. Many of the strategies described in this chapter, which are useful in the elevated mood states, are also useful for the depressed phase of the illness. CBT has long been a staple of depression treatment and can be effectively used in the depressed phase of bipolar illness, as well as with major depressive episodes. CBT has no incidence of either bipolar exacerbation or any increased incidence of hypomania with its use. Likewise, it is easily adaptable for use on its own or in combination with medication.

Light therapy in depressed mood

Patients and clinicians have known that a period of early morning awakening may provide a transient boost in mood that usually lasts no more than several hours or part of a day. Recently Benedetti et al. (16) extended this concept by treating 60 inpatients with drug-resistant bipolar depression with 1 week of repeated total sleep deprivation and light therapy combined with ongoing antidepressants and lithium. Their chronotherapy consisted of a series of three consecutive cycles of total sleep deprivation for a period of 36 hours (days 1, 3, and 5). They were then allowed to sleep during the nights of days 2, 4, and 6. In addition, they were exposed to an artificial light source (400 Lux green light) for a 30-minute period during the sleep deprivation and in the morning after recovery sleep. On this protocol, 70% of patients with non–medication-resistant bipolar disorder and 44% of medication-resistant patients achieved at least a 50% reduction in Hamilton Rating Scale for depression ratings. This response was significant, particularly for drug-resistant patients. When these patients were followed for a 9-month period, 57% of the nonresistant responders and 17% of the drug-resistant responders were euthymic at 9 months. Although not a useful treatment over an extended period, chronotherapeutic interventions do merit further investigation for bipolar depression, particularly when medicines are less than fully successful.

Can light (or lack of it) help elevated mood?

Although it has long been known that the addition of bright artificial light may be of significant benefit to patients with seasonal affective disorder, it is only recently that the effect of light has been studied in elevated mood. Barbini et al. (16) undertook a pilot study to study the inverse, that is, whether enforced darkness could lessen manic symptoms. In this study, 16 manic patients with bipolar disorder underwent 14 hours per day of enforced darkness and rest for 3 consecutive days. Their mania ratings decreased significantly faster than controls and they were discharged from the hospital 9 days earlier than controls. The results are somewhat confounded by the fact that the patients who underwent "dark therapy" slept an average of 4 hours longer than the control subjects, so the improvement in mania could also be a function of improved and longer sleep rather than increased exposure to darkness alone.

The bottom line

- Several psychotherapeutic approaches have shown value in the treatment of elevated mood. These include the following:
  ○ Cognitive behavioral therapy
  ○ Psychoeducation
  ○ Family-focused therapy
  ○ Interpersonal/social rhythm therapy
  ○ Prodrome detection
- The common elements of these approaches include the following:
  ○ Identifying signs of relapse and having plans for a treatment response
  ○ Educating about elevated mood and why treatment is necessary
  ○ Emphasizing the need to continue medication even when euthymic
  ○ Focusing on stress management and problem solving
  ○ Monitoring regular daily rhythms of sleep, exercise, eating, and activities.
- Analogies to commonly understood scenarios help patients comprehend and comply with treatment.
- "Re-viewing" the patient's history and family history can be very helpful as part of treatment.
- Charting of moods on a daily, monthly, and life-long basis will facilitate pattern identification and treatment response.
- Use of web sites and books on bipolar disorder can be helpful to some patients, although instructions must be given as to how to use this information.
- Therapists can be directive in providing techniques to help patients slow down and decrease the stimulation in their environment.
- Patients can often identify with celebrities, athletes, or politicians who have publicly acknowledged bipolar disorder.
- Self-soothing techniques such as deep muscle relaxation, yoga, mediation, and abdominal breathing are useful to hypomanic individuals.

REFERENCES

1. Otto MW, Miklowitz DJ. The role and impact of psychotherapy in the management of bipolar disorder. *CNS Spectr.* 2004;9(11 Suppl 12):27–32.
2. http://www.psycheducation.org/depression/Psychotherapy.htm. 2006.
3. Basco MR, Rush AJ. *Cognitive therapy for bipolar disorder.* New York: Guilford Press; 1996.
4. Fava GA, Bartolucci G, Rafanelli C, et al. Cognitive-behavioral management of patients with bipolar disorder who relapsed while on lithium prophylaxis. *J Clin Psychiatry.* 2001;62:556–559.
5. Cochran SD. Preventing medical noncompliance in the outpatient treatment of bipolar affective disorders. *J Consult Clin Psychol.* 1984;52:873–878.

6. Otto MW, Reilly-Harrington N, Sachs GS. Psychoeducational and cognitive-behavioral strategies in the management of bipolar disorder. *J Affect Disord*. 2003; 73:171–181.
7. Steinhauer E. Psychosocial treatment of bipolar disorder. FRCP(C). *Medscape Psychiatry Ment Health*. 2003;8(1). http://www.medscape.com/viewarticle /457054.
8. Ball JR, Mitchell PB, Corry JC, et al. A randomized controlled trial of cognitive therapy for bipolar disorder: Focus on long-term change. *J Clin Psychiatry*. 2006;67:277–286.
9. Colom F, Vieta E, Martinez-Aran A, et al. A randomized trial on the efficacy of group psychoeducation in the prophylaxis of recurrences in bipolar patients whose disease is in remission. *Arch Gen Psychiatry*. 2003;60(4):402–407.
10. Frank E, Swartz HA, Mallinger AG, et al. Adjunctive psychotherapy for bipolar disorder: Effects of changing treatment modality. *J Abnorm Psychol*. 1999; 108:579–587.
11. Frank E, Kupfer DJ, Thase ME, et al. Two-year outcomes for interpersonal and social rhythm therapy in individuals with Bipolar 1 disorder. *Arch Gen Psychiatry*. 2005;62:996–1004.
12. Frank E, Swartz HA, Kupfer DJ. Interpersonal and social rhythm therapy: Managing the chaos of bipolar disorder. *Biol Psychiatry*. 2000;48:593–604.
13. Perry Alison, Tarrier Nicholas, Morriss Richard, et al. Randomised controlled trial of efficacy of teaching patients with bipolar disorder to identify early symptoms of relapse and obtain treatment. *Br Med J*. 1999;318:149–153.
14. Doran CM. *Prescribing mental health medication: The practitioner's guide*. Routledge; 2003:393–394.
15. Miklowitz DJ, Wisniewski SR, Miyahara S, et al. Perceived criticism from family members as a predictor of the one-year-course of bipolar disorder. *Psychiatry Res*. 2004;136(2–3):101–111.
16. Barbini B, Benedetti F, Colombo C, et al. Dark therapy for mania: A pilot study. *Bipolar Disord*. 2005;7(1):98–101.

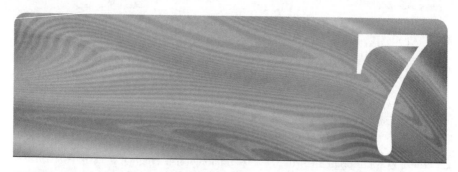

TREATMENT OF ELEVATED MOOD WITH MEDICATION

- General issues
- How much medication is enough?
- The steroid analogy
- Can't I just be a little manic?
- Medication research considerations
- Primary factors in choosing medication
    - Target symptoms
    - Prior response
    - Medical comorbidity
- Secondary considerations in medication choice
- Hypomania versus mania medication choice
- Treating to remission
- Off-label prescribing
- FDA-approved antimanic treatments
    - Overlapping terms
    - Consensus guidelines
    - Lithium
    - Carbamazepine
    - Divalproex
    - Antipsychotics
- Side effect considerations with atypical antipsychotics
    - Metabolic considerations
    - Seizures
    - QTc prolongation
    - Hyperprolactinemia
    - Pregnancy and lactation

    Affective switches and cycle acceleration
- Combination treatments for elevated mood
    - Benzodiazepines
- Medications in psychotic mania
- Choosing medication by temperament
- Treatment of bipolar depression with medication
- The ideal standard for a bipolar spectrum patient with depression
    - Types of evidence
- Overriding principles of treating depression in bipolar disorder
    - Expert consensus guideline
    - TIMA guidelines
    - American Psychiatric Association and British Association for Psychopharmacotherapy guidelines for depressive episodes
    - Canadian Network for Mood and Anxiety Treatment (CANMAT) guidelines for the management of patients with bipolar disorder
    - Consolidating the guidelines
- Use of antidepressants in bipolar depression—the great debate
- Why is there controversy?

- Consolidated recommendations for the use of traditional antidepressants
- Integrating temperament into bipolar depression treatment
- Electroconvulsive therapy
- The bottom line
- *References*

General issues

As described elsewhere (1), prescribing mental health medication is unlike prescribing other types of medication, for example, antihypertensives or antibiotics. Both patient and practitioner beliefs can dramatically color the prescribing process. On the basis of a family member's experience with psychotropics, shared family beliefs, professional hearsay or media presentations about psychotropics, patients and even some practitioners may have biased viewpoints. Despite gradually improving teaching about mental health and psychiatry, many beliefs about what causes mental illness and what constitutes appropriate treatment can significantly affect the prescribing process. Patients have preconceived notions about what mental health medications can or cannot do, and what risks are involved. Some of the myths related to mental health medications are listed in Table 7.1.

Although these myths will not be explored in detail in this text, the reader is referred to the author's other writings for specific discussion. Suffice it to say that in our population, belief in these myths abounds; and dealing with these misconceptions becomes an essential part of medication treatment of elevated mood. These general myths are further complicated by specific myths related to elevated mood, which are listed in Table 7.2.

TABLE 7.1
Myths about mental health medication

Mental health medication is a placebo
Mental health medication is addictive
Mental health medication will change personality
Mental health medicine must be stopped as soon as possible
Mental health medication will overcome bad habits
If side effects occur, the medication must be working
Taking mental health medication means a personal weakness or failure
Alcohol is prohibited when taking psychotropic medicine
A person must be substance-free to be assessed/treated accurately for mental illness

TABLE 7.2

Common beliefs about medication and elevated mood

Medication for elevated mood will

- take away creativity, cognitive skills, or ability to have fun
- make a person depressed, "flat," or boring
- cause dangerous side effects
- make permanent brain changes
- be appropriate only for hospitalized or "crazy" people
- require life-long treatment

As part of any initial treatment session that involves medication prescription, it is wise for the clinician to ask the patient about concerns or questions before making specific recommendations. This can be phrased as follows:

> *If I were to suggest that medication would be helpful in treating the problems for which you came today, do you have any specific concerns about taking medication based on what you've read or what you've been told by your family and friends?*

Although it is generally unnecessary to ask about each of the concerns mentioned in Table 7.2, when specific questions or concerns are raised, it is essential that they be addressed before the actual prescription is made.

Sample responses to each of the concerns listed in Table 7.2 are as follows:

> ***Concerns about creativity, cognitive skills, or enjoyment.*** *This is a common concern about mood medication. You are a person who has shown creativity, energy, and the ability for significant accomplishment. Clearly, we intend to keep those skills intact. Our goal will be to further enhance your creativity and productive activity by allowing you to be more consistent in mood and to channel your energies productively. We also want to target some of the more problematic behaviors such as ... (Here, list presenting complaints such as irritability and anger, depressed episodes, impulsive behavior, or difficulty with relationships). Medication is not going to negatively affect your cognitive abilities or intelligence. In fact, if you are feeling consistently better, I would expect you would be able to use your innate traits more efficiently. Individuals who have problems with their moods can often increase their enjoyment of life when they can depend on their body and brain to regulate mood in a predictable and consistent manner.*

Causing depression. *Although my assessment is that you have been somewhat overly active and "over-revved" recently, there would be no benefit in allowing you to become depressed. Our goal is to gradually bring down this level of overactivity to a pace that is comfortable for you and the others around you. Together we will be watching for any signs of depression to make sure that it does not happen.*

Concerns about making personality flat or boring. *Any treatment that would make you flat or boring is certainly not desirable and not something I expect for you. Some people with elevated mood are exceptionally talkative and overly energetic. Medication we use would help you to be more stable and consistently productive. Those individuals who are used to living life in "overdrive" do find that they talk less to some extent and find it less desirable to work exceptionally long hours. The benefit, though, is that they also become better listeners and conversationalists, and often find themselves more productive in the hours that they work. Between the two of us, we will keep close watch on any changes that would occur from medication because our overall goal is to have you feel better and function better; being flat or boring doesn't accomplish anything.*

Concerns about dangerous side effects. *Fortunately, side effects that occur with mood medications are more annoying than serious or life-threatening. If we start medication, we will discuss any side effects that are common and any unusual side effects that are significant. Most importantly, I want us to stay in contact and, if you have any concerns about negative effects from the medication, let me know so we can discuss them.*

Concerns about permanent brain changes. *We have virtually no evidence to suggest that medications for elevated mood will in any way permanently affect your neurochemistry or brain structure. Although sometimes symptoms recur when medications are stopped, you are unlikely to have irreversible behavioral changes.*

Concerns about strong medication only for "crazy" people. *When some of the medicines we use now were introduced 30 or 40 years ago, they were used primarily for hospitalized, very ill individuals in large doses. We have now come to understand that many of the same medicines in smaller doses can be useful for people with mild-to-moderate symptoms. Many productive and admired individuals take mental health medications, and those around them are not even aware of it. The most important thing now is to help you feel well and stable.*

Concerns about lifelong medication. *Although there are individuals who benefit from taking medication long term, that is not our plan initially. If we agree to start medication, we would do so for a defined period of time after which, together, we would decide to gradually decrease the dose and ultimately stop the medication.*

What we do from that point forward depends on how you respond to stopping medication. For now, the decision to start medication is not a decision to take it indefinitely.

How much medication is enough?

In a patient with elevated mood, the estimate of how much medication is sufficient must be judged individually for each patient. The bottom line answer to this question is *that amount of medication that can be mutually negotiated between clinician and patient.* Some of the negotiation between clinician and therapist about necessary levels of medication may involve a reevaluation and potential redefinition of what is normal. Many hypomanic patients have been functioning at an accelerated pace for months or years. Mood stabilizing or modulating medications may make them feel that they are being "slowed down," although by society's standards, they are only becoming "normal" with treatment.

The steroid analogy

A useful analogy during this stage of negotiations is that of an athlete who uses steroids.

A person with chronically elevated mood is similar to an athlete who has been using anabolic steroids over an extended period of time. Such a person may have become accustomed to levels of activity, strength, and performance that are "supernormal." They often ignore the negative aspects of steroids, such as hormonal changes, rage episodes, liver damage, skin changes, baldness, feminization (for men)/masculinization (for women), depression, and erectile dysfunction. Used long enough, the person may even believe that it is "normal" to be able to run as fast, hit a ball as far, or lift as much weight as they can when they are taking steroids. When the steroids are stopped, they may feel somewhat slowed down or less strong, but there are significant positive trade-offs. Many of the side effects mentioned disappear and the risk of life-threatening conditions such as liver or prostate cancer are significantly reduced. Most individuals find that even if their athletic performance is lessened to some degree from not using steroids, their overall health, happiness, and functioning is considerably enhanced. The trade-off is well worth any diminished athletic activity. Similarly, with elevated mood, you may have been used to functioning at "120 miles per hour" throughout much of your life. Even if treatment does slow you to "100 miles per hour," there will be significant enhancements to your overall functioning from this minimal "loss of speed."

Can't I just be a little manic?

This analogy is often followed by questions such as, "Can't I just be a little manic?" or "Isn't there a way to keep me going 120 miles an hour without the risk?" The best reply is *"That is a very common request but something I do not know how to do. It is no more possible than safely driving city streets at excessive speed, or using steroids without the health risks."*

No matter what amount of medication the therapist thinks is ideal, it is only with the concurrence and agreement of the patient that the ultimate regimen can be defined and maintained. When treating patients with seriously elevated mood or full mania, the amount of medication is often determined by what medication levels are necessary for minimizing a variety of reckless, dangerous, or impulsive behaviors. Safety, recklessness, and impulsivity are not always seen in a similar light by the patient, his family, or the clinician. With less severely ill elevated mood patients, the appropriate level of medication may be that which minimizes the presenting complaints but still permits some elevated mood or overactivity. In this case, target symptoms need to be identified and medications specifically aimed at minimizing or eliminating these target symptoms. Depending on the particular medication and the breadth of its effectiveness, any one medication may or may not treat other target symptoms or incidental manifestations of elevated mood.

Lastly, clinicians may view medication amounts as being optimal when it slows the patient's speed of thought down to a level that permits psychotherapeutic intervention. If a patient is talking, thinking, and behaving so rapidly that they cannot listen to or incorporate psychotherapeutic interventions, medication levels are likely insufficient.

What is not a part of the equation when deciding how much medication is enough is the outdated notion that side effects must be evident in order to indicate that the medication is working. This old notion suggested that medications were ineffective unless doses that produced side effects were reached. Modern psychopharmacology, however, sees side effects as totally unwanted unless they can be serendipitously useful to the patient's functioning and overall treatment (such as sedation from a mood stabilizing medication that might be useful in helping a patient with insomnia).

The art of medication management of individuals with elevated mood requires tact, skill, and often repetitive discussions to negotiate and renegotiate what is the appropriate and optimal level of medication.

Medication research considerations

In summarizing the current literature on the treatment of elevated mood with medication, there are several caveats and general issues to be taken into consideration by the clinician. These include the following:

- Most research has been conducted on patients with bipolar I disorder exclusively or mixed groups of bipolar I and bipolar II. Evidence of effectiveness in bipolar I episodes of mania may or may not generalize to treatment of hypomania.
- Although there are more randomized placebo-controlled studies (Class A data) for the treatment of elevated mood than there are for depressed mood

in bipolar disorder, clinicians are often guided by consensus guidelines from various groups. Consensus guidelines are those recommendations formulated from the opinions of national experts. These can be obtained in two different ways. The first, as exemplified by the Expert Consensus Guidelines, is a pure tabulation of the answers to mailed questionnaires. It is then an opinion poll and not "evidence" per se. It does, however, reflect how major thought leaders practice. The second form of consensus guidelines involves a gathering of experts coming together to present and discuss their recommendations in a group. The resulting document (e.g., the Texas Implementation of Medication Algorithms or TIMA guidelines) is the end product of their discussions. Here the experts may present data to back up their opinion. The group can interact and challenge one another in order to arrive at consensus. When consensus is not reached, a hierarchy of recommendations and divergent opinion is presented. Although it is not true "evidence" in the sense of a randomized, controlled trial, the process will produce recommendations that will carry more import than an opinion poll.

- Because research on elevated mood is likely to have been performed on heterogeneous groups of patients as discussed in Chapter 2, even our current data may be on a somewhat shaky foundation.

Primary factors in choosing medication

Despite limitations and confounding factors, research does give us useful clinical guidelines for the management of elevated mood with medication. This portion of the chapter will be divided into several sections. The text will first focus on the general issues in regard to choosing medication, then review the consensus guidelines from various professional groups. This will be followed by discussion of the advantages and disadvantages of individual antimanic medications. Lastly, additional considerations affecting the choice of medications such as medication safety, tolerability, and side effects as well as choosing medications based on underlying temperament will be outlined.

When choosing medication treatment for elevated mood, the choice is determined by a variety of factors that may be different for individual patients (Table 7.3). Simply knowing that a medication is effective is, of course, vital. Other factors, however, as discussed subsequently can significantly alter a clinician's pharmaceutical choice.

Target symptoms

On the basis of our theoretical assumptions, recent clinical practice has assumed that antimanic medications for elevated mood have effectiveness on the constellation of manic/hypomanic symptoms with equal effectiveness. Medication research has grouped patients with bipolar I and bipolar II disorders together regardless of the intensity of specific symptoms within the diagnosis. Someone with a predominant irritable elevated mood, therefore,

TABLE 7.3
Primary factors in choosing medication for mood
• Target symptoms of the current episode
• Medication response in prior episodes
• Safety of the pharmaceutical
• Tolerability of the pharmaceutical (side effects)
• Other concurrent medications taken by the patient
• Ongoing medical conditions
• Patient temperament

would be included in the same research protocol group with a patient who has primarily grandiose euphoric mania. Broad-based conclusions of medication effectiveness in an overall elevated mood group may or may not reflect equal effectiveness within subgroups of this population. Although there is limited research on which to firmly base clinical decisions at present, it is hoped that ongoing research will begin to separate phenotypic differences in ways that permit the clinician to identify the most appropriate treatment for specific target symptoms. Armed with this information, clinicians can more specifically choose the most effective medicine for the specific symptomatology such as irritability, sleeplessness, overactivity, grandiosity, impulsivity, and other symptoms of elevated mood. Steven Stahl's concept that individual symptoms are determined by abnormalities in specific brain neurocircuitry, symptoms, and circuits fosters this manner of thinking (2).

Prior response

As is the case in treating all psychiatric conditions with recurrent episodes, a prior history of positive response in a previous elevated mood episode will direct a clinician to strongly consider restarting the efficacious medication. This general principle may, however, be modified if the positive response was complicated by significant and/or serious side effects. If tolerability was impaired, another medication with a different side effect profile might be chosen. Also if a previously used medication was helpful for a period of time but then lost effectiveness, it may not be the best first choice for a symptomatic recurrence.

Medical comorbidity

Ongoing medical conditions or concurrent treatment with nonpsychiatric medications may also affect the choice of antimanic pharmaceuticals.

Such situations can direct a clinician toward a particular medication choice as well as away from a particular medication selection. For example, a patient who presents with elevated mood and a seizure disorder might preferentially be treated with an anticonvulsant that has antimanic properties such as sodium valproate, carbamazepine, or lamotrigine. A patient with ongoing hepatic dysfunction may have a less complicated course if lithium or lamotrigine is used to treat their elevated mood because both are excreted renally. Although the calcium channel blocker verapamil is not high on the list of antimanic treatments, it may become more desirable in a patient who suffers from hypertension or cardiac arrhythmia, in that both medical and mental health conditions may be treated simultaneously with one medication. Unstable type 1 diabetic patients with frequent fluctuations in salt and fluid balance might be more prone to changes in serum lithium levels, and therefore lithium might not be the best tolerated first choice for treatment of elevated mood in these patients.

Safety and tolerability of medications are of crucial importance in choosing pharmaceuticals to treat elevated mood and will be discussed in more detail later in the chapter.

Using the patient's underlying temperament to help determine the choice of medication is a relatively new concept. It makes sense however to utilize the broad panorama of the patient's overall mood pattern to help determine the optimal treatment for a current index episode of elevated mood. This topic too will be discussed subsequently.

Secondary considerations in medication choice

Although not as important as the considerations mentioned earlier, other factors may also influence a clinician's selection of medication as noted in Table 7.4.

In 21st century psychopharmacology, it is common to have information about first-degree biological relatives who may have been treated for mood conditions. Although a clinician would not automatically choose a medication

TABLE 7.4
Secondary factors in medication choice

- Family history of response to specific pharmaceuticals
- Monotherapy versus combination therapy
- Expense and generic availability
- Insurance formulary issues
- Patient preference

just because a close biological relative had responded to it, this history might be the deciding factor between two equivalently effective medications for the identified patient. Beyond the possible genetic underpinnings and biological likelihood of response, the presence of a positive response in a close family member may favorably predispose the patient psychologically toward this choice. The opposite is also true. If a family member had not had any response or significant side effects to a specific pharmaceutical, the patient may be biologically and/or psychologically negatively predisposed to such a choice.

Monotherapy is always preferential to combination therapy if the therapeutic effects are roughly equivalent. Modern treatment of elevated mood, however, is rarely accomplished through monotherapy. Intelligent, carefully selected combinations of treatments may provide significantly better treatment response than what one agent can provide. The "treat to remission" concept discussed in the subsequent text gives strong credence to the recommendation that combination therapy be used when significant mood symptoms are not ameliorated by one agent. In general, therapeutic advantages outweigh the disadvantages of combination treatment, such as an increased likelihood of side effects, poorer compliance, and increased expense. Specific combination treatments for elevated mood are difficult to evaluate from hard evidence. There is scant class A evidence comparing various combinations of treatment to each other except as compared to against monotherapy.

The cost of the newest (and often more effective) pharmaceuticals is significant and a factor that we must take into account when choosing a treatment. The availability of less expensive generic formulations, resources to pay out of pocket, as well as inclusion on insurance formularies become significant, although bothersome, factors affecting the clinician's choice. Our most elegant diagnostic formulations and treatment regimens are useless if the patient cannot afford or cannot access the medications that we recommend and prescribe.

Lastly, patient preference is becoming a larger factor in the choice of pharmaceuticals. Whether it is because of family response or nonresponse, articles from the media and Internet, or discussion with other patients, patients come to treatment with specific biases for or against various medications for elevated mood. Although a secondary factor, clinicians cannot ignore that patients are much more favorably disposed to medications that they have positive expectations about and negatively predisposed to medications they fear or have heard will cause significant problems. Media advertising is common practice for antidepressant medication. Recently, the media has also begun advertising for bipolar medications. Such advertising may affect consumer expectation or feelings about a particular pharmaceutical choice.

Hypomania versus mania medication choice

Few would argue that effectiveness is of first and primary importance in choosing any pharmaceutical. Whether a patient is mildly to moderately hypomanic or fully manic, no ineffective medication would be a sensible choice. Choosing medication for milder elevated mood states however, is perhaps much more influenced by considerations of tolerability than treatment of mania that often begins in the hospital and is instituted in inpatient settings. Hypomanic patients (who are often outpatients, and may have been overly active) may be much more attuned to issues of annoying side effects. They are also more likely to be noncompliant if side effects are prominent. Given that their hypomanic elevated mood states may be seen as a value and asset (at least when not out of control), they often are skeptical of the necessity for medicine at all. They will clearly be negatively predisposed to medication treatments that cause significant side effects.

This is not to say that treatments for full mania are not, and should not be, influenced by possible side effects. When these treatments are undertaken in a controlled setting such as a hospital, it is often possible to monitor side effects more closely and if they are mild, continue treatment until they abate or are modified by changes in therapeutic regimen. The irony, therefore, is that in mildly elevated mood states, medication tolerability may be almost as important as effectiveness. A well-tolerated medicine that has a slightly decreased efficacy may be more acceptable to a hypomanic patient than a statistically more effective medication that has annoying side effects.

Treating to remission

A well-rooted concept in the literature of depression/anxiety treatment is that clinicians should not settle for *improvement*, but strive for *elimination* of all target symptoms. The literature is now replete with studies that suggest that when significant symptomatology is left untreated, the likelihood of symptomatic relapse is higher. This concept has only recently begun to be applied to bipolar disorder and elevated mood.

Information from the large national Systematic Treatment Enhancement Program for Bipolar Disorder (STEP-BD) gives strong support to the concept that "treating to remission" is necessary in bipolar disorder as well (3). A subset of the total number of patients focused on the 1,469 patients who had participated in the program for at least 2 years and had achieved recovery. While not specifically studying patients who achieved full remission per se, 48.5% of patients of this subgroup who had achieved recovery experienced relapse within a 2-year window despite the highest quality evidence-based care. This does not prove that treatment to remission would have lessened the frequency of these relapses, but it emphasizes the prevalence of recurrences and the need for aggressive, thorough treatment of symptoms.

Short-term, 3- to 4-week medication trials often do not permit full treatment of symptoms to remission. Comparing studies is confounded by the fact that different studies use different definitions of remission. Most investigators use a cutoff score (e.g., ≤12 on the Young Mania Rating Scale [YMRS]) for several weeks. Despite this lack of direct and comparable data, most reasonable clinicians assume that the treatment that relieves the maximum number of symptoms most completely is desirable in this highly recurrent disease.

Off-label prescribing

As in all of psychiatry, prescribing medications for non-FDA approved, off-label uses is more the rule rather than the exception. Anticonvulsants, atypical antipsychotics, antidepressants, and benzodiazepines are all frequently prescribed for one or more symptoms of bipolar disorder with frequency, without a formal U.S. Food and Drug Administration (FDA) indication. In some cases, this is forward thinking, intelligent prescription, based on clinical experience that may precede formal studies and trials. At other times, however, it represents practice based on habit or hearsay with minimal clinical logic. Such off-label prescription is likely to continue in the foreseeable future, but can be made safer and more justified if the seven steps listed here are followed.

Seven steps to safer, more effective off-label prescribing (4):

1. **Be familiar** with evidence-based findings/guidelines.
2. **Clarify** your rationale for off-label prescription.
3. **Obtain** second opinion if indicated.
4. **Perform** risk–benefit analysis.
5. **Obtain** informed consent from patient or appropriate surrogate.
6. **Document** steps 1 through 5 in the patient's record.
7. **Monitor** for known and unexpected adverse effects.

Following evidence-based guidelines such as those reviewed in this text is essential to understanding what has proved to be effective and what may not. Although it is not inappropriate to use medications for off-label indications, clinicians should be clear about why they are doing it. This may include lack of efficacy of on-label medications, a past history of response to the off-label drug or the presence of medical or comorbid conditions that make on-label medications less desirable. Although many off-label prescriptions are in common usage and can be justified on the basis of the clinician's judgment alone, when an unusual or potentially risky choice is made, a second opinion supporting the decision may be useful. It is important to document the clinician's thinking in the written record on any off-label prescription including the fact that the patient was informed of the off-label use with its potential risks and rewards. As with any medication, the patient should be monitored for side effects or untoward responses as there may be some additional clinician liability when serious untoward reactions occur in an off-label prescription.

FDA-approved antimanic treatments

Before considering the recommendations of various expert groups the reader must be familiar with those compounds that have FDA approval

TABLE 7.5

FDA-approved medications for the treatment of mania

Agents	Mania	Mixed episodes	Maintenance
Mood stabilizer			
Lithium (Eskalith, Lithobid)	✓	—	✓
Divalproex (Depakote)	✓	✓	—
Lamotrigine (Lamictal)	—		✓
Carbamazepine ER (Equetro)	✓	✓	—
Antipsychotics			
Chlorpromazine (Thorazine)	✓	—	
Risperidone (Risperdal)	✓	✓	—
Olanzapine (Zyprexa)	✓	✓	✓
Quetiapine (Seroquel)	✓	—	—
Ziprasidone (Geodon)	✓	✓	—
Aripiprazole (Abilify)	✓	✓	✓

From Thompson PDR. *The physician's desk reference*, 60th ed. Thompson PDR; 2006, (5).

for treating the elevated mood states of bipolar disorder. These are shown in Table 7.5.

Overlapping terms

Before discussing specific recommendations for specific phases of bipolar disorder, it is crucial to identify some terms that have been variously applied to mood states of elevation and depression. The term *elevated mood* is a generic one and includes those states of mania, hypomania, and mixed mania, both syndromal and subsyndromal.

As we discuss specific medications, some terms bear definition. Ketter and Calabrese have proposed a nomenclature using "above-baseline" states to refer to diagnosable elevated mood conditions and "below baseline" to refer to depressive states (6,7). Other thought leaders have used the term *treating from above* to mean medications which have more prominent effects on elevated mood states than on depressed states. *Treating from below* then means medications that preferentially treat depressed mood states. Ketter and Calabrese label these as stabilization from above-baseline mood states and stabilization from below-baseline mood states. Other potential mood labels include *up-dominated mood patterns* and *down-dominated mood patterns*. The former refers to a phenotypically bipolar person who has predominantly elevated mood episodes and the latter to an individual who has predominantly depressive mood episodes.

Consensus guidelines

Four separate guidelines will be summarized here, followed by the author's consolidated recommendation regarding individual agents.

Texas Implementation of Medication Algorithms (TIMA) guidelines

The Texas Consensus Conference Panel on medication treatment of bipolar disorder devised the Texas Implementation of Medication Algorithms (TIMA Guidelines). Initially published in 2002, they have been updated in 2006. The recommendations for the treatment of above-baseline mood episodes, that is, hypomanic, manic, and mixed episodes in bipolar I disorder are summarized in Table 7.6.

This algorithm is divided into four stages and separates at Stage 1 into treatments recommended for euphoric elevated mood and those recommended for mixed elevated mood. Stage 1 recommends lithium, valproate, aripiprazole, quetiapine, risperidone, or ziprasidone as first-line treatment for euphoric mania, with olanzapine or carbamazepine also considered first line, but separated because of their side effect burden.

For mixed mania, valproate, aripiprazole, risperidone, and ziprasidone are first-line treatments. When there is no response to one or more of the stage 1 treatments, the patients are moved to stage 2.

This stage incorporates two-drug combinations that include lithium plus valproate, lithium plus an atypical antipsychotic, or valproate plus an antipsychotic. Specifically the recommended antipsychotics are olanzapine, quetiapine, risperidone, and ziprasidone. Aripiprazole was not identified in this stage because of the absence of evidence at the time of these recommendations.

Failure to respond to stage 2 therapies lead to the recommendations in stage 3, in which any two drugs from the list of lithium, valproate, atypical antipsychotics, carbamazepine, oxcarbazepine, and typical antipsychotics can be combined as long as it is not two atypical antipsychotics together and not clozapine.

When stage 3 treatments are ineffective, the recommendations are for the use of electroconvulsive therapy (ECT), adding clozapine to the combinations in stage 3 or using three-drug combinations from the list in stage 3.

Expert consensus guideline

Published in 2000 by Keck et al. and updated in 2004 (8), this guideline is a composite of questionnaires returned by 47 experts in the field of the

TABLE 7.6

Treatment of acute manic/hypomanic/mixed episodes in bipolar I disorder

Treatment in stages	Euphoric	Mixed

Stage 1
Monotherapy
	Li, VPA, ARP, QTP, RIS, ZIP [a,b]
	OLZ [c] or CBZ [c]
	If nonresponse, try alternate
	  choices
	Response → continue
	Partial response or no response ↓
		VPA, ARP, RIS, ZIP [a,b]
		OLZ [c] or CBZ [c]
		If nonresponse, try
		  alternate choices
		Response → continue
		Partial response or no
		  response ↓

Stage 2 Two-drug combination [b]	Li VPA AAP Choose two (not two AAPs, not ARP or CLOZ) Response → continue	Response → continue
	Partial response or no response ↓	Partial response or no response ↓
Stage 3 Two-drug combination [b]	Li VPA AAPs CBZ OXC TAP Choose 2 (not 2 AAPs, not CLOZ) Response → continue	Response → continue
	Partial response or no response ↓	partial response or no response ↓
Stage 4	ECT or add CLOZ or Li plus (VPA or CBZ or OXC) plus AAP	

AAP, atypical antipsychotic; ARP, aripiprazole; CLOZ, clozapine; CBZ, carbamazepine; ECT, electroconvulsive therapy; Li, lithium; OLZ, olanzapine; OXC, oxcarbazepine; QTP, quetiapine; RIS, risperidone; TAP, typical antipsychotic; VPA, valproic acid; ZIP, ziprasidone.
[a] It is appropriate to try more than one combination at a given level.
[b] Use targeted adjunctive treatment as necessary before moving to the next stage, such as sedatives or clonidine for agitation or aggression, benzodiazepines or gabapentin for anxiety or hypnotics for insomnia.
[c] Safety and other concerns led to placement of OLZ and CBZ as alternative choices in the first stage.
Adapted from Suppes T, et al. The Texas medication algorithm project. *J Clin Psychiatry.* 2005;66:870–886, (9)

treatment of bipolar disorder. They were asked to rate mood medications on a scale of 1 to 9, with

- 1 being extremely inappropriate;
- 2 and 3 being usually inappropriate treatment, rarely used;
- 4 to 6 being equivocal, a second-line treatment;
- 7 to 8 being a first-line treatment that would often be used;
- 9 being a treatment of choice.

Specifically in regard to elevated mood, the experts were asked to separate out treatments for acute mania from maintenance treatment for bipolar I disorder.

TABLE 7.7

Expert consensus guideline: initial treatment for first manic episode

Clinical presentation	Preferred initial strategies	Alternative strategies
Euphoric (classic) mania	MS alone MS + AAP Add a BZD	AAP alone
Dysphoric mania or true mixed mania	MS + AAP MS alone	Add a BZD AAP alone Combination of two MSs
Mania with history of rapid cycling	MS + AAP MS alone	Combination of two MSs Add a BZD AAP alone
Mania with psychosis	MS + AAP AAP alone	Add a BZD MS alone

MS, mood stabilizer; AAP, atypical antipsychotic; BZD, benzodiazepine.

On the basis of clinical presentation of the initial manic episode, the responses were divided into preferred and alternate strategies for initial and maintenance therapies as shown in Tables 7.7 and 7.8.

For purposes of these tables, a *mood stabilizer* is defined as an agent that had been previously defined in 2000 in the first version of these guidelines. Specifically, carbamazepine, lithium, and valproate are listed as "mood stabilizers." Although the categories are broken out into classic euphoric mania, mixed mania, mania with a history of rapid cycling, and mania with psychosis, many of the preferred treatments are similar. Specifically, the

TABLE 7.8

Expert consensus guideline: preferred agents

Clinical presentation	Preferred	Alternate
Choice of MS		
Euphoric mania	Lithium, divalproex	
Psychotic mania	Divalproex, lithium	
Mixed mania or mania—rapid cycling	Divalproex	Lithium, CBZ
Choice of AAP		
Euphoric, psychotic or mixed mania	Olanzapine Risperidone Quetiapine	Aripiprazole Ziprasidone

AAP, atypical antipsychotic; MS, mood stabilizer; CBZ, carbamazepine.

TABLE 7.9

Expert consensus guideline: maintenance strategies after a manic episode

Acute-phase treatment	Preferred continuation treatment	Alternate strategy
MS	Continue MS at same dose Add psychotherapy [a]	Continue MS at lower dose
AAP	Continue AAP at same dose	Add psychotherapy Continue AAP at lower dose
MS + AAP	Continue at same doses Add psychotherapy [a]	Taper and discontinue AAP Continue at lower doses

MS, mood stabilizer; AAP, atypical antipsychotic.
[a] Very high second line (rated first line by more than two thirds the number of the experts)

preferred mood stabilizers are divalproex or lithium with carbamazepine as an alternative. When atypical antipsychotics are used, olanzapine, risperidone, and quetiapine are preferred with aripiprazole and ziprasidone as alternatives. Classic euphoric mania can be treated with a mood stabilizer alone, a mood stabilizer plus an atypical antipsychotic, or with possible short-term augmentation with benzodiazepines. An alternative to these preferred strategies is an atypical antipsychotic alone.

The Expert Consensus Guidelines for maintenance strategies are shown in Table 7.9.

As shown in the preceding text, the preferred maintenance strategies depend on the response to acute-phase treatment. If a patient responded to a mood stabilizer alone, it is to be continued with the possibility of adding psychotherapy, and possibly lowering the dose of the mood stabilizer over time. If an atypical antipsychotic was used alone, there is a parallel strategy to continue the atypical antipsychotic, while at the same time adding psychotherapy or lowering the atypical antipsychotic over time. When a mood stabilizer plus an atypical antipsychotic is used in the acute-phase treatment, the preferred strategy is to continue both at the same dosage and add psychotherapy. Alternatively the patient could have the atypical antipsychotic tapered and discontinued over time while maintaining the mood stabilizer.

American Psychiatric Association and British Association for Psychopharmacology guidelines

The guidelines developed by the American Psychiatric Association (APA) and the British Association for Psychopharmacology (BAP) are shown in Table 7.10. They are grouped together because they made their guidelines on the basis of level of severity of the symptoms, which is different than the other guidelines.

Although there are some differences, these two guidelines have significant agreement and in many ways agree with the Expert Consensus guidelines. Specifically for severe illness, a combination therapy of lithium or divalproex plus an antipsychotic are the preferred treatments with carbamazepine as an alternative. Benzodiazepines can be added as a short-term adjunctive therapy.

Maintenance treatments following an initial episode of mania are shown in Table 7.11.

Again there is considerable overlap and agreement between these two guidelines and the Expert Consensus guidelines for maintenance treatment. Of note is the addition of ECT in both the APA and BAP guidelines if the acute response is inadequate. Also psychosocial interventions are specifically added by both bodies.

Having discussed the various guidelines formulated by official and expert bodies, we will now look at the various individual medications in their treatment of acute mania.

Lithium

As one of the oldest medications available to treat bipolar disorder and having been in clinical usage for over 50 years, lithium has abundant data support for its usefulness in acute mania and remains one of the first-line agents in this phase of the illness. Response rates (defined as >50% improvement in manic symptoms) fall between 49% and 70% (10). Bowden et al. showed lithium's effectiveness as compared to placebo as early as day 10 (11). These are several of many studies showing lithium's effectiveness. Although lithium has proven therapeutic effect, it is used as monotherapy for a relatively small group of patients with bipolar disorder because of side effects or comorbid medical conditions. Polyuria, polydipsia, hand tremor, and long-term effects on kidneys and thyroid are known complications. The narrow therapeutic index makes lithium toxicity a significant possibility if lithium levels are not followed carefully. Lithium has been shown to be specifically effective under the following conditions (12,13):

- It is begun during the first few episodes of the illness.
- Depressive symptoms do not accompany mania.
- Comorbid medical or psychiatric problems are absent.
- A family history is positive for lithium-responsive bipolar disorder.

A further advantage of lithium is that it decreases the risk of suicidal behavior in individuals with bipolar disorder. That is particularly important in a bipolar population that has elevated suicide rates particularly during the early phases of the illness (13).

TABLE 7.10

Evidence-based treatment guidelines for acute mania or mixed episode [a]

Level of intervention	APA	BAP
First-line treatment		
Severe illness	Combination therapy: lithium or divalproex plus antipsychotic [b]	Monotherapy: antipsychotic [b] or divalproex
With agitation	Parenteral antipsychotic if severely agitated	Parenteral antipsychotic and benzodiazepines if severely agitated
Less severe illness	Lithium, divalproex, or atypical antipsychotic [c] Alternatives: carbamazepine or oxcarbazepine in lieu of lithium or divalproex	Lithium or carbamazepine
Short-term adjunctive therapy	Benzodiazepines	Benzodiazepine (e.g., clonazepam, lorazepam)
Antidepressants	Should be tapered and discontinued	Should be tapered and discontinued
Differences in management of mixed state	Valproate preferred to lithium	Valproate in irritable dysphoric states only
Breakthrough episode while on therapy		
Manic or mixed episode	Optimize medication dose Introduce or resume atypical antipsychotic	Optimize medication dose Initiate antipsychotic or divalproex
Severely ill or agitated	Short-term adjunctive therapy with antipsychotic or benzodiazepine	Not addressed
Inadequate symptom control with first-line treatment	Add another first-line medication Alternatives: carbamazepine or oxcarbazepine; atypical antipsychotic; switch from one atypical antipsychotic to another (e.g., clozapine) Consider ECT	Consider lithium or divalproex plus antipsychotic Consider ECT

APA, American Psychiatric Association; BAP, British Association for Psychopharmacology; ECT, electroconvulsive therapy.

[a] Based on American Psychiatric Association and Goodwin (14,15)

[b] Atypical antipsychotics are preferred over conventional antipsychotics because of their more benign side effect profile.

[c] Olanzapine or risperidone; alternatives with less supporting evidence for manic or mixed states include ziprasidone and quetiapine.

Adapted from American Psychiatric Association. Practice guideline for the treatment of patients with Bipolar Disorder [Revision]. *Am J Psychiatry.* 2002;159(Suppl 4):1–50; Goodwin GM. Consensus Group of the British Association for Psychopharmacology. Evidence-based guideline for treatment Bipolar Disorder: Recommendations from the British Association for Psychopharmacology. *J Psychopharmacol.* 2003;17:149–173.

TABLE 7.11

Long-term treatment for bipolar I disorder: evidence-based recommendations [a,b]

Level of intervention	APA	BAP

Initial monotherapy	Lithium or divalproex
	Alternatives: lamotrigine,
	  carbamazepine,
	  oxcarbazepine
	ECT if it elicited response in
	  acute episode
		Lithium (preferred)
		Alternatives: divalproex,
		  olanzapine,
		  carbamazepine,
		  oxcarbazepine, lamotrigine
		ECT if it elicited response in
		  acute episode and patient
		  does poorly on oral agents

Failure to respond to
  monotherapy
	Consider combination
	  therapy; add atypical
	  antipsychotic or
	  antidepressant
		If mania predominates,
		  lithium or divalproex plus
		  atypical antipsychotic
		If depression predominates,
		  lamotrigine, or
		  antidepressant plus lithium
		  or divalproex
		Consider clozapine

Role of atypical
  antipsychotic
	Reassess need for ongoing
	  antipsychotic if used for
	  acute episode
		Helps prevent manic relapse

Adjunctive therapy	Psychosocial intervention	Psychosocial intervention

APA, American Psychiatric Association; BAP, British Association for Psychopharmacology; ECT, electroconvulsive therapy.
[a] Based on American Psychiatric Association.
[b] Both the APA and the BAP recommend maintenance medication following a single manic episode.
Practice guideline for the treatment of patients with Bipolar Disorder [Revision]. *Am J Psychiatry.* 2002;159(Suppl 4):1–50; Goodwin GM. Consensus Group of the British Association for Psychopharmacology. Evidence-based guideline for treatment Bipolar Disorder: Recommendations from the British Association for Psychopharmacology. *J Psychopharmacol.* 2003;17:149–173.

Carbamazepine

Interest in the use of the carbamazepine molecule has been long standing and second only to lithium. Although several studies were conducted in the 1980s regarding the usefulness of carbamazepine (16,17), a resurgence of its popularity has emerged with the use of carbamazepine extended-release monotherapy under the trade name of Equetro. In a study by Weisler et al. (18), carbamazepine showed a 41.5% response rate with manic and mixed mania patients as compared to 22.4% for placebo. Response was defined as ≥50% decrease in the YMRS. Whether in the traditional or extended-release forms, the usage of carbamazepine has been complicated by the fact that the molecule induces metabolism of many other agents based on P450 mechanisms. Liver toxicity, agranulocytosis, and Stevens-Johnson syndrome are infrequent, but known serious complications of the use of carbamazepine.

Oxcarbazepine, the keto- analog of carbamazepine (sometimes dubbed son of Tegretol) under the brand name Trileptal has shown possible efficacy, but has not been proved in randomized controlled trials (RCTs). Its demonstrated effectiveness, therefore, remains questionable. It does have a side effect advantage over carbamazepine in that it does not appear to carry the risk of liver toxicity, induction of the cytochrome P450 system, or leukopenia. It does, however, have a slightly increased incidence of hyponatremia.

Divalproex

Sodium valproate in the divalproex formulation has been commonly used over the past 12 years in the acute treatment of mania or mixed mania. In the initial studies leading to its approval, Bowden et al. showed improvement in manic symptoms as compared to placebo as early as day 5 as measured by the SADS-C(Schedule of Affective Disorders and Schizophrenia-Change Version) (11). Although initially thought to be more effective in patients with rapid cycling (19), more recent data (20) suggests that divalproex may be no more effective than lithium in persons with rapid cycling. Other populations in which divalproex is thought to have an advantage over lithium include the presence of depressive features during mania (21) and bipolar disorder complicated by comorbid alcohol dependence (22–24). A further advantage of this compound is that it can be given as a loading dose (20 to 30 milligrams per kilogram of body weight). This is particularly useful for severely ill hospitalized manic patients. Common side effects include nausea, diarrhea, weight gain, sedation, hair loss and thrombocytopenia. Pancreatitis is a rare but serious side effect.

Antipsychotics

Although first-generation antipsychotics have long been used for rapid treatment of psychosis and agitation in severe mania, these medications have been largely supplanted by the second-generation antipsychotics that have distinct safety advantages and some therapeutic advantages beyond antipsychotic activity. Because of the blockade of the postsynaptic 5HT2A receptor and agonism at the 5HT1A receptor, these agents have active enhancement of serotonin levels leading to positive mood effects and beneficial effects on the negative symptoms of psychosis (12,25). All five of the newest second-generation antipsychotics, aripiprazole, olanzapine, quetiapine, risperidone, and ziprasidone have shown statistically significant efficacy as compared to placebo when used as monotherapy to treat acute mania (26). In addition, both olanzapine and aripiprazole have indications for maintenance treatment for bipolar disorder. In studies conducted with hospitalized bipolar I patients with manic episodes, all of these atypical antipsychotics decreased the components of the manic syndrome in roughly the same percentage when compared to placebo.

Olanzapine

Olanzapine was the first atypical antipsychotic to receive FDA approval for mania. In doses of 15 mg per day, there was a statistical advantage over placebo in the treatment of mania with increasing rapidity of response with higher increasing dosages (27,28).

Quetiapine

In addition to its effect on bipolar depression as noted later in this chapter, quetiapine has been shown to be effective in the treatment of acute mania both as monotherapy and as combination therapy with mood stabilizers. It has been shown to have equivalent efficacy to lithium after 4 weeks of treatment as monotherapy in doses starting at 300 mg per day moving up to 600 mg per day (29). It has also been useful as an add-on therapy to mood stabilizers (30,31).

Risperidone

Used as both monotherapy and combination therapy with lithium or valproate in the treatment of acute and mixed episodes of mania, risperidone has shown significant benefits as compared to placebo as early as day 3 of treatment. In doses averaging 4 mg per day, cumulative improvement was shown with further therapy (32). Risperidone plus mood stabilizer was roughly equivalent to haloperidol plus mood stabilizer (33). Risperidone monotherapy has also been FDA approved for mania treatment (32,34).

Ziprasidone

Particularly when aggressively titrated, ziprasidone has shown rapid onset of action in acute mania when compared to placebo (35). Beginning at 80 mg on day 1 and 160 mg on day 2, 50% of the patients taking ziprasidone responded, as defined by a $\geq$50% decrease in YMRS) (36,37). Ziprasidone monotherapy shows virtually no change in weight or cholesterol level (38). When combined with lithium, ziprasidone offsets some of the weight gain usually associated with lithium (39).

Aripiprazole

The latest atypical antipsychotic to receive FDA approval for the treatment of acute mania and mixed affective episodes is aripiprazole. Separating from placebo on day 4, aripiprazole patients in the study by Keck et al. showed a ≥50% reduction in YMRS as compared to placebo (40% versus 19%) (40). Because the patients in this study were acutely manic hospitalized patients, the initial target dose was 30 mg per day. Outpatients with less severe symptomatology may be begun on lower doses from 2.5 to 10 mg per day. A follow-up study carried out to 26 weeks with a bipolar I population by Keck, Calabrese et al. showed that aripiprazole 15 to 30 mg was superior to placebo in maintaining efficacy in patients who had been stabilized and maintained on aripiprazole during the initial 6-week study as shown by a longer time to relapse (41). The latter study was part of the data that led to the FDA approval for this agent in maintenance treatment for bipolar patients. A larger study involving 347 patients by Sanchez et al. compared aripiprazole monotherapy with haloperidol in a randomized double-blind 12-week study of patients with acute manic or mixed episode (42). Significantly, more aripiprazole patients responded to treatment and also had a lower incidence of side effects as compared to haloperidol.

In summary, all five of the atypical antipsychotics have shown efficacy in treating mania and mixed mania in monotherapy. Meta-analysis of the randomized placebo-controlled trials (43) and attempts to compare various one-drug studies within the group (44–46) suggest that the overall efficacy of these agents is roughly equivalent. From the standpoint of therapeutic effectiveness, therefore, any of the agents could be chosen with clinical confidence. Because these agents have different side effect profiles (see below), this parameter may be used to intelligently select first-line monotherapy for mania and mixed mania.

Side effect considerations with atypical antipsychotics

The side effect profiles of the various anticonvulsants have already been discussed previously. This section therefore focuses on the side effect considerations in choosing the atypical antipsychotic. The previous section documents their effectiveness in the elevated mood pole of bipolar disorder. A subsequent portion of the chapter will also document their potential effectiveness on the depressed phase of bipolar disorder. This class of medicines, therefore, is becoming a valuable component in the arsenal to manage both elevated and depressed mood states. Although these agents have roughly comparable effectiveness, they have significantly different neuroreceptor profiles and significantly different propensity to induce side effects. As a group, they also have a significantly lessened incidence of some side effects traditionally associated with first-generation antipsychotics, namely extrapyramidal symptoms (EPS), tardive dyskinesia (TD), and neuroleptic malignant syndrome (NMS). The relatively small differences between these agents in this constellation of symptoms will not be discussed here.

The agents will be analyzed in reference to six major classifications of side effects specifically:

- Metabolic effects including weight gain, dyslipidemia and glucose abnormalities
- Sedation, EPS, seizures, NMS, and neurological complications
- Cardiovascular complications
- Hyperprolactinemia
- Reproductive health and safety, pregnancy, and lactation
- Precipitation of switches in mood state

Metabolic considerations

A major focus of clinical research and discussion over the past 10 years has been the propensity for atypical antipsychotics to alter patient weight, lipid profile, and serum blood sugar. These concerns have been of major importance to clinicians in selection of agents for treatment of psychoses and bipolar disorder. Research in this area has been complicated by the fact that obesity and overweight are epidemic in the American population in recent years. It is well known that obesity itself increases the incidence of diabetes mellitus, coronary artery disease, hypertension and dyslipidemia. Particularly confounding is the fact that obesity is present in up to 35% of patients with bipolar disorder (47). Although obesity likely has multiple etiologic factors, sedentary lifestyle, comorbid binge eating as well as medication-induced weight gain contribute to the problem. Bipolar patients with obesity also have a higher proportion of centrally distributed adiposity that is known to be a major risk factor for coronary artery disease (47). Multiple reviews have investigated the connection between the use of atypical antipsychotics and weight gain and attempted comparison of the various agents (48–52). Summary statements about weight gain with use of atypical antipsychotics are as follows:

- Weight gain as measured by increased body mass index is a strong predictor of noncompliance. Obese patients are twice as likely to have lessened adherence to medication treatment.
- Although weight gain is a possible side effect for any atypical antipsychotic medication, there is a clear differentiation between the various agents as shown in Table 7.12.

Clozapine and its chemical congener olanzapine have consistently shown the highest amount of weight gain. Quetiapine and risperidone have less incidence of this side effect, although it is moderately significant for some patients. Aripiprazole and ziprasidone have consistently shown the lowest incidence of weight gain in this category.

Although elevations of serum lipids, specifically triglycerides and low density lipoproteins, are also associated with atypical antipsychotics, it is unclear how much of these elevations are a direct effect of the medication or

TABLE 7.12

Atypical antipsychotics and metabolic abnormalities adapted from the American Diabetic Association

Drug	Weight gain	Risk for diabetes	Worsening lipid profile
Clozapine	+++	+	+
Olanzapine	+++	+	+
Risperidone	++	D	D
Quetiapine	++	D	D
Ziprasidone	+/−	−	−
Aripiprazole	+/−	−	−

D, discrepant results. Symbols: + indicates increased effect, − indicates no effect.

are precipitated by increased weight and/or increased incidence of diabetes. In general, the pattern of risk for dyslipidemia follows the pattern for weight gain. Clozapine and olanzapine are most noted for this problem, and ziprasidone and aripiprazole have the least incidence. Risperidone and quetiapine have somewhat discrepant results, although some authors have suggested that their incidence is intermediate between the highest and lowest incidence. In general, the studies on dyslipidemia in psychiatric patients have been undertaken on those with schizophrenia rather than on those with bipolar disorder. Most experts assume, though, that the risk ladder translates to bipolar patients.

Alterations in glucose metabolism have multiple etiologies, one of which is excess weight. Case reports, peer reviews, and epidemiologic studies have suggested that atypical antipsychotics have effect on glucose metabolism, although there are relatively few rigorous studies. These are summarized in several recent reports that suggest that the pattern of potential risk for diabetes follows the ladder for weight gain and dyslipidemia mentioned in the preceding text (53,54). Given this information, the FDA requested that a warning for possible increase in hyperglycemia and diabetes mellitus be added to all atypical antipsychotics as a class effect. Although this class effect warning does apply to aripiprazole and ziprasidone, virtually every comparative study has shown that these two agents have minimal propensity to elevate glucose levels or induce diabetes mellitus.

Seizures

The only increased risk of seizures with the atypical antipsychotic group involves dose-dependent increase in seizure risk with larger dosages of clozapine and olanzapine (55–57).

QTc prolongation

Although initially raised as a potential issue with the use of ziprasidone, most experts agree that any such elevation with ziprasidone or other atypical antipsychotics is relatively minimal and not likely to be significant in clinical practice (58). None of the agents prolong the QTc interval by >16 ms, and coadministration of metabolic inhibitors with each of the agents did not lengthen the prolongation.

Hyperprolactinemia

Elevation of the hormone prolactin has been associated with a variety of symptoms including irregular menses, breast tenderness, infertility, and galactorrhea. Estrogen deficiency symptoms such as hot flashes in women and decreased libido, erectile dysfunction, gynecomastia, and galactorrhea in men have also been associated with prolactin elevation (45,59,60). Only one of the atypical antipsychotics, risperidone, has been associated with significant prolactin elevations in patients. A variety of studies have shown that risperidone increases prolactin at doses of 6 mg per day or greater, but hyperprolactinemia has also been shown in lower doses in some patients (61,62).

Pregnancy and lactation

As yet there are minimal databases on which to make significant recommendations regarding the safety of atypical antipsychotics in pregnancy. They are all currently labeled as pregnancy category C. Although evidence for risperidone, quetiapine, ziprasidone, and aripiprazole is too small for recommendations to be made, the olanzapine database is somewhat larger. It suggests that this agent is not associated with a rate of major congenital abnormality above baseline (63,64).

In lactation, as with virtually all psychotropics, it can be assumed that atypical antipsychotics do appear in some small amounts in breast milk. Although no specific reports of fetal toxicity have been demonstrated, atypical antipsychotics have not been cleared of the possibility that they may be associated with the possibility of toxicity (65).

Affective switches and cycle acceleration

In contrast to traditional antidepressants that are discussed later in the chapter and have been potentially associated with cycle induction and mood switches, atypical antipsychotics reveal limited, but relatively reassuring data. Randomized double-blind, placebo-controlled trials of olanzapine and quetiapine in bipolar depression did not show evidence of switches into mania. Maintenance studies conducted with aripiprazole, olanzapine, risperidone, and ziprasidone have not demonstrated aggravation of mania or depression and/or cycle acceleration (66–68). The lack of affective switches and cycle acceleration make this class of agents prime candidates for treatment of elevated and depressed mood in bipolar patients where affective switches and cycle acceleration are of prominent concern.

Combination treatments for elevated mood

As can be discerned from the practice guidelines, monotherapy, although desirable, is not always effective in the treatment of elevated mood. The more serious the severity of elevated mood, the more likely that combination treatment will be necessary to achieve adequate therapeutic success (69). Severe bipolar mania or mania with rapid cycling disease often requires that combination therapy be instituted simultaneously. With milder elevated mood, monotherapy is initially instituted and augmentation with a second agent is only considered when therapeutic results are insufficient. Mildly to moderately hypomanic patients may be more resistant to taking multiple medications than monotherapy.

For the treatment of elevated mood, most intelligent combinations involve the use of medications with different mechanisms of action. Typically this involves two mood stabilizers which act differently (e.g., lithium, divalproex and/or carbamazepine.) A similarly intelligent combination involves an atypical antipsychotic with one of the mentioned mood stabilizers earlier. This latter practice is becoming increasingly common and well tolerated. As many as 90% of patients with acute mania receive a mood stabilizer–antipsychotic combination (70,71). Although no single atypical antipsychotic has demonstrated significantly increased effectiveness when combined with a mood stabilizer, there are at least six double-blind placebo-controlled trials that have consistently found positive outcomes in subjects with acute bipolar mania who have adjunctive atypical antipsychotics added to their mood stabilizer regimen when compared to mood stabilizer monotherapy (72). This particular combination of medication for acute mania has shown that the dosage of the atypical antipsychotic used for augmentation therapy can often be lower than that necessary when it is used as monotherapy. The side effects of the antipsychotic, therefore, may be decreased at lower doses and the ultimate side effect burden is equal to or less than high doses of atypical antipsychotic monotherapy. Because of their potential effectiveness in both elevated mood and depressed mood, mood stabilizer/atypical antipsychotic combinations may be particularly effective maintenance treatments. Risperidone, olanzapine, quetiapine and ziprasidone all have randomized placebo-controlled studies of their effectiveness as augmentation treatment. Although aripiprazole has no specific augmentation studies, its usefulness in acute mania and maintenance treatment as monotherapy makes it a likely candidate for positive augmentation therapy as well.

Benzodiazepines

Benzodiazepines have had a checkered history in the treatment of elevated mood and bipolar disorder. Despite this history of somewhat contradictory evidence, benzodiazepines are still commonly used by many practitioners in the treatment of elevated mood. As recently as 2004 a population of New Hampshire Medicaid beneficiaries with bipolar disorder and substance use disorder showed a 75% usage of benzodiazepines over a 5-year period. This figure was higher than that in patients who had bipolar disorder without a substance use disorder (58%) (73). In developing intelligent guidelines for the use of benzodiazepines in elevated mood patients it is important to carefully evaluate when in the course of the disorder benzodiazepine use is studied. Multiple studies (74–76) show that high potency benzodiazepines such as clonazepam or lorazepam are useful adjunctive treatments in the early phases of an acute manic episode. In general, these studies have evaluated the use of benzodiazepines in addition to mood stabilizers such as lithium, or valproate, or antipsychotics. Benzodiazepines alone, however, are not overly efficacious in the treatment of acute mania compared to mood stabilizer alone or an intramuscular antipsychotic alone such as olanzapine (77,78). Longer-term maintenance studies of the use of high potency benzodiazepines in the prophylaxis of mood episodes have resulted in negative outcomes. Either as monotherapy or as adjunctive therapy benzodiazepines do not confer prophylactic benefits against the recurrence of either manic or depressive episodes (78,79).

Benzodiazepines, despite their potential disadvantages (see Chapter 8), do have significant usefulness in the treatment of anxiety as well as insomnia. In the acute phase of mania, benzodiazepines can be used for anxiety control and/or insomnia. In less frequent circumstances when there are no contraindications, longer-term use of these agents for these specific indications may also be appropriate.

Beyond lack of efficacy in maintenance treatment of elevated mood itself, clinicians need be acutely aware of the patient's substance abuse history because abuse of benzodiazepines is common in this population (73,80). The abuse of benzodiazepines alone or in combination with abuse of alcohol or other drugs substantially increases the presence of overall mood and anxiety symptoms and low ratings for general quality of life. Interestingly, benzodiazepine use is unrelated to remission of the substance use disorder or frequency of hospitalization when compared to those who were not prescribed benzodiazepines (80).

Medications in psychotic mania

More than half the number of manic episodes in bipolar disorder are accompanied by psychotic features (81). Grandiose delusions are the most common psychotic symptom, followed by formal thought disorder, hallucinations, and catatonia. Specific studies on the treatment of psychotic features of elevated mood with medication are limited to treating acute mania (82). Lithium or divalproex plus an atypical antipsychotic is the preferred regimen. Alternatives to lithium or divalproex are carbamazepine and oxcarbazepine. Typical antipsychotics, most notably haloperidol, have also been shown to be effective in acute psychotic mania (76,83). As has been noted earlier in this section, all five atypical antipsychotics, aripiprazole, olanzapine, quetiapine, risperidone, and ziprasidone have shown significant efficacy and are FDA approved for acute mania. Because they also have been approved for the psychotic symptoms of schizophrenia, one would expect that they would be particularly efficacious on the psychotic symptoms of bipolar disorder although most studies do not identify specific efficacy on psychotic symptoms in the bipolar patients studied. Within the first 3 to 6 weeks of treatment, hospitalized patients with acute mania of moderate or greater severity with psychotic symptoms show greater initial response rates with combination treatment of atypical antipsychotics plus a mood stabilizer than with monotherapeutic strategies (84).

Choosing medication by temperament

Although there is relatively little direct evidence to support specific choice of antimanic medications on the basis of the patient's underlying temperament, clinical experience and extrapolation from limited data would suggest that utilizing the context of the patient's baseline temperament is one factor in choosing medication. A patient who has a hyperthymic temperament who experiences a hypomanic or manic episode might preferentially be treated with medications that have the strongest antimanic evidence such as lithium, valproate, carbamazepine, or any of the atypical antipsychotics. Precipitation of a depressed episode or increasing mood cycling is less of a concern in this population.

In patients with a cyclothymic temperament and dysthymic temperament, the choice of antimanic agents may be similar; however, the clinician needs to be aware of the possibility of future depressed episodes as a response to treatment. In these instances, lowering the dose of the antimanic agent or the possibility of adding an agent which could counteract depressive symptomatology (e.g., lamotrigine) is advised. The use of temperament in choosing antimanic agents is a less significant consideration in treating an elevated mood episode than in treating a depressed episode in a bipolar patient. This will be discussed in more detail later in this chapter.

Treatment of bipolar depression with medication

Many areas of elevated mood are complex and controversial. However, nowhere is this complexity and potential controversy more evident than in the medication treatment of bipolar depression. Until relatively recently, this has been a vastly understudied area of research, perhaps, in part, complicated by issues of diagnosis and the consistent identification of patient cohorts for study (see Chapters 1 and 2). This section seeks to clarify the current state of both the science and the art of treating bipolar depression with medication and examine the potential controversies. Despite our increasing level of evidence-based data, there remains considerable latitude for clinical judgment and variable treatment regimens for individual patients. As with every area of psychopharmacology, the art of practice can at times be as important as the science of practice.

The ideal standard for a bipolar spectrum patient with depression

Although we do not yet have an ideal gold-standard medication for bipolar depression, it is important to identify those characteristics that would characterize such a medication. These are listed in Table 7.13.

As we will see from the evidence in the following sections, there are current medications that meet some, but not all, of these conditions.

Types of evidence

When reviewing the treatments for bipolar depression, several types of evidence present themselves, as noted in Table 7.14.

There is little doubt that the RCTs are the most desirable kinds of evidence on which to base treatment recommendations. There are, however, far fewer RCTs for bipolar depression than for acute bipolar mania. In general, the depression studies also have smaller samples and, therefore, the conclusions reached may have less general applicability.

As discussed earlier in the section on medication for elevated mood, the second type of data is an expert consensus guideline. The Expert Consensus Guidelines for the Treatment of Bipolar Disorder is, for example, purely a survey of 50 leading experts in the field of bipolar disorder. The results of their responses to a questionnaire are then tabulated and summarized so that it essentially is an expert opinion poll without evidence. The other four guidelines cited (from the APA, BAP, Canadian Network for Mood and Anxiety Treatment [CANMAT] and TIMA) are also a result of a summation of expert opinions; however, in these cases, the experts sit down

TABLE 7.13

Characteristics of an ideal medication for depression within the bipolar spectrum

- Useful as monotherapy
- Effective on the depressed phase of the condition
- Does not destabilize the patient, causing excessive cycling or hypomania/mania
- Would prevent or delay further episodes of mania
- Would prevent or delay further episodes of depression
- Would have a benign side effect profile
- Would be easily combined with other medications, when necessary

TABLE 7.14
Types of medication evidence

- Randomized, controlled clinical trials of monotherapy (RCT)
- Randomized, controlled clinical trials of combination therapy (RCT)
- Expert consensus guidelines
  - Expert Consensus Guidelines for the Treatment of Bipolar Disorder (December 2004)
  - Texas Implementation of Medication Algorithms Guidelines (TIMA), (June 2005) British Association for Psychopharmacotherapy Practice Guidelines for Bipolar Disorder,
  - American Psychiatric Association Guidelines April 2002, (Updated 2006)
  - Canadian Network for Mood and Anxiety Treatments Guidelines of Management for Patients with Bipolar Disorder: Consensus and Controversies CANMAT, (2005)

in groups to discuss the evidence and come to a summary report. In some cases, considerable consensus is achieved; in other circumstances, there are significantly dissenting opinions. Although helpful in bridging the gap from the limited class A evidence of RCTs, such guidelines can form an extension of the data by revealing what the experts in the field judge to be most helpful in treating a particular condition.

Several other issues confound both the study design and the evaluation of study results. These are listed in Table 7.15.

No matter when RCTs are designed and completed, the extensive length of time before such studies are published and the results promulgated to practicing clinicians ensures that there is a gap of several years between clinical practice and the best Class A evidence. Even when the evidence is

TABLE 7.15
Confounding factors in bipolar research

- Peer-reviewed articles are significantly delayed for publication
- Placebo-controlled studies have a trade-off between internal validity and external validity
- The definition of a mood stabilizer is not uniformly accepted
- Maintenance or prophylactic studies are expensive and require a long follow-up
- Newer agents always receive more Class A studies than older agents
- Possible bias in publication

Djulbegovic B, Lacevic M, Cantor A, et al. The uncertainty principle and industry-sponsored research. *Lancet.* 2000;356:635–638; Baker CB, Johnsrud MT, Crismon ML, et al. Quantitative analysis of sponsorship bias in economic studies of antidepressants. *Br J Psychiatry.* 2003;183:498–506.

promulgated, it often takes a significant time for some clinicians to incorporate the results of these studies into their prescribing behavior.

Those studies with the highest quality, namely placebo-controlled studies, have somewhat less applicability to general clinical practice. "There is a trade-off between internal validity (success of the study itself) and external validity (of the study results to clinical practice)" (85). Although it may be less of an issue in studies of true hypomania, placebo-controlled studies also require relatively stable, compliant patients. Thus, the most severely ill patients are often excluded from studies, although such patients may make up a sizeable percentage of patients seen in clinical practice.

Maintenance or prophylactic studies are also complicated by several factors, most notably, the long period of follow-up necessary to come to adequate conclusions, the complex study design, and extra expense required. Although of great clinical value, the number of such studies is limited.

Because the definition of what constitutes a "mood stabilizer" has been a matter of considerable debate and disagreement, studies have shied away from using this term. There are virtually no RCTs that truly prove "mood stabilization." A more measurable quantity is the interval between remission and a relapse of symptomatology with longer intervals indicating therapeutic effect of delaying relapse. Therefore, the RCTs till date have been approved for "maintenance treatment" rather than mood stabilization.

Because many of the studies useful in bipolar disorder have been funded by the pharmaceutical industry, they focus on newer agents that the companies wish to test and market. There are, therefore, fewer studies that evaluate monotherapy or combination therapy with older agents or comparative studies between newer agents and older agents.

Lastly, in what has been dubbed the *file drawer effect*, studies showing positive effect are more likely to be published than those with negative effects, particularly if they are industry sponsored. Therefore, the evidence available to the clinician may show a bias toward certain agents (85,86).

Overriding principles of treating depression in bipolar disorder

As noted earlier, there is far less class A data for the treatment of depression in bipolar disorder than there is for acute mania. Therefore, a great need still exists for evidence-based approaches to this common clinical disorder. Most of the recommendations come less from RCTs than from practice guidelines and consensus guidelines. Unfortunately, some consensus guidelines disagree with other guidelines. A further consideration is that most RCTs contain research subjects that are a mixture of patients with bipolar I and bipolar II disorder. Expert opinion tabulated in these guidelines generally recommends similar approaches for treating Bipolar II disorder as those recommended for Bipolar I disorder. These conclusions may or may not apply to each subgroup.

This can result in skewed recommendations based on the severe behavioral sequelae of full mania rather than the lesser behavior sequelae of hypomania. This may be particularly important when viewing recommendations for treatment of depression in patients who have only experienced hypomania versus patients who have experienced full-blown manic episodes. Lastly, the research on the medication treatment of depression in bipolar disorder is a highly active area of interest. RCTs and revisions of clinical guidelines are being made frequently and repeatedly. It is, therefore, incumbent on the clinician to stay educated about the most up-to-date information and not perseverate on recommendations made even 3 to 4 years ago.

The information and evidence for the use of various psychotropic medications in the treatment of bipolar depression will be presented in several ways in this chapter. First, we will review those elements of existing clinical guidelines, specifically as they refer to treating bipolar depression. Secondly, each individual medication will be reviewed with the evidence for its usefulness. Lastly, the author will provide consolidated recommendations in an attempt to provide usable clinical guidelines for the practitioner.

Expert consensus guideline

Published in 2004 (87), the Expert Consensus Guidelines/recommendations for treatment of bipolar depression are summarized in Table 7.16.

TABLE 7.16

Expert consensus guideline: choice of medication for bipolar depression

Clinical presentation	Preferred initial strategies	Alternate strategies
Mild to moderate depression	Lamotrigine alone Lithium alone	AD + lithium Lithium + lamotrigine AD + divalproex
Severe non psychotic depression	AD + lithium Lithium + lamotrigine Lamotrigine [a]	Lithium alone AD + divalproex AD + AAP Divalproex + lamotrigine
Severe psychotic depression	AD + AAP Lithium + AAP Lamotrigine + AAP	Divalproex + AAP
Depression with history of AD-induced mania or rapid cycling	Lamotrigine alone Lithium + lamotrigine	Lithium alone Divalproex + lamotrigine Lamotrigine + AAP

AD, antidepressant; AAP, atypical antipsychotic.
[a] Very high second line (rated first line by more than two thirds of the experts)

Of particular note in this chart is that mild-to-moderate depressions are not treated with an antidepressant other than lamotrigine, except as an alternate strategy. Severe depressions, both psychotic and nonpsychotic, are treated either with a combination of lithium plus lamotrigine, lamotrigine alone, or lithium plus an antidepressant. Preferred treatments for a psychotic depression include lamotrigine plus an atypical antipsychotic, lithium plus an atypical antipsychotic, or an antidepressant plus an atypical antipsychotic. Taking into account the controversies of using an antidepressant (discussed later in the chapter), this expert consensus guideline lists lamotrigine, bupropion, citalopram, escitalopram, and sertraline as first-line antidepressants. Second-line antidepressants include paroxetine, fluoxetine, venlafaxine, and duloxetine. A significant omission from this list is the olanzapine/fluoxetine combination (OFC). Because this is the only FDA-approved product for bipolar depression, one must assume that this medication drops toward the bottom of recommendations advocated by experts because of the side effect profile, specifically weight gain, increased incidence of dyslipidemia, and metabolic syndrome caused by the olanzapine component of this combination.

This guideline does not recommend the use of an atypical antipsychotic alone as treatment for bipolar depression. Olanzapine, quetiapine, risperidone, and aripiprazole are all potential recommendations for treatment of a bipolar depression in combination with an antidepressant.

The expert consensus guideline further specifies maintenance strategies as noted in Table 7.17.

In summary, these maintenance strategies are dependent on the treatment used in the acute phase. The preferred continuation treatment—a mood stabilizer plus an additional agent (an atypical antipsychotic, lamotrigine,

TABLE 7.17

Expert consensus guideline: maintenance strategies after a depressive episode

Acute-phase treatment	Preferred continuation treatment	Alternate strategy
AAP + MS	Taper and discontinue AAP, continue MS Add psychotherapy	Continue regimen at same dose Continue regimen at reduced dose
MS + lamotrigine	Continue regimen at same dose	Add psychotherapy
AAP + lamotrigine	Continue regimen at same dose	Add psychotherapy Taper and discontinue AAP, continue lamotrigine Cont. regimen at reduced dose

AAP, atypical antipsychotic; MS, mood stabilizer.

or an antidepressant)—all specify that the additional agent be gradually tapered and discontinued. The maintenance treatment then consists of the mood stabilizer alone, with or without additional psychotherapy. When the acute-phase treatment involves an atypical antipsychotic or lamotrigine with an additional antidepressant, the antidepressant is tapered and discontinued, and the atypical antipsychotic or lamotrigine as monotherapy is the primary maintenance therapy with the possible addition of psychotherapy.

TIMA guidelines

The TIMA guidelines categorize data into three segments, with type A data being the most powerful and type C being the least influential:

- Type A data—randomized, blinded, placebo-controlled trials
- Type B data—open, controlled trials, large case series and/or large retrospective analyses
- Type C data—preliminary unconfirmed findings from small case reports, case series, and expert consensus

The stage 1 or most preferred treatment recommendations for an acute depression are shown in Table 7.18.

The recommendations are divided by whether the patient is currently on an antimanic agent or has a recent history of severe mania. In this case, lamotrigine is added to the antimanic agent. If the patient has no antimanic agent currently, or has no history of severe and/or recent mania, lamotrigine monotherapy is the preferred treatment.

Stage 2 therapy for those patients who do not respond to, or are intolerant of, stage 1 treatments are placed on either quetiapine or the OFC.

Third stage treatment is recommended if both stages 1 and 2 treatments are ineffective or are not tolerated. In this circumstance, a combination of agents including lithium, lamotrigine, quetiapine, or the OFC are used in combination at the clinician's discretion.

Stage 4 treatment utilizes the four medications mentioned in stage 3 and adds that the combination therapy might also include valproic acid or carbamazepine and an antidepressant (an selective serotonin reuptake inhibitor [SSRI], bupropion, or venlafaxine). ECT is also a strong consideration for patients who have not responded to a variety of medication combinations. Reflecting the controversy of whether or not to use an antidepressant for bipolar depression, there was a minority opinion that stage 4 treatment, particularly as it refers to the use of a primary antidepressant, should precede stages 2 and 3.

The fifth and final stage of their recommendations is to use monoamine oxidase inhibitors (MAOIs), tricyclic antidepressants (TCAs), pramipexole, other atypical antipsychotics not previously mentioned. Oxcarbazepine, inositol, stimulants, and thyroid preparations could be added in a combination therapy. The consensus group notes that the treatments in stage 5 are largely recommended despite limited empirical data. They are supported more by

TABLE 7.18

Treatment algorithm for acute depression in bipolar I disorder

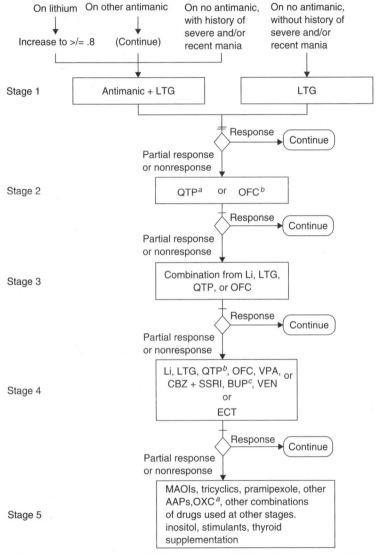

AAP, atypical antipsychotic; BUP, bupropion; CBZ, carbamazepine; ECT, electroconvulsive therapy; Li, lithium; LTG, lamotrigine; MAOI, monoamine oxidase inhibitor; OFC, olanzapine-fluoxetine combination; OXC, oxcarbazepine; QTP, quetiapine; SSRI, selective serotonin reuptake inhibitor; VEN, venlafaxine; VPA, valproate.
c SSRIs include citalopram, escitalopram, fluoxetine, paroxetine, sertraline, and fluvoxamine.
Adapted from Suppes T, et al. The Texas medication algorithm project. *J Clin Psychiatry.* 2005;66:870–886, (9)

TABLE 7.19

Maintenance treatment of depression in bipolar disorder if the most recent episode is depressed

Level I	Patients with recent and/or severe history of mania All other patients	Lamotrigine combined with an antimanic agent Lamotrigine monotherapy
Level II	Lithium	
Level III	Combination of an antimanic and antidepressant that has been effective in the past, including olanzapine–fluoxetine combination [a]	
Level IV	Valproate, carbamazepine, aripiprazole [b], clozapine, olanzapine [a], quetiapine [b], risperidone [b], ziprasidone [b]	
Level V	Typical antipsychotics [a], oxcarbazepine [b], ECT	

- Well-tolerated, effective, acute-phase treatments are reasonable and acceptable options for maintenance treatment
- Antidepressant monotherapy is not recommended

[a] Safety issues warrant careful consideration of this option for potential long-term use.
[b] Relatively limited information is currently available on this agent in long-term use.
Adapted from Suppes T, et al. The Texas medication algorithm project. *J Clin Psychiatry.* 2005;66:870–886.

expert opinion and clinical consensus rather than by randomized, controlled trials. The maintenance recommendations for patients who have experienced an acute depressive episode are listed in Table 7.19.

Preferred maintenance treatment is lamotrigine monotherapy or lamotrigine combined with an antimanic agent; level 2 is lithium; level 3 is combination of an antimanic and an antidepressant agent that has been previously effective (including the OFC); level 4 recommendations involve valproate, carbamazepine, aripiprazole, clozapine, olanzapine, quetiapine, risperidone, and ziprasidone. Finally, level 5 treatments include typical antipsychotics, oxcarbazepine, and ECT.

American Psychiatric Association and British Association for Psychopharmacotherapy guidelines for depressive episodes

The 2002 American Psychiatric Association Guidelines and the 2003 British Association for Psychopharmacology Guidelines in the treatment of acute depressive episodes with bipolar disorder are summarized in Table 7.20.

Although the APA guidelines use lithium or lamotrigine as monotherapy and only add an antidepressant as an add-on to lithium or divalproex, the British guidelines use an SSRI plus lithium, divalproex, or an antipsychotic as first-line treatment. In both cases, as with other guidelines, antidepressant monotherapy is not recommended. ECT is strongly considered for more severely ill or treatment-resistant patients.

TABLE 7.20

Evidence-based treatment guidelines for acute depressive episodes [a]

Level of intervention	APA	BAP
First-line treatment	Therapy: lithium or lamotrigine Antidepressant monotherapy not recommended; consider SSRIs as add-on to lithium or divalproex	Combination therapy: SSRI plus lithium, divalproex, or an antipsychotic for patients with history of mania; antidepressant monotherapy not recommended
More severely ill	Lithium plus antidepressant Consider ECT	Consider ECT
Less severe illness	Not addressed.	Consider lamotrigine, lithium or divalproex initially, despite limited evidence
With psychotic features	Atypical antipsychotic usually required Alternative: ECT	Consider adding atypical antipsychotic
Breakthrough depressive episode during maintenance	Optimize dose of maintenance medication Add lamotrigine, bupropion, or paroxetine Alternative: add different SSRI, venlafaxine, or MAOI	Optimize dose of maintenance medication Address current stressors, if any Ensure current medication (e.g., lithium, divalproex, atypical antipsychotic) protects from manic relapse Initiate antidepressant (or consider augmentation/change if currently receiving) Consider SSRI or lamotrigine if prior antidepressant provoked mood instability [b]
Severe	Consider ECT	Add antidepressant to lithium, divalproex, or atypical antipsychotic
Treatment-resistant	Consider ECT	Not addressed

APA, American Psychiatric Association; BAP, British Association for Psychopharmacology; ECT, electroconvulsive therapy; MAOI, monoamine oxidase inhibitor; SSRI, selective serotonin reuptake inhibitor.

[a] Based on American Psychiatric Association and Goodwin.

[b] Antidepressants are less likely to induce mania when added to lithium, divalproex, or an antipsychotic.

Adapted from American Psychiatric Association. Practice guideline for the treatment of patients with Bipolar Disorder [Revision]. *Am J Psychiatry.* 2002;159(Suppl 4):1–50; Goodwin GM. Consensus Group of the British Association for Psychopharmacology. Evidence-based guideline for treatment Bipolar Disorder: Recommendations from the British Association for Psychopharmacology. *J Psychopharmacol.* 2003;17:149–173.

Canadian Network for Mood and Anxiety Treatment (CANMAT) guidelines for the management of patients with bipolar disorder

This guideline emanating from the bipolar subcommittee of CANMAT studied over 500 peer-reviewed articles, proceedings, and articles in press to make their recommendations. They made an assessment of the quality of evidence using the Periodic Health Examination classification rating. These were as follows:

• Type A evidence had good support for the intervention considered in clinical practice.
• Type B had fair support for the intervention to be considered in clinical practice.
• Type C had poor support for the intervention to be considered in clinical practice.
• Type D showed that there was fair support for the intervention to be *excluded* in clinical practice.
• Type E data showed good support for the intervention to be *excluded* in clinical practice.

These guidelines were published in 2005 (88). Of note, is that this guideline is the only one to adequately distinguish treating bipolar II depression from bipolar I depression, suggesting that the former is "associated with significant rates of rapid cycling and suicide and a comparable degree of psychosocial impairment as seen with bipolar I disorder." The guidelines for bipolar II depression are somewhat less than specific, as the authors feel there is limited evidence for those treatments. Nevertheless, their somewhat qualified recommendations for bipolar II depression include lithium, lamotrigine, lithium or valproic acid with an antidepressant, and an atypical antipsychotic with an antidepressant. They also suggest the adjunctive use of the dopamine agonist pramipexole and adjunctive gabapentin and topiramate, on the basis of relatively small studies. Maintenance treatment for bipolar II depression lists first-line choices as lithium or lamotrigine, second-line options as an antimanic agent with an antidepressant or combination treatment including two agents from a list that includes lithium, lamotrigine, valproic acid, and an atypical antipsychotic.

The CANMAT recommendations for acute bipolar I depression endorse a mood stabilizer/antidepressant combination as first line despite the risk of switching into mania. Other first-line choices include lithium, lamotrigine, lithium/lamotrigine combination, and olanzapine plus an SSRI. Their recommendations for maintenance treatment of a patient with bipolar depression heavily emphasize psychoeducation and psychotherapy including the various schools of treatment mentioned in Chapter 6 of this text. The authors suggest that lithium is more powerful at preventing mania than depression and that lamotrigine is more effective at preventing depression than mania.

Olanzapine was found to be effective against further outbreaks of both depression and mania. In a somewhat complicated set of recommendations, a variety of combinations are recommended. Antidepressant monotherapy was specifically contraindicated.

Consolidating the guidelines

Although the guidelines are not totally consistent, particularly in the order the treatments mentioned earlier are recommended, there are some generalizations that can be made that are helpful to the clinician in the treatment of depression in patients with elevated mood.

- *Lamotrigine.* At least four studies (89–92) have shown lamotrigine to be robust in its ability to provide maintenance treatment for bipolar disorder, primarily based on delaying time to depression. It has been FDA approved for the maintenance of bipolar I disorder since 2003 and has been in wide usage for bipolar depressed individuals both as monotherapy and as combination therapy with a variety of mood stabilizers and atypical antipsychotics. Lamotrigine is considered primarily for use in treatment of patients with depression who have a history of current or past elevated mood. Lamotrigine has an additional advantage in being metabolized by glucuronic acid conjugation with excretion through the kidney. Therefore, it is one of the useful treatments for bipolar depression that does not involve liver metabolism. It also has a relatively positive profile in pregnant patients. Typical therapeutic doses are between 50 and 250 mg per day with the higher dosage based on maintenance studies.
- *Quetiapine.* Quetiapine has been used for several years in the treatment of acute mania; however, a recent large scale study has shown the effectiveness of quetiapine for bipolar depression in 300 and 600 mg doses (93). Quetiapine has also been shown to be an effective add-on in combination medication treatment of bipolar disorder (94). As a relatively sedative medicine, it can also be useful to treat the sleep problems of bipolar disorder.
- *Olanzapine/fluoxetine combination (OFC).* OFC was the first FDA-approved treatment for depressive episodes in bipolar disorder. The response rate of 56.1% in the 833 patients who were randomly assigned to three treatment groups (olanzapine alone, OFC and placebo) was significantly higher than the rate for olanzapine alone and for placebo (95). Although quality of life in patients with bipolar disorder was also improved with OFC (96), its use has been hampered by the side effect profile of the olanzapine element of the combination. Weight gain, dyslipidemia, and tendency to induce the metabolic syndrome have been significant considerations. The combination drug appears to have similar rates of

these significant side effects to olanzapine alone. As a combination drug, OFC has advantages of increased compliance (in which one pill is taken rather than two) and disadvantages (inflexible dosage combinations). Typical therapeutic doses of OFC are 6 to 12 mg of olanzapine and 25 to 50 mg of fluoxetine.

- **Lithium.** Lithium has a long and distinguished track record in the treatment of bipolar disorder and has been FDA-approved for long-term treatment. Lithium has been considerably effective in both acute treatment of mania and maintenance treatment to prevent manic or hypomanic relapses. Its effect on acute depression treatment or as maintenance treatment to prevent depressive relapses, however, has been minimal. It does have usefulness in the treatment of bipolar depression in combination with other treatments, specifically lamotrigine, quetiapine, and atypical antipsychotics. It is the only mood stabilizer with the apparent ability to minimize suicide attempts in bipolar patients. It has been shown to have less suicide attempts than carbamazepine-treated or divalproex-treated hospitalized patients (97). In randomized studies, lithium was minimally better than placebo and inferior to TCAs in treating depression. Many of these studies, however, were conducted >25 years ago and included mixed samples of bipolar and unipolar depressed patients, which hamper the interpretation of data for elevated mood patients. There is some evidence that blood levels of >0.8 meq per L of lithium may be more effective than lower levels. Typical effective doses yield a blood level of between 0.6 and 1.2 meq per L, although several studies have suggested that 0.7 to 0.8 meq per L is generally satisfactory.

- **Sodium valproate.** The divalproex formulation of valproic acid was evaluated in two placebo-controlled trials of patients with acute bipolar depression (98,99) with mixed results. Divalproex monotherapy for bipolar depression is not recommended, although it may be useful as part of a combination treatment. In the study by Davis et al. (99), the sample size was small (25 outpatients), but this pilot study did show that divalproex was effective in reducing the symptoms of depression and anxiety in the depressed phase of patients with bipolar I disorder. Another small study on divalproex monotherapy in bipolar II patients with depression (98) showed 63% of 19 patients to have had antidepressant response from valproate monotherapy. The third study (99) did show improvements in (Hamilton Rating Scale for Depression) HAM-D scores of 43% as compared to placebo's 27%, although the difference was not statistically different.

- **Other agents.** There are several other pharmacologic agents that have relatively small studies suggesting possible efficacy with bipolar depression.
  - There have been two studies of the use of pramipexole as an augmentation agent in the treatment of bipolar depression (100,101). Pramipexole, a dopamine agonist, has only been evaluated as an add-on agent and not in monotherapy but has shown improvement in depressive symptoms in the studied groups.

○ Zonisamide, an anticonvulsant that is structurally similar to serotonin, has been shown to facilitate dopaminergic and serotonergic transmission. It has been evaluated in an open-label study of bipolar depression (102) and a retrospective chart review (103). If these initial studies are further validated, zonisamide may have usefulness in the treatment of bipolar disorder because it may also have mood stabilizing properties at higher doses and has the beneficial side effect of weight loss similar to topiramate.

Use of antidepressants in bipolar depression—the great debate

Perhaps nowhere in the field of mood disorders is there greater complexity and controversy than the issue of whether antidepressants are appropriate treatment for episodes of bipolar depression. Although there have been multiple studies over the past 25 years, there are remarkably few randomized, placebo-controlled (A level) trials. As with other situations where the evidence is limited, clinicians frequently fall back on expert consensus guidelines and the recommendations of thought leaders. Unfortunately, in this area too, there are contradictory recommendations. It remains controversial where, if at all, antidepressants should be used in the pyramid of treatments. Multiple studies can be cited to support a reluctance to use antidepressants whereas other studies can be used to justify their early usage (104–124).

Why is there controversy?

There are a variety of reasons why there is such divergence of opinion. These include the following:

• Acute-phase studies of depression (typically 8 to 12 weeks in duration) do not measure the same effects as maintenance studies of 6 to 12 months in duration.
• Different studies have looked at the effects of different classes of antidepressants (TCAs, MAOIs, SSRIs, serotonin-norepinephrine reuptake inhibitors [SNRIs] and dopamine/norepinephrine reuptake inhibitors such as bupropion).
• Efficacy studies from the use of antidepressants in unipolar depression have been widely promulgated both by academicians and by the pharmaceutical industry to clinicians, although it is not clear that efficacy in unipolar depression has significant validity for depression in bipolar illness.
• The vast majority of studies that have looked at bipolar depression have not segregated patients with bipolar I disorder from those with bipolar II disorder. The authors conclude that their results apply to both groups, although this may not in fact be true.
• All of the reasons listed in Chapter 1 as to why hypomania is overlooked or misdiagnosed by clinicians are true for research populations. Many so-called

"unipolar" depressed patients may, in fact, be bipolar in disguise with subsyndromal hypomanic elements. Unipolar depressed sample population may, in fact, not be pure from a research standpoint.

- Even if, from a phenotypic standpoint, one makes the assumption that patients with bipolar I and bipolar II disorders belong to distinct categories, it is unclear whether these two patient groups would have differing responses to antidepressants. Given the recent emphasis on bipolar spectrum disorders, as discussed in Chapter 1, the situation is clouded further.

Considerations when using antidepressants are fivefold. They include the following:

- Antidepressant efficacy in acute-phase depressions in patients with bipolar disorder
- Prophylactic efficacy of antidepressants in preventing recurring depressions
- The possibility that antidepressants increase the switch rate into hypomania or mania
- The possibility that antidepressant precipitates mixed affective episodes with the negative connotations of these mixed episodes (see Chapter 8)
- The possibility and frequency with which antidepressants increase cycle frequency and/or rapid cycling

Are antidepressants effective in the acute phase of depression in patients with bipolar disorder? Several studies have shown that antidepressants were as effective in this group as mood stabilizers. No studies, however, have found them to be more effective than mood stabilizers in acute bipolar depression (105). Two randomized, double-blind, placebo-controlled studies looked at the use of antidepressants in bipolar depression (106,107). The larger of these two studies failed to show a difference when paroxetine or imipramine was added to lithium as compared with placebo added to lithium, although this was the purported intent of the study. Interestingly, the subset of the data showed that antidepressants were effective in patients with a lithium level <0.8 mEq per L and not effective as compared to placebo with therapeutic lithium levels >0.8 mEq per L. It is unclear whether this signifies that add-on antidepressant therapy is not necessary when patients can tolerate higher lithium plasma levels or that elevated lithium levels in some way counteract the therapeutic effects of the antidepressants, perhaps by decreased side effects or by another as-yet-unknown mechanism. Cohn et al. looked at the addition of fluoxetine in a randomized, controlled trial that did show positive affect but of modest intensity as compared to imipramine and placebo (108). A dose escalation study of venlafaxine in a small group of patients, some of whom had unipolar disorder and some of whom had bipolar II disorder with major depressive episodes, showed similar efficacy in reducing baseline HAM-D scores by 50% for 3 months (109).

For maintenance therapy in patients with bipolar disorder, antidepressants have not shown efficacy in preventing future bipolar episodes in seven specific trials. Three were placebo-controlled combinations of TCAs with lithium or adding TCAs to lithium. Two were specifically in patients with bipolar type II disorder; however, the data was obtained from post hoc analysis of unipolar depression trials and retrospective assessments of "manic switches" (110–115).

Two studies by Altshuler et al. looked at the impact of antidepressant continuation versus antidepressant discontinuation at 1-year follow-up (116,117). These patients had responded to a combination of mood stabilizer and antidepressants in the Stanley Foundation Bipolar Network. Rapid cycling patients were excluded from the study and none of the patients had switched into hypomania/mania. Those who stopped antidepressants in <6 months showed a 70% relapse rate and those who were maintained on antidepressants for 1 year showed a 24% relapse rate. This data suggested that some patients who responded to antidepressants were at significant risk for relapse if the antidepressant was discontinued and were unlikely to relapse if the antidepressant was continued. This group also revealed a relatively low rate of switch into hypomania or mania.

MAOIs have also shown effectiveness acutely in bipolar depression (12,13,16,17) but are difficult to use clinically. There has been no study as yet of patients with bipolar disorder with the selegiline patch.

The frequency with which bipolar depressed patients are "switched" into hypomania or mania by antidepressants has been a long-standing issue of debate and some controversy as to the frequency of this occurrence, as well as which antidepressant agents may be more likely to cause switching (118,119). Most clinicians have seen one or more patients switch into an elevated mood state while on an antidepressant; however, the level of severity of these switches has often not been quantified. Stoll et al. (119) opine that most switches into hypomania or mania are mild and less intense than spontaneous hypomanias/manias, whereas other researchers have seen more serious manic or hypomanic switches. A further confounding factor is that the definition of a "switch" and whether mood stabilizers were used concurrently or not differs from study to study. Ghaemi (117) suggests that switch rates with TCAs and MAOIs are approximately 40%, whereas with newer antidepressants (SSRIs, SNRIs, and bupropion) are approximately 20%.

The most recent evidence (120) compared the switch rates of sertraline, bupropion, and venlafaxine in 159 patients with bipolar I or bipolar II disorder, 25% of whom had a history of rapid cycling. Patients were observed over an initial 10-week acute-phase treatment and then followed in a 1-year continuation phase. There were 11% switches into hypomania and 8% switches into mania during the acute phase, and 22% into hypomania and 15% into mania in the 1-year continuation phase. In this group only 23% of patients in the continuation phase maintained a sustained antidepressant response without a switch. This data also revealed significant differences between the three antidepressants in that venlafaxine showed a considerably higher switch rate than the other two compounds with twice the rate of sertraline and three times the rate of bupropion, which was the lowest in terms of switch rates. Because there was no placebo arm, however, it is difficult to generalize this information to all patients with bipolar disorder. Goldberg and Truman from their work (121) suggest that paroxetine, sertraline, and bupropion have less risk of switching into elevated mood than other antidepressants.

The possibility that an antidepressant will precipitate a mixed affective state is of particular concern because, as will be seen in Chapter 8, mixed states are more difficult to treat, longer in duration, and have a higher incidence of suicidality. There have been several reports of precipitating mixed states with various antidepressants (122).

A final concern with antidepressant use in elevated mood is the possibility that antidepressants increase cycle acceleration and may promote rapid cycling. A 10-year prospective, double-blind study of 51 rapid cycling patients by the National Institute of Mental Health showed that 20% of these patients developed rapid cycling as a result of taking TCAs (118). Ghaemi (117), referencing several studies, opines that a similar cycle acceleration occurs with SSRIs in approximately 20% of patients. Amsterdam et al. in a 12-week, open-label phase of a double-blind relapse prevention study showed that fluoxetine caused a manic switch in 3.8% of patients with bipolar II disorder and 0.3% of unmatched patients with unipolar depression (123). A second study by Amsterdam et al. (124) showed that fluoxetine was effective in 38% of bipolar II depressed patients with a 7.3% hypomanic switch rate occurring in this study group over an 8-week period. Another confounding variable, which would be significantly important to patients with hypomania (i.e., Bipolar II patients), is whether the switch rate is significantly different for patients with bipolar II disorder when compared with those with bipolar I disorder. There is some evidence to suggest that that is the case (125,126). Other evidence (117,127,128) suggests that short-term mood destabilization and early loss of response may characterize the use of antidepressants in a significant portion of these patients, although the exact prevalence is difficult to determine.

Despite the rather universal prohibition from most thought leaders that antidepressant monotherapy is contraindicated in bipolar depression, ongoing research of the use of traditional antidepressants in this population continues. A recent study (129) involved the use of adjunctive escitalopram on patients with bipolar disorder who were maintained on a consistent mood stabilizer at therapeutic doses (lithium, valproic acid or carbamazepine). This 12-week, open-label, uncontrolled study used escitalopram at 10 mg and the patients were followed for 12 weeks. The population of 20 patients excluded anyone with mixed or manic episodes, psychotic features, or a history of alcohol or substance abuse within the past 6 months. There was a clinically meaningful improvement in depressive symptoms with half the number of the responders meeting criteria for full remission of the depressive episode and a mean drop in the HAM-D scores of over 12 points. One of the 20 patients became manic and two developed hypomanic symptoms. Side effects were not insignificant with

75% of the subjects experiencing some mild-to-moderate side effects, most notably headache, somnolence, insomnia, nausea, and sexual dysfunction. One might expect that a longer-term trial of escitalopram or any traditional antidepressant would reveal more episodes of switch into hypomania or mania. It is relatively clear, however, that, at least in this study, a significant response to a major depressive episode in the context of bipolar disorder can frequently be achieved with the addition of a traditional antidepressant.

Consolidated recommendations for the use of traditional antidepressants

With this array of disparate and sometimes contradictory evidence, what clinical recommendations can be made for the use of traditional antidepressants in bipolar depression? These can be summarized in Table 7.21.

The one caveat that is espoused by virtually all experts in this field is that patients with elevated mood should not be treated with traditional antidepressant monotherapy. Unfortunately, with the underdiagnosis of bipolar disorder and overdiagnosis of major depressive episodes, this is exactly what happens in many cases of depression treatment. Both psychiatrists and primary care practitioners cannot be guided simply by old habits and a comfort with traditional antidepressants. Knowledge of mood stabilizers and possible combinations of medications is essential in treating bipolar depression. Although class A research remains minimal in quality and quantity, clinicians should make an effort to follow the ongoing literature as it emerges, such that clinical decisions can be influenced as much as possible by evidence-based conclusions.

When traditional antidepressants are used in patients with bipolar disorder, it is essential that the clinical course of the patient is monitored carefully

TABLE 7.21
Guidelines for usage of traditional antidepressants in elevated mood patients

- Avoid antidepressant monotherapy
- Follow the literature—it is constantly changing
- Judge the needs of each patient individually
- Carefully follow a patient's course with history provided by outside observers
- A short-term, positive response to antidepressants does not indicate the need for chronic antidepressant therapy
- Patients who respond to the use of antidepressants but relapse when they are discontinued may need chronic maintenance treatment with antidepressants and mood stabilizers

by the clinician using the input of family members or other outside sources, mood charting, and a watchful eye for the emergence of mood cycling or mixed affective states. Likewise, if antidepressants have not been used but other treatments including mood stabilizers alone or in combination are not adequately treating depressed symptoms, clinicians should be willing to consider their use at least acutely. Each patient must be evaluated individually both when initially seen as well as over time, to determine the proper use or avoidance of traditional antidepressants as the patient's clinical course dictates. Clinicians cannot take an "all-or-nothing" or "black-and-white" approach toward the use of traditional antidepressants, because current evidence suggests they can be both useful and potentially harmful to different individuals.

There are some patients who appear to benefit from the chronic use of traditional antidepressants in combination with one or more mood stabilizers. Patients who are candidates for this chronic antidepressant–mood stabilizer therapy include those who

- have responded acutely to the use of antidepressants;
- have relapsed one or more times when the antidepressant is withdrawn;
- do not show evidence of increased cycling or mixed affective states;
- show improved behavioral and functional capacity when antidepressants are used.

Any patient who meets these guidelines and is treated with antidepressants on a maintenance basis, but continues to have recurrent depressive episodes may be a candidate for multiple antidepressants or the use of increased doses of mood stabilizer or multiple mood stabilizers.

Lastly, finances sometimes play a role in clinical decisions. Clinicians who practice in low income clinics and/or see patients without health insurance may be forced to initiate treatment plans that are less than ideal. More expensive, branded preparations that show clinical evidence of effectiveness with bipolar depression (e.g., lamotrigine or quetiapine) may simply be unavailable to certain patients for financial reasons. Such a patient may require the use of generic medications regardless of clinical guidelines under the maxim that "some treatment is better than no treatment." The combination of a generic mood stabilizer (e.g., lithium, valproate, or carbamazepine) with a generic SSRI (e.g., fluoxetine, sertraline, paroxetine, citalopram, or fluvoxamine) may be the only treatment with which the patient can be reasonably expected to comply because of cost, although the long-term use of such a combination may have its downsides.

Integrating temperament into bipolar depression treatment

The clinical guidelines that have been cited earlier in this chapter give road maps to the treatment of depression in patients with elevated mood.

However, to date, such guidelines have not taken into account newer data on the bipolar spectrum and affective temperament. Taking into account the recommendations from these guidelines and factoring in the patient's underlying temperament, the following additional recommendations are also made:

1. When treating an acute depression in a patient who has a history of elevated mood, the patient's preexisting temperament may influence the choice of treatment strategies. Although there is little hard evidence to guide the clinician, certain common sense assumptions may help in making treatment decisions, especially when expert consensus guidelines offer multiple possible treatments. It is the author's recommendation that patients with an acute depression who have had a dysthymic temperament but a history of mildly elevated mood are going to require more antidepressant effect and may be less at risk for increased cycling or the induction of mixed episodes, whereas those with cyclothymic temperaments or a hyperthymic temperament before the acute episode may be more at risk for induction of cycling or the induction of mixed episodes when antidepressant treatment is initiated.

2. In acute bipolar depressions with a history of dysthymic temperament, first-line treatment is lamotrigine monotherapy, quetiapine monotherapy or OFC. Level 2 treatment is lamotrigine plus an SSRI, bupropion, venlafaxine, or duloxetine. Level 3 treatment is a combination of lithium, lamotrigine, quetiapine, OFC, plus a traditional antidepressant. Level 4 treatment is any combination from level 3 plus aripiprazole, ziprasidone, olanzapine, or ECT.

3. In an acute depression presenting in a patient with cyclothymic or hyperthymic temperament, level 1 treatment consists of lamotrigine monotherapy or lamotrigine plus an antimanic agent (lithium, valproate, carbamazepine or atypical antipsychotic). Level 2 treatment is combination of lithium, lamotrigine, quetiapine, or OFC. Level 3 treatment is a combination of lithium, lamotrigine, quetiapine, OFC plus an SSRI, an SNRI, or bupropion. Level 4 treatment is any of the combinations in Level 2 treatment plus MAOIs, tricyclics, or ECT.

Electroconvulsive therapy

Although not a "medication" *per se*, physical treatment of elevated mood must include the use of electroconvulsive therapy (ECT). Although it is likely not a treatment used in milder elevated mood states, ECT can be extraordinarily efficacious and truly lifesaving for patients with severe elevated mood. ECT is also a truly bimodal treatment, effective in the treatment of both acute mania and the depression of bipolar disorder. Mukherjee et al. in their review of 50 years of clinical experience with ECT for acute mania suggests that as many as 80% of patients treated showed marked clinical improvement (129). Other studies (130–132) suggest that many manic patients respond relatively quickly to ECT in comparison to mood stabilizer medication treatment. ECT

TABLE 7.22

Indications for use of electroconvulsive therapy in elevated mood

Significant acute mania accompanied by the following:

• Pregnancy

• Manic delirium with severe hypothermia

• Neuroleptic Malignant Syndrome

• Catatonia

• Comorbid general medical conditions

• Intolerance of or non response to psychopharmacologic agents

Adapted from Small JG, Klapper MH, Kellams JJ, et al. Electroconvulsive treatment compared with lithium in the management of manic states. *Arch Gen Psychiatry.* 1988;45:727–732.

is also often useful in patients who have been refractory to pharmacotherapy. Although rigorous studies are scarce, most experts agree that ECT is also effective in rapid cycling bipolar disorder as well as in non–rapid cycling disorder. It has been suggested by Mukherjee et al. that bilateral ECT is superior to unilateral ECT in the treatment of acute mania (129). The primary indications for ECT in a patient with elevated mood are shown in Table 7.22.

Other considerations when using ECT in acute mania are that lithium be temporarily discontinued to avoid the rare but serious complications of delirium and status epilepticus (133–136). In order to ensure that seizures do not occur during the ECT benzodiazepines or anticonvulsants should also be discontinued. Acutely manic patients need a minimum of six treatments and may require as many as ten to fifteen treatments. A patient who has responded well to a course of ECT may also be considered for ongoing maintenance ECT treatments (130,137,138).

Patient acceptance of the need for ECT is often poor. There are commonly held misconceptions about what is involved in the treatment, the potential side effects, and the ultimate clinical state of a person who experiences ECT. This is commonly known as the "*One Flew Over the Cuckoo's Nest*" Syndrome. Many of the problematic issues associated with ECT as it was administered 50 to 60 years ago have been resolved through scientific advances, particularly involving the use of unilateral treatments.

Short-term memory loss is a well-known side effect. Most patients will have a loss of memory for the period surrounding the treatments themselves and may have some loss of prior memories, although this is less common. Impairment of the *capacity* for memory rarely occurs, although it has been reported. In general, most patients return to their normal ability to remember concepts and experiences within several weeks of stopping the treatments.

The bottom line

- Many factors can affect the clinician's choice of medication to treat an elevated mood episode. There are primary factors including the following:
  - Target symptoms
  - Prior medication response
  - Safety
  - Tolerability
  - Ongoing medical issues
  - Temperament
- There are also secondary factors in choosing medication:
  - Known response in blood relatives
  - Expense
  - Insurance formulary coverage
  - Patient preferences
- Medication guidelines can provide helpful information for selection of medications; however, such guidelines are not universally consistent.
- In the treatment of acute mania, there are multiple on-label approvals by the FDA for treatment, although off-label uses of medication are common.
- The more severe the elevated mood episode, the more likely it is that combination therapy of a mood stabilizer plus an atypical or typical antipsychotic will be necessary.
- Hypomanic patients are more likely to be acceptive of monotherapy rather than combination therapy. Side effect profile and intensity are almost as equally important for these patients as efficacy.

REFERENCES

1. Doran CM. *Prescribing mental health medication.* Routledge; 2003:1–16.
2. Stahl SM. *Essential pharmacology neuroscientific basis and practical applications,* 2nd ed, Cambridge University Press; 2000.
3. Perlis RH, Ostacher MJ, Patel JK, et al. *Predictors of recurrence Bipolar Disorder: Primary outcomes from the systematic treatment enhancement program for Bipolar Disorder (STEPBD).* Am J Psychiatry. 2006;163(2):217–224.
4. Kramer SI, McCall WV. Off-label prescribing: more effective treatment. *Curr Psychiatry.* 2006;5(4):41–46.
5. Thompson PDR. *The physicians desk reference,* 60th ed. Thompson PDR; 2006.
6. Stein BJ, Kupfer DJ, Schatzberg AF. *Textbook of mood disorders.* American Psychiatric Publishing; 2006:464–465.
7. Ketter TA, Calabrese JR. Stabilization of mood from below versus above baseline in Bipolar Disorder: A new nomenclature. *J Clin Psychiatry.* 2002;63:146–151.
8. Keck PE, Perlis RH, Otto MW, et al. *Postgrad med special report.* 2004:1–120.
9. Suppes T, Dennehy EB, Swann AC, et al. The Texas medication algorithm project. *J Clin Psychiatry.* 2005;66:870–886.
10. Jefferson J. Lithium is not a fad whose time came and went. It is a valuable medication that belongs in psychiatry's arsenal for Bipolar Disorder. *Curr Psychiatry.* 2002;1:19–24.

11. Bowden CL, Brugger AM, Swann AC, et al. Depakote Mania Study Group. Efficacy of divalproex vs lithium and placebo in the treatment of mania. *JAMA*. 1994;271–918:24.

12. Goldberg JF, Citrome L. Latest therapies for Bipolar Disorder. Symposium on Bipolar Disorder. *Postgrad Med*. 2005;117(2).

13. Goodwin FK, Jamison KR. *Manic depressive illness*. New York: Oxford University Press; 1990.

14. American Psychiatric Association. Practice guideline for the treatment of patients with Bipolar Disorder [Revision]. *Am J Psychiatry*. 2002;159(Suppl 4):1–50.

15. Goodwin GM. Consensus Group of the British Association for Psychopharmacology. Evidence-based guideline for treatment Bipolar Disorder: Recommendations from the British Association for Psychopharmacology. *J Psychopharmacol*. 2003;17:149–173.

16. Post RM, Uhde TW, Roy-Byrne PP, et al. Correlates of anti manic response to carbamazepine. *Psychiatry Res*. 1987;21:71–83.

17. Lerer B, Moore N, Myendorff E, et al. Carbamazepine versus lithium in mania: A double-blind study. *J Clin Psychiatry*. 1987;48:89–93.

18. Weisler R, Kalali A, Ketter T. The SPD417 Study Group. A multi center, randomized, double-blind, placebo-controlled trial of extended-release carbamazepine capsules as monotherapy for Bipolar Disorder patients with manic or mixed episodes. *J Clin Psychiatry*. 2004;65:478–484.

19. Calabrese JR, Markovitz PJ, Kimmel SE, et al. Spectrum of efficacy of valproate in 78 rapid-cycling Bipolar Patients. *J Clin Psychopharmacol*. 1992; 12(1 Suppl):53–6S.

20. Shelton MD III, Rapport DJ, Youngstrom EA, et al. Is rapid cycling a predictor of non response to lithium? Poster NR759. *Presented at the 157th American Psychiatric Association Annual Meeting*. New York: May 1–6, 2004.

21. Swann AC, Bowden CL, Morris D, et al. Depression during mania: Treatment response to lithium or divalproex. *Arch Gen Psychiatry*. 1997;54(1):37–42.

22. Salloum IM, Cornelius JR, Daley DC, et al. Efficacy of valproate maintenance in patients with Bipolar Disorder and alcoholism. *Arch Gen Psychiatry*. 2005;62(1):37–45.

23. LeFauve CE. Valproate reduces alcohol consumption in people with comorbid alcohol dependency and Bipolar Disorder. *Evid Based Ment Health*. 2005;8:79.

24. Goldberg JF, Garno JL, Leon AC, et al. A history of substance abuse complicates remission from acute mania in Bipolar Disorder. *J Clin Psychiatry*. 1999;60:733–740.

25. Citrome L, Volavka J. The promise of atypical antipsychotics: Fewer side effects mean enhanced compliance and improved functioning. *Postgrad Med*. 2004; 116(4):49–63.

26. Yatham LM. Acute and maintenance treatment of Bipolar mania: The role of atypical antipsychotics. *Bipolar Disord*. 2003;5(Suppl 2):7–19.

27. Tohen M, Sanger TM, McElroy SL, et al. Olanzapine versus placebo in the treatment of acute mania. *Am J Psychiatry*. 1999;156(5):702–709.

28. Tohen M, Jacobs TG, Grundy SL, et al. Efficacy of olanzapine in acute Bipolar mania. *Arch Gen Psychiatry*. 2000;57(9):841–849.

29. Bowden CL, Grunze H, Mullen J, et al. A randomized, double-blind, placebo-controlled efficacy and safety study of quetiapine or lithium as

monotherapy for mania in Bipolar Disorder. *J Clin Psychiatry.* 2005;66(1):111–121.

30. Sachs G, Chengappa KNR, Suppes T, et al. Quetiapine with lithium or divalproex for the treatment of Bipolar mania: A randomized, double-blind, placebo-controlled study. *Bipolar Disord.* 2004;6:213.
31. Sajatovic M, Brescan DW, Perez DE, et al. Quetiapine alone and added to a mood stabilizer for serious mood disorders. *J Clin Psychiatry.* 2001;62(9):728–732.
32. Hirschfeld R, Keck PE, Kramer M, et al. *Presented at ACNP.* 2002.
33. Sachs GS, Grossman F, Ghaemi SN, et al. Combination of a mood stabilizer with risperidone or haloperidol for treatment of acute mania: A double-blind, placebo-controlled comparison of efficacy and safety. *Am J Psychiatry.* 2002;159:1146–1154.
34. Yatham LN, Grossman F, Augustyns I, et al. Mood stabilizers plus risperidone or placebo in the treatment of acute mania: International, double-blind, randomized controlled trial. *Br J Psychiatry.* 2003;182:141–147.
35. Keck PE Jr, Versiani M, Potkin S, et al. Ziprasidone in Mania Study Group. Ziprasidone in the treatment of acute Bipolar mania: A three-week, placebo-controlled, double-blind randomized trial. *Am J Psychiatry.* 2003;160:741–748.
36. Data on file Pfizer Inc.
37. Mamo D, Kapur S, Shammi CM, et al. A PET study of dopamine D2 and serotonin 5-HT2 receptor occupancy in patients with schizophrenia treated with therapeutic doses of ziprasidone. *Am J Psychiatry.* 2004;161:818–825.
38. Keck PE, Versiani M, Potkin S, et al. Ziprasidone in the treatment of acute bipolar mania: a three-week, placebo-controlled, double-blind, randomized trial. *Am J Psychiatry.* 2003;160(4):741–748.
39. Weisler RH, Warrington L, Dunn J, et al. *Presented at APA.* 2004.
40. Keck PE, Marcus R, Tourkodimitris S, et al. Aripiprazole Study Group. A placebo-controlled, double-blind study of the efficacy and safety of aripiprazole in patients with acute Bipolar mania. *Am J Psychiatry.* 2003;160:1651–1658.
41. Keck PE, Calabrese JR, McQuade RD, et al. A randomized, double-blind, placebo-controlled 26-week trial of aripiprazole in recently manic patients with Bipolar I Disorder. *J Clin Psychiatry.* 2006;67:626–637.
42. Sanchez R, Bourin M, Auby P. Aripiprazole vs haloperidol for maintained treatment effect in acute mania. *Presented at the 5th International Conference on Bipolar Disorder.* Pittsburgh, PA: June 12–14, 2003.
43. Perlis RH, Welge JA, Vornik LA, et al. Atypical antipsychotics in the treatment of mania: a meta-analysis of randomized, placebo-controlled trials. *J Clin Psychiatry.* 2006;67:4.
44. Keck PE. *The role of second-generation antipsychotic monotherapy in the rapid control of acute Bipolar mania. J Clin Psychiatry.* 2005;66(3):5–11.
45. Chue P, Kovacs CS. Safety and tolerability of atypical antipsychotics in patients with Bipolar Disorder: Prevalence, monitoring and management. *Bipolar Disord.* 2003;5(suppl 2):62–79.
46. Davis JM, Chen N, Glick ID. Subjecting meta-analyses to closer scrutiny: Little support for differential efficacy among second-generation antipsychotics at equivalent doses. [Letter to the editor]. *Arch Gen Psychiatry.* 2006;63:937–939.
47. Poirier P, Despres JP. Waist circumference, visceral obesity and cardiovascular risk. *J Cardiopulm Rehabil.* 2003;23:161–169.

48. McIntyre RS, McCann SM, Kennedy SH. Antipsychotic metabolic effects: Weight gain, diabetes mellitus, and lipid abnormalities. *Can J Psychiatry*. 2001;46:273–281.

49. Nemeroff CB. Safety of available agents used to treat Bipolar Disorder: Focus on weight gain. *J Clin Psychiatry*. 2003;64:532–539.

50. Allison DB, Mentore JL, Heo M, et al. Antipsychotic-induced weight gain: A comprehensive research synthesis. *Am J Psychiatry*. 1999;156:1686–1696.

51. Case DE, Haupt DW, Newcomer JW, et al. Antipsychotic-induced weight gain and metabolic abnormalities: Implications for increased mortality in patients with schizophrenia. *J Clin Psychiatry*. 2004;65(Suppl 7):4–18.

52. American Diabetes Association, American Psychiatric Association, American Association of Clinical Endocrinologists, North American Association for the Study of Obesity. Consensus development conference on antipsychotic drugs and obesity and diabetes. *Diabetes Care*. 2004;27:596–601.

53. McIntyre RS, Konarski JZ. Tolerability profiles of atypical antipsychotics in the treatment of Bipolar Disorder. *J Clin Psychiatry*. 2005;66(Suppl 3):28–36.

54. Keck PE, Potkin S, Warrington LE, et al. Efficacy and safety of ziprasidone in Bipolar Disorder: Short- and long-term data [poster]. *Presented at the 157th Annual Meeting of the American Psychiatric Association*. New York, NY: May 1–6, 2004.

55. *Clozaril [package insert]*. East Hanover, NJ: Novartis Pharmaceutical Corp; 2003.

56. Frye MA, Ketter TA, Altshuler LL, et al. Clozapine in Bipolar Disorder: Treatment implications for other atypical antipsychotics. *J Affect Disord*. 1998;48:91–104.

57. Amann BL, Pogarell O, Mergl R, et al. EEG abnormalities associated with antipsychotics: A comparison of quetiapine, olanzapine, haloperidol and healthy subjects. *Hum Psychopharmacol*. 2003;18:641–646.

58. Harrigan EP, Miceli JJ, Anziano R, et al. A randomized evaluation of the effects of six antipsychotic agents on QTc, in the absence and presence of metabolic inhibition. *J Clin Psychopharmacol*. 2004;24:62–69.

59. Aran GW. An overview of side effects caused by typical antipsychotics. *J Clin Psychiatry*. 2000;61(suppl 8):5–11.

60. Maguire GA. Prolactin elevation with antipsychotic medications: Mechanisms of action and clinical consequences. *J Clin Psychiatry*. 2002;63(suppl 4):56–62.

61. Clevenger CV, Furth PA, Hankinson SE, et al. The role of prolactin in mammary carcinoma. *Endocr Rev*. 2003;24:1–27.

62. Cavallaro R, Cocchi F, Angelone SM, et al. Cabergoline treatment of risperidone-induced hyper prolactinemia: A pilot study. *J Clin Psychiatry*. 2004;65:187–190.

63. Goldstein DJ, Corbin LA, Fung MC. Olanzapine-exposed pregnancies and lactation: Early experience. *J Clin Psychopharmacol*. 2000;20:399–403.

64. Chaudron LH, Jefferson JW. Mood stabilizers during breastfeeding: A review. *J Clin Psychiatry*. 2000;61:79–90.

65. Gentile S. Clinical utilization of atypical antipsychotics in pregnancy and lactation. *Ann Pharmacother*. 2004;38:1265–1271.

66. Tohen M, Chengappa KNR, Supper T, et al. Relapse prevention in Bipolar I Disorder: 18-month comparison of olanzapine plus mood stabilizer v. mood stabilizer along. *Br J Psychiatry*. 2004;194:337–345.

67. McIntyre RS, Mancini DA, Srinivasan J, et al. The antidepressant effects of risperidone and olanzapine in Bipolar Depression. *Can J Clin Pharmacol.* 2004; 11:e218–e226.

68. Keck PE Jr. Evaluation and management of breakthrough depressive episodes. *J Clin Psychiatry.* 2004;65(Suppl 10):11–15.

69. American Psychiatric Association. Practice guideline for the treatment of patients with Bipolar Disorder [revision]. *Am J Psychiatry.* 2002;159 (Suppl 4):1–50.

70. Yatham LN, Grossman F, Augustyns I, et al. Mood stabilizers plus risperidone or placebo in the treatment of acute mania: International, double-blind, randomized controlled trial. *Br J Psychiatry.* 2004;182:141–147.

71. Miller DS, Yatham LN, Lam RW. Comparative efficacy of typical and atypical antipsychotics as add-on therapy to mood stabilizers in the treatment of acute mania. *J Clin Psychaitry.* 2001;62:975–980.

72. Bowden CL. Atypical antipsychotic augmentation of mood stabilizer therapy in Bipolar Disorder. *J Clin Psychiatry.* 2005;66(Suppl 3):12–19.

73. Clark RE, Xie H, Brunette MF. Benzodiazepine prescription practices and substance abuse in persons with severe mental illness. *J Clin Psychiatry.* 2004;65(2): 151–155.

74. Bowden CL, Brugger Am, Swann AC, et al. Efficacy of divalproex vs lithium and placebo in the treatment of mania. *JAMA.* 1994;271(12):918–924.

75. Bradjewn J, Shriqui C, Kosycki D, et al. Double-blind comparison of the effects of clonazepam and lorazepam in acute mania. *J Clin Psychopharmacol.* 1990;10:403–408.

76. Lenox RH, Newhouse PA, Creelman WL, et al. Adjunctive treatment of manic agitation with lorazepam versus haloperidol: A double-blind study. *J Clin Psychiatry.* 1992;53(2):47–52.

77. Meehan K, Zhang F, David S, et al. A double-blind, randomized comparison of the efficacy and safety of intramuscular injections of olanzapine, lorazepam, or placebo in treating acutely agitated patients diagnosed with Bipolar mania. *J Clin Psychopharmacol.* 2001;21(4):389–397.

78. Aronson TA, Shukla S, Hirschowitz J. Clonazepam treatment of five lithium-refractory patients with Bipolar Disorder. *Am J Psychiatry.* 1989;146:77–80.

79. Winkler D, Willeit M, Wolf R, et al. Clonazepam in the long-term treatment of patients with unipolar depression, Bipolar and schizoaffective disorder. *Eur Neuropsychopharmacol.* 2003;13(2):129–134.

80. Brunette MF, Noordsy DL, Xie H, et al. Benzodiazepine use and abuse among patients with severe mental illness and co-occurring substance use disorders. *Psychiatr Serv.* 2003;54(1):1395–1401.

81. Dunayevich E, Keck PE. Prevalence and description of psychotic features in Bipolar mania. *Curr Psychiatry Rep.* 2000;2(4):286–290.

82. Work Group on Bipolar Disorder. Quetiapine monotherapy for mania associated with Bipolar Disorder: Combined analysis of two international, double-blind, randomized, placebo-controlled studies. *Curr Med Res Opin.* (2002);21(6):923–934.

83. Chou JC, Czobor P, Charles O, et al. Acute mania: Haloperidol dose and augmentation with lithium or lorazepam. *J Clin Psychopharmacol.* 1999;19(6):500–505.

84. Keck PE. Combination vs single medication treatment of Bipolar Disorder. *Medscape Psychiatry Ment Health.* 2005.

85. Djulbegovic B, Lacevic M, Cantor A, et al. The uncertainty principle and industry-sponsored research. *Lancet.* 2000;356:635–638.

86. Baker CB, Johnsrud MT, Crismon ML, et al. Quantitative analysis of sponsorship bias in economic studies of antidepressants. *Br J Psychiatry.* 2003;183:498–506.

87. Keck PE, Perlis RH, Otto MW, et al. Expert consensus guideline: Choice of medication for Bipolar Depression. *Postgrad Med Special Report.* 2004;Dec: 1–120.

88. Yatham LN, Kennedy SH, O'Donovan C, et al. Canadian Network for Mood and Anxiety Treatment s (CANMAT) guidelines for the management of patients with Bipolar Disorder: Consensus and controversies. *Bipolar Disord.* 2005; 7(Suppl 3):5–69.

89. Goodwin GM, Bowden CL, Calabrese JR, et al. A pooled analysis of 2 placebo-controlled 18-month trials of lamotrigine and lithium maintenance in Bipolar I Disorder. *J Clin Psychiatry.* 2004;65:432–441.

90. Calbrese JR, Bowden CL, Sachs GS, et al. Lamictal 602 Study Group. A double-blind placebo-controlled study of lamotrigine monotherapy in outpatients with Bipolar I depression. *J Clin Psychiatry.* 1999;60:78–88.

91. Bowden CL, Calabrese JR, Sachs G, et al. Lamictal 606 Study Group. A placebo-controlled 18-month trial of lamotrigine and lithium maintenance treatment in recently manic or hypomanic patients with Bipolar I Disorder. *Arch Gen Psychiatry.* 2003;60:392–400.

92. Calabrese JR, Bowden CL, Sachs G, et al. Lamictal 605 Study Group. A placebo-controlled 18-month trial of lamotrigine and lithium maintenance treatment in recently depressed patients with Bipolar I Disorder. *J Clin Psychiatry.* 2003; 64:1013–1024.

93. Calabrese JR, Keck PE, MacFadden W, et al. A randomized, double-blind, placebo-controlled trial of quetiapine in the treatment of Bipolar I or II depression. *Am J Psychiatry.* 2005;162:1351–1360.

94. Milev R, Abraham G. Add-on quetiapine for Bipolar Depression: Twelve months open label prospective trial. *Ann Gen Psychiatry.* 2006;5(Suppl 1):5196.

95. Tohen M, Vieta E, Calabrese J, et al. Efficacy of olanzapine and olanzapine-fluoxetine combination in the treatment of Bipolar I depression. *Arch Gen Psychiatry.* 2003;60:1079–1088.

96. Shi L, Namjoshi MA, Swindle R, et al. Effects of olanzapine alone and olanzapine/fluoxetine combination on health-related quality of life in patients with Bipolar Depression: Secondary analysis of a double-blind, placebo-controlled, randomized clinical trial. *Clin Ther.* 2004;26(1):125–134.

97. Goodwin FK, Fireman B, Simon GE, et al. Suicide risk in Bipolar Disorder during treatment with lithium and divalproex. *JAMA.* 2003;290:1467–1473.

98. Sachs GS, Collins MA, Altshuler LL, et al. Divalproex sodium versus placebo for the treatment of Bipolar Depression. *Presented at: 40th Annual Meeting of the American College of Neuropsychopharmacology.* Waikoloa, Hawaii: December 10, 2001.

99. Davis LL, Bartolucci A, Petty F. Divalproex in the treatment of Bipolar Depression: A placebo-controlled study. *J Affect Disord.* 2005;85:259–266.

100. Sporn J, Ghaemi SN, Sambur MR, et al. Pramipexole augmentation in the treatment of unipolar and Bipolar Depression: A retrospective chart review. *Ann Clin Psychiatry.* 2000;12(3):137–140.

101. Zarate CA Jr, Payne JL, Singh J, et al. Pramipexole for Bipolar II depression: A placebo-controlled proof of concept study. *Biol Psychiatry.* 2004;56:54–60.

102. Anand A, Bukhari L, Jennings SA, et al. A preliminary open-label study of zonisamide treatment for Bipolar Depression in 10 patients. *J Clin Psychiatry.* 2005;66(2):195–198.

103. Baldassano CF, Ghaemi SN, Chang A, et al. Acute treatment of Bipolar Depression with adjunctive zonisamide: A retrospective chart review. *Bipolar Disord.* 2004;6(5):432–434.

104. Young LT, Joffe RT, Robb JC, et al. Double-blind comparison of addition of a second mood stabilizer versus an antidepressant to an initial mood stabilizer for treatment of patients with Bipolar Depression. *Am J Psychiatry.* 2000;157:124–126.

105. Cohn JB, Collins G, Ashbrook E, et al. A comparison of fluoxetine, imipramine and placebo in patients with Bipolar Depressive Disorder. *Int Clin Psychopharmacol.* 1989;4(4):313–322.

106. Nemeroff CB, Evans DL, Gyulai L, et al. Double-blind, placebo-controlled comparison of imipramine and paroxetine in the treatment of Bipolar Depression. *Am J Psychiatry.* 2001;158(6):906–912.

107. Cohn JB, Collins G, Ashbrook E, et al. A comparison of fluoxetine, imipramine and placebo in patients with Bipolar Depressive Disorder. [Abstract]. *Int Clin Psychopharmacol.* 1989;4:313–322.

108. Amsterdam JD, Garcia-Espana F. Venlafaxine monotherapy in women with Bipolar II and unipolar depression. *J Affect Disord.* 2000;59(3):225–229.

109. Megna JL, Devitt PJ. Treatment of Bipolar Depression with twice-weekly fluoxetine: Management of antidepressant-induced mania. *Ann Pharacotherapy.* 2001;35(1):45–47.

110. Amsterdam JD. Efficacy and safety of venlafaxine in Bipolar type-II major depressive episode. *J Clin Psychopharmacol.* 1998;18(6):414–417.

111. Ghaemi SN, Lenox MS, Baldessarini RJ. Effectiveness and safety of long-term antidepressant treatment in Bipolar Disorder. *J Clin Psychiatry.* 2001; 62(7):565–569.

112. Altmann LS. Antidepressants for Bipolar Depression: Tips to stay out of trouble. When it makes sense to use them and for how long. *Current Psychiatry.* 2005;4(7):15–20.

113. Amsterdam JD, Garcia-Espana F, Fawcett J, et al. Efficacy and safety of fluoxetine in treating Bipolar II major depressive episode. *J Clin Psychopharmacol.* 1998;18:435–440.

114. Amsterdam JD, Garcia-Espana F. Venlafaxine monotherapy in women with Bipolar II and Unipolar major depression. *J Affect Disord.* 2000;59:225–229.

115. Altshuler L, Kiriakos L, Calcagno J, et al. Impact of antidepressant discontinuation versus antidepressant continuation at 1-year risk for relapse of Bipolar Depression: A retrospective chart review. *J Clin Psychiatry.* 2001;62:612–616.

116. Altshuler L, Suppes T, Black D, et al. Impact of antidepressant discontinuation after acute Bipolar Depression remission on rates of depressive relapse at 1-year follow-up. *Am J Psychiatry.* 2003;160:1252–1262.

117. Ghaemi SN, Rosenquist KJ, Ko JY, et al. Antidepressant treatment in Bipolar versus unipolar depression. *Am J Psychiatry.* 2004;161:163–165.

118. Wehr TA, Sack DA, Rosenthal NE, et al. Rapid cycling affective disorder: Contributing factors and treatment responses in 51 patients. *Am J Psychiatry.* 1988;145:179–184.

119. Stoll AL, Mayer PV, Kolbrener M, et al. Antidepressant-associated mania: A controlled comparison with spontaneous mania. *Am J Psychiatry.* 1994;151: 1642–1645.
120. Leverich GS, Altshuler LL, Frye MA, et al. Risk of switch in mood polarity to hypomania or mania in patients with Bipolar Depression during acute and continuation trials of venlafaxine, sertraline and bupropion as adjuncts to mood stabilizers. *Am J Psychiatry.* 2006;163:232–239.
121. Goldberg JF, Truman CJ. Antidepressant-induced mania: An overview of current controversies. *Bipolar Disord.* 2003;5:407–420.
122. Zubieta JK, Demitrack MA. Possible bupropion precipitation of mania and mixed affective state. *J Clin Psychopharmacol.* 1991;11(5):327–328.
123. Amsterdam JD, Garcia-Espana F, Fawcett J, et al. Efficacy and safety of fluoxetine in treating Bipolar II major depressive episode. *J Clin Psychopharmacol.* 1998;18:435–440.
124. Amsterdam JD, Shults J, Brunswick DJ, et al. Short-term fluoxetine monotherapy for Bipolar type II or Bipolar NOS major depression—low manic switch rate. *Bipolar Disord.* 2004;6:75–81.
125. Dunner DL, Stallone F, Fieve RR, et al. Lithium carbonate and affective disorders: A double-blind study of prophylaxis of depression in Bipolar illness. *Arch Gen Psychiatry.* 1976;33:117–120; Correction 1982;39:1344–1345.
126. Fieve RR, Kumbaraci R, Dunner DL. Lithium prophylaxis of depression in Bipolar I, Bipolar II, and Unipolar patients. *Am J Psychiatry.* 1976;133:925–929.
127. Joffe RT, MacQueen GM, Marriott M, et al. Induction of mania and cycle acceleration in Bipolar Disorder: Effect of different classes of antidepressant. *Acta Psychiatr Scand.* 2002;105:427–430.
128. Sharma V. Loss of response to antidepressants and subsequent refractoriness: Diagnostic issues in a retrospective case series. *J Affect Disord.* 2001;64:99–106.
129. Mukherjee S, Sackheim HA, Schnur DB. Electroconvulsive therapy of acute manic episodes: A review of 50 years' experience. *Am J Psychiatry.* 1994;151:169–176.
130. Small JG, Klapper MH, Kellams JJ, et al. Electroconvulsive treatment compared with lithium in the management of manic states. *Arch Gen Psychiatry.* 1988;45:727–732.
131. Prudic J, Sackeim HA, Devanand DP. Medication resistance and clinical response to electroconvulsive therapy. *Psychiatry Res.* 1990;31:287–296.
132. Kusumakar V, Yatham NY, Haslam DRS, et al. Treatment of mania, mixed state, and rapid cycling. *Can J Psychiatry.* 1997;42(Suppl 2):79S–86S.
133. Small JG, Kellams JJ, Milstein V, et al. Complications with electroconvulsive treatment combined with lithium. *Biol Psychiatry.* 1985;20:125–134.
134. Rudorfer MV, Linnoila M, Potter WZ. Combined lithium and electroconvulsive therapy: Pharmacokinetic and pharmacodynamic interactions. *Convuls Ther.* 1987;3:40–45.
135. El-Mallakh RS. Complications of concurrent lithium and electroconvulsive therapy: A review of clinical material and theoretical considerations. *Psychopharmacol Bull.* 1987;23:595–601.
136. Black DW, Winokur G, Nasrallah H. Treatment of mania: A naturalistic study of ECT vs lithium in 438 patients. *J Clin Psychiatry.* 1987;48:132–139.
137. McCabe MS, Norris B. ECT vs chlorpromazine in mania. *Biol Psychiatry.* 1977;12:245–254.
138. Small JG, Klapper MH, Kellarns JJ. ECT compared with lithium in the management of manic states. *Arch Gen Psychiatry.* 1988;45:727–732.

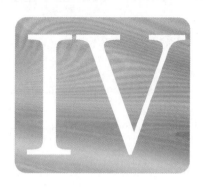

Special Situations

MIXED EPISODES
AND RAPID CYCLING

The identification of mixed affective states is one of the most critical items related to hypomania that has only recently begun receiving attention. Mixed affective states (sometimes referred to as mixed episodes, mixed states or mixed mood episodes) are those in which depressive and/or manic/hypomanic symptoms simultaneously occur. Although described by Kraeplin in the 19th century, the presence and importance of mixed affective states had been lost over the past 40 years as our diagnostic categories have focused on polarity—the presence of pure depression and pure mania isolated from one another.

Although included in the *Diagnostic and Statistical Manual of Mental Disorders* (DSM-IV) text revision (TR), the understanding of mixed episodes has evolved such that many real-world symptomatic episodes that contain simultaneous elements of both depression and hypomania are excluded by the current definition. According to DSM-IV TR, mixed episodes require that full criteria for a manic episode as well as a major depressive episode be fulfilled for most days during a one-week period (see Table 8.1). Although, some patient's symptoms may fit this criterion, such categorization is one of the least likely presentations of mixed states.

A mixed episode must also be sufficiently severe to cause marked impairment in social or occupational functioning, or necessitate a hospitalization to prevent self-harm. This definition excludes those patients regularly seen in an

TABLE 8.1

Diagnostic and Statistical Manual of Mental Disorders-IV text revision criteria for mixed episode

A. These criteria are met both for a manic episode and for a depressive episode (except for duration) nearly every day during at least a 1-week period

B. The mood disturbance is sufficiently severe to cause marked impairment in occupational functioning or in usual social activities or relationships with others, or to necessitate hospitalization to prevent harm to self or others, or there are psychotic features

C. The symptoms are not due to the direct physiologic effects of a substance (e.g., a drug of abuse, a medication, or other treatment) or a general medical condition (e.g., hyperthyroidism)

Note: Mixed-like episodes that are clearly caused by somatic antidepressant treatment (e.g., medication, electroconvulsive therapy, light therapy) should not count toward a diagnosis of bipolar I disorder.

outpatient practice who may have less than full manic criteria interspersed with depressive symptoms. Also, patients whose symptoms may cause some measure of impairment, but not to the required level of "marked impairment" are frequently seen. Lastly, the criteria require that the symptoms are not the direct effect of a substance, including drugs of abuse, alcohol, or other medications. Because mixed affective states frequently overlap with substance abuse, significant problems exist in distinguishing dysphoria coexisting with substance abuse from underlying mixed affective states unrelated to substance abuse. DSM-IV TR criteria appear, therefore, to be exclusionary rather than inclusionary, omitting patients with symptoms shown in Table 8.2.

Recent evidence suggests that mixed episodes occur frequently and may be far more common than formerly believed. Bauer et al. (1) in a survey of bipolar outpatients in the hypomanic state showed that 94.1% of these patients also had significant depressive symptoms, although only 17.6% met DSM-IV

TABLE 8.2

Mixtures of elevated and depressed mood states not identified by current *Diagnostic and Statistical Manual of Mental Disorders* criteria of a mixed episode

• Episodes with subsyndromal mood symptoms that do not meet full manic or major depression criteria

• Episodes lasting less than 1 week

• Episodes causing limited impairment

• Episodes clouded by the presence of substance abuse

TR criteria for a mixed affective state. Also, in this study, 70.1% of those in a depressive episode had clinically significant coexisting manic symptoms (108 out of 154).

Newer perspectives on mixed affective states

The exact number of symptoms necessary to qualify as a mixed affective episode in a purely phenotypic nosology system remains hotly debated (2–5). For purposes of this text, mixed affective states are more broadly defined as any episode lasting 2 or more days that includes a mixture of three or more depressed symptoms and three or more hypomanic/manic symptoms, as suggested by Benazzi (2,3). Although this debate persists, it is clear that many patients identified by this definition fall short of the current DSM-IV TR criteria for a mixed affective episode. Nonetheless, such patients present with significant distress and are seen frequently in a variety of clinical settings. This mixed affective state definition subsumes several other diagnostic labels, including dysphoric mania, agitated depression, energized depression, mixed hypomania, and dysphoric hypomania that may or may not be discrete entities.

Two particularly common clinical presentations of mixed affective states are defined as follows:

- A person with primarily depressive complaints, who has two or more hypomanic symptoms occurring simultaneously (such as goal-directed hyperactivity, grandiosity, racing thoughts, hypersexuality, pressured speech, reduced need for sleep, or severe aggressiveness)
- An individual with primarily elevated mood symptoms who also has interspersed two or more depressed symptoms (depressed mood, suicidal ideation, lack of interest in activities, or hypersomnia).

The definition of a mixed affective state and its clinical recognition is more than simply a theoretical interest. Patients experiencing mixed episodes tend to be chronic and difficult to treat (6) . Of specific concern to clinicians is the level of suicidality in these patients with mixed affective episodes. Suicidality has been noted to be significantly higher in elevated mood patients with mixed mania when compared with nonmanic patients (54.5% vs. 2%) (7–9).

Characteristics of mixed affective states

Demographic elements of mixed affective states have been further elucidated, as shown in Table 8.3.

A number of sources have suggested that mixed states are more common in women than in men, particularly during the postpartum period (10–14). For women, also, the incidence of depressive symptoms generally increases with the severity of hypomania; there is a similar, but weaker relationship, shown in men. In women, however, it is a nonlinear response, showing that at the highest levels of hypomania the rate of mixed symptoms declines, whereas the relationship for men is linear throughout.

TABLE 8.3

Demographic elements of mixed affective states

1. Incidence significantly greater in women than in men

2. Common comorbidities of substance abuse and other psychiatric conditions

3. More incidence of earlier depressive episodes than manic episodes

4. A family history with predominantly depressive, rather than manic episodes.

5. Men with high incidence of irritability and agitation

6. High suicide risk

Adapted from Freeman MP, McElroy SL. Clinical picture and etiologic models f mixed states. *Psychiatr Clin North Am.* 1999;22[3]:535–546, vii; Akiskal HS, Hantouche EG, Bourgeois ML, et al. Gender, temperament, and clinical picture in dysphoric mixed mania: Findings from a French national study [EPIMAN]. *J Affect Disord.* 1998;50:175–186; Perugi G, Akiskal HS, Micheli C, et al. Clinical characterization of depressive mixed state in bipolar I patients. *J Affect Disord.* 2001;57:105–114, (10–12).

An important clue

A diagnostic clue to the presence of a mixed affective state may occur when a mood stabilizer is used to treat a misdiagnosed bipolar disorder without recognition of the mixed state. Patients quickly report feeling "much worse" on mood stabilizer monotherapy. In this case, the mood stabilizer (e.g., lithium, valproic acid, or carbamazepine—all of which are more effective on elevated mood symptoms than on depressed symptoms) may decrease or eliminate hypomanic elements seen clinically, leaving only the depressed elements. This can lead to the patient feeling significantly more depressed (see Figures 8.1 and 8.2). Patients with mixed states have a mixture of hypomanic and depressed symptomatology. In Figure 8.1, the hypomanic symptoms are in white and the depressive symptoms in crosshatch. Although they are of varying intensities, the symptoms coexist. Figure 8.2 represents the clinical picture after treatment with a mood stabilizer. Here the hypomanic symptoms are lessened considerably, leaving the depressive symptoms more prominent although their absolute severity may be roughly equivalent to that before mood stabilization. The patient perceives this as "increased depression" when, in fact, it is a dampening of the hypomanic symptoms, leaving a picture of predominant depression.

Subsequently, these patients often have a significant aversion to a specific medication, which in their opinion, made them feel worse. It takes some skill on the part of the clinician to convince the patient that although uncomfortable, this reaction carries useful diagnostic information, confirming a mixed affective state. In some cases, the clinician may recommend continued mood stabilizer treatment in combination with an antidepressant. In other cases, it may be more useful to utilize a medication listed in Chapter 7 (e.g.,

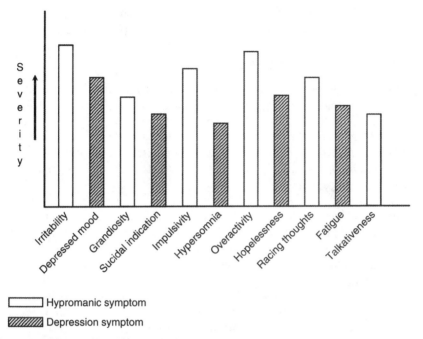

Figure 8.1 Mixed affective state before treatment.

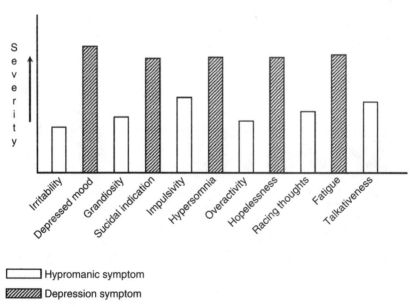

Figure 8.2 Mixed affective state after mood stabilizer.

lamotrigine, fluoxetine/olanzapine combination or an atypical antipsychotic), which may treat both elements of the mixed state more effectively.

Treatment of mixed affective states

Although there is no reference literature on the nonmedication treatment of mixed affective states, education and psychotherapeutic strategies, as outlined in Chapter 6, are likely to be useful techniques.

Despite a more chronic and poorer prognosis, there are a variety of medications that have been shown to be beneficial when treating mixed affective states. The principles guiding the use of medication to treat mixed affective states are listed in Table 8.4.

Although patients with mixed affective states may present with primarily elevated mood and few depressive symptoms, they present more typically with a chief complaint of depressed mood but also have a mixture of accelerated or hypomanic traits. It has been common practice for clinicians to treat this latter group of patients with antidepressants, often because mixed affective state has been undiagnosed. Although there is limited evidence for some beneficial use of antidepressants in treating bipolar depression (15,16), there is virtually no evidence that the use of antidepressants in mixed states is beneficial. A randomized study of the use of imipramine in patients with mixed episodes found no benefit (17) . The Systematic Treatment Enhancement Program for Bipolar Disorder (STEP-BD) Project likewise found no benefit in the use of newer antidepressants in the depressive aspect of mixed affective state (18) . Additionally, there is some suggestion that antidepressants frequently appear to *cause* mixed episodes in bipolar patients (19) . Depressive symptoms did not improve in these patients and manic symptoms worsened (18) . Despite this cited evidence, antidepressants are more frequently prescribed for mixed episodes than for pure mood episodes in the hospital (20) .

Considering this, antidepressants should not be the first-line treatment for individuals diagnosed with a mixed affective state, even if the patient's

TABLE 8.4

Principles in medication treatment of mixed states

- Antidepressant monotherapy is not useful in mixed state treatment and may worsen the prognosis. If antidepressants are considered, use them cautiously after mood stabilization

- Anticonvulsant mood stabilizers, particularly valproic acid, carbamazepine, and lamotrigine, are the cornerstone of mixed affective state treatment

- Lithium, although more effective than placebo, is less helpful than anticonvulsant mood modulators

- All atypical antipsychotics have been shown to be useful as adjunctive treatments or monotherapy in mixed states

- Polypharmacy is often necessary to achieve full stability in mixed affective states

primary complaints are of a depressive nature. Mood stabilizers are the recommended treatment and the core of potential combination treatments. Although lithium is an effective mood stabilizer in prophylaxis of depression and manic phases of bipolar disorder, it is less effective in controlling both manic and depressed symptoms in patients with mixed affective states. Studies have demonstrated that lithium is almost twice as effective in pure manic episodes than in mixed affective episodes (21–24). Valproate has repeatedly been shown useful in a variety of studies when compared to placebo or lithium (25,26). In a study of 179 patients with mixed mania, 72% of patients responded to sodium valproate as compared to 37% to lithium. In fact, the presence of depressive mood symptoms present during mania may be predictive of response to valproate (27).

Carbamazepine, in its newest formulation (Equetro), has also received U.S. Food and Drug Administration (FDA) approval for treatment of mixed affective episodes (28). Because the research into its effectiveness on mixed episodes has only been done with the extended-release compound, it is unclear whether the underlying molecule, carbamazepine, is similarly effective.

Lamotrigine, also an anticonvulsant, has also been shown to be useful in mixed affective states and is particularly effective with depressed symptoms in this diagnosis (29).

Atypical antipsychotics

Atypical antipsychotics are clinically effective in mixed state treatment. Aripiprazole, olanzapine, risperidone, and ziprasidone have all received FDA approval for the treatment of mixed episodes.

Aripiprazole has been shown to be both a treatment for acute mania and a treatment for mixed episodes (30–32). Clinical global improvement scores improved in patients treated with aripiprazole and having mixed episode states with a bipolar I diagnosis.

Olanzapine has also shown benefit in the treatment of mixed mania when compared to sodium valproate (33,34). In 251 manic or mixed patients, those treated with olanzapine showed significantly greater improvement in Young Mania Rating scores (YMRS) as compared to patients taking sodium valproate. Olanzapine patients also experienced a greater improvement in depression as measured by Hamilton Rating Scale for Depression (HAM-D) scores. A recent study demonstrated the efficacy of olanzapine in preventing relapse of all mood states of bipolar disorder. This was the first study that presented data regarding the use of olanzapine versus placebo in specifically preventing mixed affective states (31) .

Risperidone has been effective both as monotherapy and as an augmentation agent for manic and mixed symptoms. Because it has also shown some efficacy in depressive symptoms, it could be considered for patients experiencing mixed episodes (35) .

In addition to its effectiveness in acute mania, *ziprasidone* has also been studied with mixed episode patients. In a 3-week study, patients treated with ziprasidone showed a statistically significant improvement compared with placebo in both YMRS and HAM-D scores (36,37).

Quetiapine, although effective for acute mania, has not been sufficiently tested in patients with mixed affective episodes. An 8-week double-blind study comparing quetiapine with placebo in patients with bipolar depression showed significant response. Additionally, quetiapine has demonstrated usefulness in rapid cycling bipolar disorder (RCBD) (36) .

As noted elsewhere in the text, effectiveness is not the only criteria in selecting an agent to treat mixed affective states. One should, therefore, also consider the following:

- Does the agent worsen depressive symptoms?
- Does the medication worsen manic symptoms?
- Does the medication have significant side effects, particularly weight gain and possible induction of metabolic syndrome?

Treatment with atypical antipsychotic medications has evidenced no exacerbation of mania or depression; however, atypical antipsychotics carry a class warning for possible induction of metabolic syndrome. Although atypical antipsychotics do affect glucose and lipid metabolism with the potential development of metabolic syndrome, clozapine and olanzapine are associated with the greatest increased risk of developing diabetes mellitus and dyslipidemia. The newest atypical antipsychotics, ziprasidone and aripiprazole, have shown virtually no increased risk of diabetes or dyslipidemia (37) .

Rapid cycling bipolar disorder

In the 19th century, Emil Kraeplin described rapid cycling bipolar disorder as follows: "At times the malady begins with a close series of very short attacks following very quickly one after the other . . . that is especially the case in a small group of youthful patients preferably, as it seems, women" (38). Kraeplin saw this as a phase of the illness and not necessarily a separate illness category. With the advent of the DSM and its revisions, rapid cycling has been a specifier that can be applied to either bipolar I or bipolar II disorder with criteria as listed in Table 8.5.

TABLE 8.5

Diagnostic and Statistical Manual of Mental Disorders (DSM-IV) text revision (TR) criteria for rapid cycling specifier

At least four episodes of a mood disturbance in the previous 12 months that meet criteria for a major depressive, manic, mixed or hypomanic episode

Note: Episodes are demarcated either by partial or full remission for at least 2 months or a switch to an episode of opposite polarity (e.g., major depressive episode to manic episode).

Although not found in the DSM, common usage has defined other rapid cycling types that include the so-called "ultra rapid" cycling having four or more episodes per *month* and ultradian cycling, in which mood cycles occur within a day at least four times per week.

Characteristics of rapid cycling

Although patients with RCBD have been studied significantly over the past three decades, precise knowledge remains limited. Generally accepted RCBD characteristics are listed in Table 8.6.

Patients who experience a period of rapid cycling some time in their disorder have a history of earlier onset, increased time ill, increased frequency of episodes, and an overall poorer prognosis. Such patients often have an onset in prepubertal or early teen years, predominately with depressed symptoms. Geller et al. have shown that as many as 87% of prepubescent and early adolescent bipolar individuals have rapid cycling (43,44). Of this group, 10% had ultrarapid cycling and 77% had ultradian cycling. In addition to early onset, patients with RCBD have a higher incidence of suicide attempts, a higher incidence of depressive symptoms in any week and more morbidity from three depressive symptoms. Of this group followed up in the Stanley Foundation Bipolar Network, 23% experienced rapid cycling, 10% ultrarapid cycling, and 20% ultradian cycling (45) .

Despite the seriousness and increased morbidity of rapid cycling periods, these episodes appear to be self-limited in time and generally resolve within a 2- to 5-year time frame (46) . Even when the rapid cycling portion resolves, the increased morbidity frequency remains lifelong.

TABLE 8.6

Characteristics of rapid cycling bipolar disorder

- Higher incidence in women
- Higher incidence in bipolar II subtype
- Earlier age of onset
- Longer duration of illness
- Higher morbidity
- Depression at onset
- Family history of major affective disorder
- Higher incidence of suicide attempt
- Poor therapeutic and prophylactic response to lithium

Adapted from (39–42).

Causes of rapid cycling

There has been considerable speculation about the etiology of rapid cycling. Some of this speculation has focused on changes in circadian rhythm including bright light and darkness exposure (47–49). There is some evidence to suggest that clinical hypothyroidism also predisposes to RCBD (50,51). The most controversial and potentially important cause or exacerbating factor for rapid cycling is the use of antidepressant medications in genetically susceptible bipolar individuals. This has been extensively discussed in chapters 4 and 7 on depression and medication treatments. Kilzieh and Akiskal (52) have also suggested that the presence of cyclothymia may be considered as a normal variant of rapid cycling. Research completed to date has not conclusively elucidated any firm conclusions that can be drawn as to the causative factors in RCBD. Unfortunately, as discussed by several authors, the severity of illness in RCBD precludes the double-blind controlled investigations that would potentially identify causative factors as well as treatment alternatives.

Medication treatment for rapid cycling

A variety of studies, with many of them having been completed during the 1970s and 1980s, suggest that lithium monotherapy, carbamazepine monotherapy, and lithium/carbamazepine combinations have poor or limited response in patients with RCBD (53–55).

On the basis of several studies conducted in the early 1990s, combinations of anticonvulsants have been considered the most useful treatment for RCBD (56–58). These conclusions, however, have been challenged by a recent large scale study of valproic acid and lithium in RCBD. An open label acute stabilization phase of treatment study that enrolled 254 patients was conducted by Calabrese et al. (59) and published in 2005. These patients were then followed up to determine the length of time until relapse. This study showed that valproic acid was no more effective than lithium in the long-term management of RCBD in preventing relapse, particularly depressive relapses. Valproic acid was however better tolerated, with fewer discontinuations for side effects.

To date, there has been only one prospective, placebo-controlled study of lamotrigine in RCBD that was conducted by Calabrese et al. (60) . In this study, 324 patients with RCBD were stabilized on a variety of psychotropic regimens to which lamotrigine was added. Once stabilized, patients were tapered off other psychotropics and randomly assigned to lamotrigine or placebo monotherapy for 6 months. Forty-one percent of the monotherapy lamotrigine patients remained stable without relapse for 6 months. Only 26% of placebo-treated patients remained stable without relapse. Although the difference between treatment groups did not achieve statistical significance in the overall efficacy population, lamotrigine did show efficacy in a significant number of patients. Given the effectiveness of lamotrigine in the depressed phase of bipolar illness and considering the frequency of depression in rapid cycling patients, this data is consistent with other studies, suggesting that lamotrigine is useful in a variety of bipolar conditions where depression is a predominant clinical factor.

Although atypical antipsychotics have emerged as very effective treatments for a variety of bipolar states, RCBD is one condition in which there is limited evidence for their usefulness (61–64). Evidence for the use of atypical antipsychotics in RCBD is primarily from secondary analyses of groupings of manic patients that included both rapid cycling and non–rapid cycling patients. These secondary analyses indicate that risperidone and olanzapine have short-term (6 weeks) efficacy that was approximately equivalent for both rapid cycling and non–rapid cycling patients. Although speculative, other atypical antipsychotics including aripiprazole, ziprasidone, quetiapine, and clozapine with their proven antimanic effects might also be useful for the manic side of rapid cycling symptoms.

Other studies have looked at the usefulness of atypical antipsychotics as add-on therapy to other psychotropic regimens in patients with RCBD. Quetiapine has been shown to be useful as add-on therapy in this group (65,66). Calabrese et al. used clozapine to treat a group of bipolar patients, including those with rapid cycling. Positive treatment effects were similar for cycling and non–rapid cycling patients (67).

Recommendations

Although limited and incomplete, the overall evidence-based medication guidelines for the treatment of RCBD are as follows:

- Anticonvulsants, in general, are poor treatments for RCBD, although valproic acid may be useful in patients with primarily manic symptomatology.
- Lamotrigine is helpful in RCBD for patients with predominantly depressive symptomatology.
- Traditional antidepressants are not useful and may actually worsen the prognosis in RCBD.
- Atypical antipsychotics may be useful add-on therapies for RCBD. Quetiapine, risperidone, and clozapine have demonstrated clinical evidence of effectiveness. Other atypical antipsychotics with favorable side effect profiles may also be beneficial.
- Lithium and carbamazepine, although helpful for pure euphoric type bipolar disorder, have less usage in rapid cycling.
- Alcohol, caffeine, stimulants, and sleep deprivation are generally negative stimuli and should be avoided.

The bottom line

- Mixed affective states are far more common than originally believed.
- The presence of mixed affective states is predictive of increased treatment difficulty and higher suicidal ideation.
- Mixed affective states are more common in women, are frequently co-morbid with substance abuse, and show more depressive than hypomanic symptoms. Men with a high incidence of irritability and agitation also show a higher incidence of mixed states.
- Mood stabilization is the cornerstone of medication treatment for mixed affective episodes.
- Antidepressant monotherapy is highly discouraged for the mixed state.

REFERENCES

1. Bauer MS. 'Bipolarity' in bipolar disorder: Distribution of manic and depressive symptoms in a treated population. *Br J Psychiatry Suppl.* 2005;198:87–88.
2. Benazzi F. *Bipolar II disorder: Current issues in diagnosis and management.* www.psychiatrictimes.com, accessed 2006
3. Benazzi F. Mood patterns and classification in bipolar disorder. *Curr Opin Psychiatry.* 2006;19:1–8.
4. Akiskal HS, Benazzi F. Toward a clinical delineation of dysphoric hypomania: Operational and conceptual dilemmas. *Bipolar Disord.* 2005;7:456–464.
5. Suppes T, McElroy SL, Altshuler LL, et al. Mixed hypomania in 908 patients with bipolar disorder evaluated prospectively in the Stanley Bipolar Treatment Network: A sex-specific phenomenon. *Arch Gen Psychiatry.* 2005;62:1089–1096.
6. McElroy SL, Keck PE, Pope HS, et al. Clinical and research implications of the diagnosis of dysphoric or mixed mania or hypomania. *Am J Psychiatry.* 1993;150(12):1907–1909.
7. Dilsaver SC, Chen YW, Swann AC, et al. Suicidality in patients with pure and depressive mania. *Am J Psychiatry.* 1994;151:1312–1315.
8. Suppes T, Mintz J, McElroy SL, et al. Mixed hypomania in 908 patients with bipolar disorder evaluated prospectively in the Stanley Foundation Bipolar Treatment Network. *Arch Gen Psychiatry.* 2005;62:1089–1096.
9. Goldberg JF, Garno JL, Leon AC, et al. Association of recurrent suicidal ideation with nonremission from acute mixed mania. *Am J Psychiatry.* 2005;155:173–1955.
10. Freeman MP, McElroy SL. Clinical picture and etiologic models f mixed states. *Psychiatr Clin North Am.* 1999;22(3):535–546, vii.
11. Akiskal HS, Hantouche EG, Bourgeois ML, et al. Gender, temperament, and clinical picture in dysphoric mixed mania: Findings from a French national study (EPIMAN). *J Affect Disord.* 1998;50:175–186.
12. Perugi G, Akiskal HS, Micheli C, et al. Clinical characterization of depressive mixed state in bipolar I patients. *J Affect Disord.* 2001;57:105–114.
13. Dell'Osso L, Placidi GF, Nassi R, et al. The manic depressive mixed state: Familial, temperamental and psychopathologic characteristics in 108 female inpatients. *Eur Arch Psychiatry Clin Neurosci.* 1991;240:234–239.
14. McElroy SL, Strakowski SM, Keck PE Jr, et al. Differences and similarities in mixed and pure mania. *Compr Psychiatry.* 1995;36:198–194.

15. Gijsman H, Geddes JR, Rendell JM, et al. Antidepressants for bipolar depression: A systematic review of randomized, controlled trials. *Am J Psychiatry.* 2004;161:1537–1547.
16. Prien RF, Himmelhoch JM, Kupfer DJ. Treatment of mixed mania. *J Affect Disord.* 1988;15:9–15.
17. Prien RF, Himmelhoch JM, Kupfer DJ. Treatment of mixed mania. *J Affect Disord.* 1988;15(1):9–15.
18. Schneck CD, Miklowitz DJ, Calabrese JR, et al. Phenomenology of rapid cycling bipolar disorder: Data from the first 500 participants in the systematic treatment enhancement program for bipolar disorder. *Am J Psychiatry.* 2004;161:1902–1908.
19. Simon NM, Otto MW, Weiss RD, et al. Pharmacotherapy for bipolar disorder and comorbid conditions: Baseline data from STEP-BD. *J Clin Psychopharamcol.* 2004;24:512–520.
20. Keck PE, McElroy SL, Arnold LM. Bipolar disorder. *Med Clin North Am.* 2001;85:645–661. RJ.
21. Keller MB, Lavori PW, Coryell W, et al. Differential outcome of pure manic, mixed cycling, and pure depressive episodes in patients with Bipolar illness. *JAMA.* 1986;255(22):3138–3142.
22. Prien RF, Himmelhoch JM, Kupfer DJ. Treatment of mixed mania. *J Affect Disord*1988;15(1):9–15.
23. Secunda SK, Swann A, Katz MM, et al. Diagnosis and treatment of mixed mania. *Am J Psychiatry.* 1987;144(1):96–98.
24. Weisler RH, Hirshfeld R, Cutler AJ, et al. *17th Annual US Psychiatric and Mental Health Congress. [Abstract 24].* San Diego, CA: November 18–21, 2004.
25. Freeman TW, Clothier JL, Pazzaglia P, et al. A double-blind comparison of valproate and lithium in the treatment of acute mania. *Am J Psychiatry.* 1992;149: 108–111.
26. Dilsaver SC, Swann AC, Shoaib AM, et al. The manic syndrome: Factors which may predict a patient's response to lithium, carbamazepine and valproate. *J Psychiatry Neurosci.* 1993;18(2):61–66.
27. Swann AC, Bowden CL, Morris D, et al. Depression during mania: Treatment response to lithium or divalproex. *Arch Gen Psychiatry.* 1997;54:37–42.
28. Shire Pharmaceuticals. *Equetro prescribing information.* Wayne, PA: Shire Pharmaceuticals. 2005.
29. Calabrese JR, Bowden CL, Sachs GS, et al. Lamictal 602 Study Group. A double-blind placebo-controlled study of lamotrigine monotherapy in outpatients with bipolar I depression. *J Clin Psychiatry.* 1999;60:79–88.
30. Gupta S, Masand P. Aripiprazole: Review of its pharmacology and therapeutic use in psychiatric disorders. *Ann Clin Psychiatry.* 2004;16(3):155–166.
31. Sachs G, Sanchez R, Marcus R, et al. Aripiprazole in the treatment of acute manic or mixed episodes in patients with bipolar I disorder: A three-week placebo-controlled study. *J Psychopharmacol.* 2006;20(4):536–546.
32. Keck PE Jr, Calabrese JR, McQuade RD, et al. Aripiprazole study placebo-controlled 26-week trial of aripiprazole in recently manic patients with bipolar I disorder. *J Clin Psych.* 2006;67:626–637.
33. Tohen M, Calabrese JR, Sachs GS, et al. Olanzapine in the treatment of bipolar I disorder: Randomized, placebo-controlled trial of olanzapine as maintenance therapy in patients with bipolar I disorder responding to acute treatment with olanzapine. *Am J Psychiatry.* 2006;163:247–256.

34. Tohen M, Ketter TA, Zarate CA, et al. Olanzapine versus divalproex sodium for the treatment of acute mania and maintenance of remission: A 47-week study. *Am J Psychiatry.* 2003;160(7):1253–1271.

35. Sachs G, Grossman F, Okamoto A, et al. Risperidone plus mood stabilizer versus placebo plus mood stabilizer for acute mania of bipolar disorder: A double-blind comparison of efficacy and safety. *Am J Psychiatry.* 2002;159:1446–1154.

36. Vieta E, Parramon G, Padrell E, et al. Quetiapine in the treatment of rapid cycling bipolar disorder. *Bipolar Disord.* 2002;4:335–340.

37. Newcomer J. Second-generation (atypical) antipsychotics and metabolic effects: A comprehensive literature review. *CNS Drugs.* 2005;19(Suppl 1):1–93.

38. Kraepelin E. *Manic depressive insanity and paranoia.* Edinburgh: Churchill Livingstone; 1921.

39. Maj M, Pirozzi R, Formicola AMR, et al. Reliability and validity of four alternative definitions of rapid cycling bipolar disorder. *Am J Psychiatry.* 1991;156:1421–1421.

40. Coryell W, Endicott J, Keller M, et al. Rapid cycling affective disorder: Demographics, diagnosis family history and course. *Arch Gen Psychiatry.* 1992;49:126–123.

41. Mackin P, Young AH. Rapid cycling bipolar disorder: Historical overview and focus on emerging treatments. *Bipolar Disord.* 2004;6:523–529.

42. Coryell W, Solomon D, Turvey C, et al. The long-term course of rapid-cycling bipolar disorder. *Arch Gen Psychiatry.* 2003;60:914–920.

43. Geller B, Sun K, Zimerman B, et al. Complex and rapid-cycling in bipolar children and adolescents: A preliminary study. *J Affect Disord.* 1995;34(4):259–268.

44. Geller B, Craney JL, Bolhofner K, et al. One-year recovery and relapse rates of children with a pre-pubertal and early adolescent bipolar disorder phenotype. *Am J Psychiatry.* 2001;158:303–305.

45. Kupka RW, Nolen WA, Altshuler LL, et al. The Stanley Foundation Bipolar Network: Preliminary summary of demographics, course of illness and response to novel treatments. *Br J Psychiatry Suppl.* 2001;178:s177–s183.

46. Coryell W. Rapid cycling bipolar disorder: Clinical characteristics and treatment options. *CNS Drugs.* 2005;19(7):557–569.

47. Leibenluft E, Albert PS, Rosenthal NE, et al. Relationship between sleep and mood in patients with rapid-cycling bipolar disorder. *Psychiatry Res.* 1996;63(2–3):161–168.

48. Wehr TA, Turner EH, Shimada JM, et al. Treatment of a rapidly cycling bipolar patient by using extended bed rest and darkness to stabilize the timing and duration of sleep. *Biol Psychiatry.* 1999;43:822–828.

49. Wirz-Justice A, Quinto C, Cajochen C, et al. A rapid-cycling bipolar patient treated with long nights, bedrest and light. *Biol Psychiatry.* 1999;45:1075–1077.

50. Cowdry RW, Wehr TA, Zis AP, et al. Thyroid abnormalities associated with rapid-cycling bipolar illness. *Arch Gen Psychiatry.* 1983;40:414–420.

51. Bauer MS, Whybrow PC, Winokur A. Rapid cycling bipolar affective disorder. I. Associate with grade 1 hypothyroidism. *Arch Gen Psychiatry.* 1990;47:427–432.

52. Kilzieh N, Akiskal HS. Rapid-cycling bipolar disorder: An overview of research and clinical experience. *Psychatr Clin North Am.* 1999;22:585–607.

53. Dunner DL, Fieve RR. Clinical factors in lithium carbonate prophylaxis failure. *Arch Gen Psychiatry.* 1974;30:229–233.

54. Okuma T. Effects of carbamazepine and lithium on affective disorders. *Neuropsychobiology.* 1993;27:138–145.

55. Koukopoulos A, Reginalsi D, Laddomada P. Course of the manic-depressive cycle and changes caused by treatments. *Pharmacopsychiatry*. 1980;13:156–167.
56. Barrios C, Chaudhry TA, Goodnick PJ. Rapid cycling bipolar disorder. *Expert Opin Pharmacother*. 2001;2:1963–1973.
57. Sharma V, Persad E, Mazmanian D, et al. Treatment of rapid cycling bipolar disorder with combination therapy of valproate and lithium. *Can J Psychaitry*. 1993;38:137–139.
58. Coryell W. Rapid cycling bipolar disorder: Clinical characteristics and treatment options. *CNS Drugs*. 2005;19:557–569.
59. Calabrese JR, Shelton MD, Rapport DJ, et al. A 20-month, double-blind, maintenance trial of lithium versus divalproex in rapid-cycling bipolar disorder. *Am J Psychiatry*. 2005;162:2152–2161.
60. Calabrese JR, Bowden CL, Sachs GS, et al. A double-blind placebo-controlled study of lamotrigine monotherapy in outpatients with bipolar I depression. Lamictal 602 Study Group. *J Clin Psychiatry*. 1999;60:79–88.
61. Ghaemi SN, Goodwin FK. Use of atypical antipsychotic agents in bipolar and schizoaffective disorders: Review of the empirical literature. *J Clin Psychopharmacol*. 1999;19(4):354–361.
62. Sajatovic M, DiGiovanni SK, Bastani B, et al. Risperidone therapy in treatment refractory acute bipolar and schizoaffective mania. *Psychopharmacol Bull*. 1996;32(1):55–61.
63. Vieta E, Goikolea JM. Atypical antipsychotics: Newer options for mania and maintenance therapy. *Bipolar Disord*. 2005;7(Suppl 4):21–33.
64. Vieta E, Gasto C, Colom F, et al. Letter to the editor: Treatment of refractory rapid cycling bipolar disorder with risperidone. *J Clin Psychopharmacol*. 1998;18(2):172–174.
65. Ghaemi SN, Katzow JJ. The use of quetiapine for treatment-resistant bipolar disorder: A case series. *Ann Clin Psychiatry*. 1999;11(3):137–140.
66. Dunayevich E, Strakowski FM. Quetiapine for treatment-resistant mania. *Am J Psychiatry*. 2000;157(8):134.
67. Calabrese JR, Kimmel SE, Woyshville MJ, et al. Clozapine for treatment-refractory depression. *Am J Psychiatry*. 1996;153(6):759–764.

9

ROUGHENING— WHEN TREATMENT FAILS

- Reevaluation
- Alcohol and recreational drugs
- Talking therapy
- Compliance

- Change medications and combination therapy
- Consultation
- The bottom line
  References

O nce patients with elevated mood are stabilized with psychotherapy, psychoeducation, lifestyle management, and medication, they may remain stable for an extended period. It is not uncommon, however, to have breakthrough mood episodes, the severity of which may vary. Breakthrough symptoms can consist of elevated mood symptoms, depressive symptoms, or mixed states. When these symptoms are significant, we label them as *relapse*; when they are mild to moderate, a descriptive, frequently used term is "*roughening*." When roughening or relapse occurs, many practitioners automatically reach for the prescription pad to change or add medication. Although an alteration of medication may remedy the problem, a structured format to assess all the possible causes for re-emergence of symptoms is desirable. The elements for this format are outlined in Table 9.1.

Although this acronym, TRACCCC, is useful to remember the elements that need to be considered, most clinicians would apply these actions in a different order of priority (**R**eevaluation, **A**lcohol, **C**ompliance, **T**alking therapy, **C**hanging medication, **C**ombination therapy, **C**onsultation).

Reevaluation

The emergence of symptoms, whether new or previously experienced, is an ideal opportunity to reconsider the clinician's initial assessment. In addition to the initial diagnosis, the patient's medication regimen, lifestyle issues, alcohol and drug use, and compliance should be addressed and reevaluated.

TABLE 9.1
Getting back on TRACCCC

Talking therapy
Reevaluation
Alcohol and drugs
Compliance
Change medication
Combination therapy
Consultation

From Doran CM. *Prescribing mental health medications: The practitioner's guide.* London: Routledge; 2003:109, (1).

The initial assessment could have been incorrect or only partially correct. In an elevated mood patient, a depressive episode, dysthymia, or mixed state may have emerged. New anxiety symptoms such as panic attacks, social anxiety, or generalized anxiety may appear. Especially if there has been a lengthy interval since the initial evaluation, the clinician should conduct a fresh assessment of symptomatology. Queries about symptoms that may have been given negative responses in the past may now be answered positively. It is surprising how often during a reevaluation the patient's recollection of his or her condition and history may be different from that initially described. There are several reasons for this:

- The patient may have developed new symptoms that were not present originally.
- The patient may have begun to reformulate ideas about certain behaviors or feelings as "symptoms" that were not identified as part of the initial symptom picture.
- Some patients may now, with increasing trust in the clinician, be willing to reveal symptoms that they were embarrassed to admit during an initial session. Suicidality, rage reactions, hypersexuality, substance abuse, or impulsive actions may have not been reported for fear that the clinician might look down on them or refuse to treat them.

The clinician will want to evaluate the time course of symptom development, especially those associated with life events. When did breakthrough symptoms begin? Was the onset sudden (more often associated with life events) or gradual (more often associated with a biologic breakthrough)?

- What are the specific symptoms the patient experiences now?
- How are these symptoms similar to previous episodes? What symptoms are new?
- What significant life stressors/changes have occurred in the patient's life during the period just before the onset of breakthrough symptoms?

Although it may seem obvious to a clinician, it is remarkable how frequently a patient may have experienced a significant life stressor, and a subsequent breakthrough mood episode, but failed to connect the two events.

When a symptomatic crisis occurs, it is essential that the clinician reevaluate the patient's medical status. Look for new medical conditions that may be interfering with the patient's stability. Common medical conditions to be considered include diabetes, hypertension, mononucleosis, and hepatitis. The clinician should also consider medical complications secondary to prescribed psychotropic medication. For example, the use of lithium may have caused decreased thyroid function. Patients can develop frank hypothyroidism from lithium treatment resulting in depressed mood, low pulse, low blood pressure, fatigue, or sensitivity to cold. Similarly, liver function abnormalities can be caused by a variety of mood stabilizers and antidepressants. Laboratory evaluation of the patient who develops a symptomatic relapse should include tests of kidney and liver function, fasting blood sugar, thyroid-stimulating hormone (TSH), complete blood count (CBC) and, when appropriate, serum blood levels of psychotropics being taken.

The patient should be specifically questioned on what medications—both prescription and over-the-counter—he or she is currently taking and inquire whether the starting times of any new medications correspond with the onset of symptomatic worsening. Patients should also be questioned about any recent changes from brand name to generic prescriptions. Although relatively uncommon, some patients do not absorb medications equally well from brand name and generic preparations. This can lead to altered serum and brain blood levels of the psychotropics, with resultant breakthrough symptoms or new side effects.

Alcohol and recreational drugs

It is necessary to inquire about the patient's use of alcohol or recreational drugs at the time of a symptomatic breakthrough. Alcohol or drug usage is one of the most common behaviors minimized by patients, either when initially evaluated or during a reevaluation. The patient may not have been using substances at the time of initial evaluation but has begun to do so, leading to a symptomatic breakthrough. If the clinician's suspicions remain high despite the patient's denial of substance usage, it may be warranted to draw a blood alcohol level, a serum Gamma-glutamyltransferase (GGT) (often the first liver enzyme to be elevated in the presence of excess alcohol usage), or a toxicology blood screen.

Talking therapy

Patients who are initially stabilized and doing well on a "medication only" regimen that develops a symptomatic crisis may need more than just medication. If psychotherapy was not provided at the outset of therapy, conditions may have changed, making psychotherapy an important recommendation. Patients with new stressors may be helped considerably by a course of individual, cognitive, couple, or family therapy. Clinicians may find that patients who were initially resistant to psychotherapy, are now more amenable to other therapeutic options.

Compliance

Lack of compliance with a previously effective medication regimen will often cause loss of response or symptom breakthrough. When evaluating this issue, it is often best to ask an open-ended question: "Tell me what medications you are taking and when you are taking them." Sometimes what the clinician is prescribing and has documented in the patient's chart is not what the patient has been taking! If non-compliance may be a significant factor in a symptomatic breakthrough, the clinician should learn how frequently there is a discrepancy between the full regimen and what the patient usually takes.

Change medications and combination therapy

If elevated mood symptoms emerge in a previously stable patient, it may be useful to change mood stabilizers in order to re-equilibrate the patient. Often the use of medications from different classes will promote synergy between the two medications, which together can restore symptomatic control. Although monotherapy is desirable, combination therapy and the use of multiple mood stabilizers, antipsychotics, and antidepressants is common. If a patient becomes hypomanic and is taking an antidepressant, it may be helpful to lower the dose or discontinue the antidepressant. In the latter case, unless the elevated mood symptoms are severe, it is best to stop the antidepressant gradually to minimize the likelihood of rebound depression. Concomitantly, especially if the elevated mood symptoms are significant, the clinician may also increase the dose of mood stabilizer.

Consultation

If, after a thorough evaluation of these elements and particularly if restabilization is proving difficult, consultation may be the most helpful next step. Consulting with a knowledgeable colleague or a psychopharmacologist may provide a "fresh look" at the patient's issues. In addition to providing the primary clinician added clinical information, such consultation can be seen as a helpful step, especially in patients who have become pessimistic about their condition. Through the process of consultation, patients often renew willingness to continue efforts toward eventual stability.

The bottom line

• Symptomatic relapse or roughening is common in patients with bipolar disorder.
• Although the addition or change of medication may be necessary, other factors must be considered in a systematic manner. These include the following:
  ○ Diagnostic reevaluation
  ○ Medication compliance and side effects
  ○ Substance use
  ○ The need for psychotherapy
• When restabilization proves difficult obtain a consultation.

REFERENCE

1. Doran CM. *Prescribing mental health medications: The practitioner's guide.* London: Routledge; 2003:109.

10

AGITATED ACTIVATION, ANXIETY, AND ELEVATED MOOD

- Anxiety and elevated mood diagnosis
- Anxiety comorbid with elevated mood
- Other anxiety connections
- Specific anxiety questions in bipolar mood disorder
- Akathisia
- Tremor
- Medication treatments for anxiety in elevated mood

Valproic acid
Carbamazepine
Lamotrigine
Atypical antipsychotics
Antidepressants
Other antiepileptics
Benzodiazepines
- The bottom line
  References

The likelihood that patients with hypomania will present for clinical care in the depressed state has been discussed in Chapter 4. This section now elaborates on another diagnostic confound, the relationship between anxiety and hypomania. A number of studies (1–6) report the high prevalence of anxiety in bipolar disorder. Although many psychiatric conditions are comorbid with bipolar disorder, 95.5% of the national comorbidity survey patients with bipolar I disorder met the criteria for three or more additional psychiatric disorders. Of these comorbid disorders, anxiety disorders were the most common. Boylan et al. (2) demonstrated that over half the number of patients with bipolar disorder had at least one comorbid anxiety disorder and a third of those patients had multiple anxiety disorders. The Systematic Treatment Enhancement Program for Bipolar Disorder (STEP-BD) found that half the number of the patients studied showed a lifetime comorbid anxiety disorder. The comorbidity was higher for patients with bipolar II than bipolar I disorder. Anxiety has multiple negative effects on the outcome and treatment response of individuals with bipolar disorder. The presence of anxiety in bipolar illness is associated with an earlier age of onset, decreased response to treatment, increased use of substances, decreased quality of life, and increased rates of suicide (6).

Anxiety and elevated mood diagnosis

Patients may present with overactivated, agitated, or anxious symptoms intermingled with mood symptoms or may present with symptoms of anxiety alone. The challenge for the clinician is to discern the cause of the activated or anxious state, one of which may be hypomania. There are, however, a number of other conditions—both psychiatric and medical—which can co-occur with hypomania. These comorbid conditions can challenge the most seasoned clinician because *anxiety and overactivation may be intrinsic parts of the elevated mood syndrome or be a separate comorbid condition.* Patients with elevated mood may present as agitated, anxious, and overactive and complain of anxiety. However, this is not universally true. Many hypomanic individuals, while overactive and hyperenergetic, neither subjectively feel anxious nor necessarily present an anxious appearance to the clinician. They may appear energized, busy, and productive, and have perceived themselves as nonanxious, mentally sharp, and "clicking on all eight cylinders". The course of treatment may be quite different for anxiety that is an intrinsic part of an elevated mood state, and anxiety that is referable to another condition. An accurate diagnosis, therefore, for anxiety is critical. Consider the causes of anxiety listed in Table 10.1.

Anxiety, as perceived by the patient and described to the clinician, may present in a variety of ways. The patient may describe feelings of mental nervousness or agitation, being emotionally "out of control," feeling mentally speeded or pressured, being unable to slow down, and having difficulty falling or staying asleep. Anxiety may present as panic attacks, internal restlessness, fidgeting/pacing, physical shakiness, or tremor. When hypomania is associated with anxiety, these symptoms rarely occur in isolation and are usually accompanied by one or more of the following:

- Rapid speech
- Increased speed of thought
- Lack of need to sleep
- Impulsive and/or dangerous behavior
- Displays of unusual energy

TABLE 10.1
Anxiety and elevated mood

When present with elevated mood, anxiety may be

- an intrinsic element of the hypomanic state
- a symptom of a primary anxiety disorder or another psychiatric condition other than hypomania
- a side effect of OTC or prescription medication
- a symptom of a medical condition

- Feelings of exceptional well-being
- Hypersexuality
- Grandiose ideation

Another cue to anxiety being part of hypomania is that the anxiety is episodic, rather than continuous, being punctuated by long periods without anxious symptoms. Anxiety, when due to hypomania, often presents a constellation of symptoms including those listed in the preceding text that recur periodically and predictably. Normal mood and energy, or even periods of anergia and nonproductivity may be present episodically, and during these times, the patient does not complain of anxiety. When antidepressants have been used to treat depression and the symptoms of hypomania and anxiety are in temporal correlation to the use of these antidepressants, there is a distinct possibility that the anxiety is a symptom of a hypomanic syndrome precipitated by antidepressant use.

Anxiety comorbid with elevated mood

As has been noted, patients with bipolar disorder or hypomania may have a variety of comorbid diagnosable anxiety disorders and, in some cases exhibit symptoms of more than one anxiety disorder. These are shown in Table 10.2.

Generalized anxiety disorder. With this comorbidity, the patients are consistently anxious, maintaining high levels of anxiety regardless of precipitants. They often worry excessively about areas of life including occupation, family relationships, finances, parenting, sexual relationships, medications, medication side effects, and potential lack of response to treatment, to name a few. Although environmental precipitants may make the anxiety worse, these patients are anxious and worried even in the absence of negative life precipitants.

Panic attacks and panic disorder. Elevated mood patients may have isolated rare panic attacks or have frequent debilitating episodes, constituting a panic disorder diagnosis. In some patients, the panic attacks are limited to the elevated mood state. For others, attacks are seemingly unrelated to any specific mood state occurring spontaneously

TABLE 10.2

Conditions that may be comorbid with hypomania

Generalized anxiety disorder
Panic disorder
Obsessive-compulsive disorder
Social anxiety disorder
Post-traumatic stress disorder
Separation anxiety disorder (in children)

in response to trigger behaviors or phobias such as flying, public speaking, highway driving, heights, closed spaces or fear of being alone. Patients with bipolar disorder may experience panic attacks as a side effect to the initiation of antidepressant medication. When this occurs, other hypomanic symptoms usually accompany the onset of panic attacks. These can include difficulty sleeping, a heightened level of mental and behavioral arousal, physical hyperactivity, and racing thoughts. On occasion, the new onset or worsening of panic attacks in a patient who has otherwise been diagnosed as having a unipolar depression may herald the necessity for a reevaluation and possible re-diagnosis to the bipolar spectrum. When such a patient has not been placed on a mood stabilizer and the antidepressant has been begun alone, the initiation of a mood stabilizer may eliminate or markedly decrease any anxious and panicky symptoms. In general, the antidepressant doses are simultaneously lowered and when possible, discontinued.

Obsessive-compulsive disorder. Elevated mood patients whose anxiety occurs in the context of obsessive thoughts or compulsive rituals may display significant anxiety when unable to complete mental or behavioral compulsions. Obsessiveness may be unrelated to mood states becoming more intense, however, unless there is satisfactory completion of prescribed rituals. Considerably increased agitation can be anticipated if such rituals are interrupted or left uncompleted.

Social anxiety disorder. It would be highly unusual for a patient with elevated mood to display symptoms of social anxiety during hypomania. In fact, elevated mood patients tend to be overly social to the point of being intrusive. It is possible, however, that in the depressed phase of a bipolar condition, patients may become socially reclusive and anxious about appearing in groups or attending social functions. Since most bipolar patients present for treatment in the depressed rather than the elevated mood phase, it is possible that these patients may present with depressed mood and symptoms of social anxiety. Such patients often describe distinct periods when social anxiety disappears and they are comfortable in groups, crowds, or situations of social scrutiny. This history of marked "on/off" social anxiety can often be a key sign to the diagnostician that a bipolar condition may be comorbid with what appears to be a social anxiety disorder.

Post-traumatic stress disorder **(PTSD)**. The trauma associated with PTSD can occur either prior to the emergence of bipolar symptoms or after bipolar symptoms reveal themselves. A variety of studies have looked at the comorbidity of PTSD and bipolar I disorder and found an incidence of between 9% and 18% of youth with bipolar I disorder having comorbid PTSD (7–9). There are a variety of potential causes for this overlap. With genetic loading, children with bipolar disorder are born in significantly higher frequency to couples where one or both parents have bipolar disorder. Such parents with bipolar disorder have an increased risk of angry, rageful or out-of-control behavior that may result in physical, emotional, and/or sexual trauma to their children. Likewise, parents with bipolar disorder have significantly increased incidence of alcohol and other substance abuse that further contributes to lack of impulse control and poor parenting, resulting in traumatic experiences for their children. These children, therefore, may be genetically vulnerable to bipolar disorder and have a high incidence of abuse leading to PTSD. These connections were borne out in a study with a primary aim to determine the relationship between trauma and attention-deficit hyperactivity disorder (ADHD), but yielded interesting information about PTSD and bipolar disorder (10). Two hundred and sixty children and adolescents with and without ADHD were studied in longitudinal fashion over 4 years. It was noted that 27% of youth with ADHD who were exposed to trauma had significantly higher baseline rates of bipolar disorder when compared to those with ADHD who were not exposed to trauma (9%). The investigators found that early bipolar disorder in children with ADHD is the most significant predictor for subsequent trauma and concluded that early bipolar disorder is an important antecedent for trauma rather than a consequent result of trauma.

In adults, it is not surprising then that comorbid PTSD and bipolar disorder are also common (11). In addition to PTSD resulting from childhood trauma described above, persons with elevated mood are also more likely to engage in impulsive, reckless, and dangerous behaviors with minimal regard for the consequences. Such risky behavior may lead to fights, provocations, sexual assaults, and accidents—all of which could result in PTSD. Military combatants with subsyndromal cyclothymia or bipolar II disorder might not only be more sensitive to the aftereffects of conflict but might also volunteer impulsively for dangerous missions, leading to postcombat PTSD.

Separation anxiety disorder (in children). As in social anxiety disorder, separation anxiety disorder in children may precede a diagnosis of a bipolar condition (12,13). Such children demonstrate recurrent, excessive worry and distress at being separated from home or people to whom they are most attached. These children are totally reluctant or refuse to attend school, are fearful about being alone, and are unable to sleep without a parent nearby. Recurrent nightmares or physical symptoms such as nausea, vomiting, stomach aches, or headaches are common when separation is anticipated or actually occurs.

Other anxiety connections

Anxiety or behaviors that are confused with anxiety may be part of other mental health conditions. Individuals with an *affective mixed state,* for example, may have considerable anxiety and agitation as part of their mixture of affective symptoms. Anxiety may also be *intermingled with depression,* anergia, crying spells, hypersomnia, and hyperphagia when the patient is in the depressed phase of a bipolar illness.

Although anxiety is not a regular feature of *attention-deficit disorder,* behaviors referable to attention deficits may confound even experienced clinicians. Pacing, fidgeting, and inability to sit still that are seen in children or adults may be mistakenly identified as bipolar-driven anxiety symptoms as opposed to ADHD-related behaviors. These can include problems sustaining attention, inability with following instructions, difficulty in organizing tasks, and easy distractibility. A cue to differentiating ADHD from anxious elevated mood is that ADHD is a continuous lifelong condition. ADHD presents itself from very early in childhood and into adult life, and is present in virtually all situations requiring concentration and attention. Anxiety associated with bipolar disorder is often episodic and punctuated by periods of anxiety-free euthymia or depressed mood. The presence of grandiosity and hypersexuality also mediates against the likelihood of an ADHD diagnosis and points more predictably to a bipolar diagnosis.

Mental anxiety and physical agitation may occur as a *side effect of pre-scription medications,* over-the-counter (OTC) medications, and commonly available substances. Any of the prescription medications listed in Table 10.3 can produce physical and mental agitation. The clinician should inquire about the use of these medications as part of a diagnostic assessment of anxiety

TABLE 10.3
Medications that can precipitate anxiety

- Antihypertensives
- Diuretics
- Corticosteroids
- Stimulants
- Bronchodilators
- Decongestants
- Histamine antagonists
- Xanthines such as theophylline
- Antidepressants
- Thyroxine
- Atypical antipsychotics
- Modafinil
- Atomoxetine

TABLE 10.4
Medical conditions associated with anxiety

- Asthma
- Chronic obstructive pulmonary disease (COPD)
- Coronary events
- Cushing disease
- Dementia
- Fibromyalgia
- Hyperthyroidism
- Pheochromocytoma

and elevated mood. Similarly, OTC medications, especially those containing caffeine such as APCs (aspirin, phenacetin, caffeine) as well as other combination products such as NoDoz or appetite reduction pills, can produce anxiety as a side effect. Caffeine ingested in coffee, tea, colas, and other caffeinated beverages may likewise produce significant anxiety in the mood-disordered patient. Lastly, alcohol tends to calm anxiety for most bipolar patients; however, particularly after heavy use, the physiologic rebound and withdrawal symptoms may cause significant anxiety.

In addition to medications, patients with elevated mood may have anxiety caused by independent medical conditions. When anxiety is present and associated with other physiologic complaints, a thorough physical examination and laboratory evaluation should be completed. Medical conditions associated with anxiety are listed in Table 10.4.

Specific anxiety questions in bipolar mood disorder

The most useful procedures to categorize anxiety in persons with elevated mood are thorough history taking and symptom screening. Targeted questions can elicit specific anxiety complaints and any associated symptomatology. It is particularly important to learn the time course of the anxiety, the pattern, if any, to the anxiety, and any physical and/or emotional etiologies consistent with anxiety.

- When does the anxiety come on?
- How long does it last?
- When does it go away?
- What factors precipitate it?
- What factors make it better?
- Is the anxiety associated with any changes in mood, activity or energy?
- Are there any particular life stressors that have accompanied the onset of anxiety?

- What medications are you taking? Prescribed? OTC? Herbal supplements?
- Have there been any recent changes in your medication regimen?
- What new medications, if any, have been associated with the onset of anxiety?
- Do any medications help the anxiety?
- What is your caffeine intake?
- How much alcohol do you drink? How often?
- Do you use recreational drugs? Are any associated with changes in anxiety level?

Akathisia

Over and above mental agitation, feeling "revved up," or physically hyperactive, further issues resulting from medication treatment that can overlap with anxiety in the elevated mood patient are akathisia and tremor.

Akathisia, an internal sense of restlessness, is a common side effect with traditional antipsychotics but may occur with atypical antipsychotics and occasionally with some antidepressants. Patients with akathisia will have difficulty describing their condition clearly, but will feel very distressed and have difficulty articulating the source of their discomfort. They will often pace and become more agitated if not permitted to do so. They may describe a sense that their intestines are agitated or moving even though there are no frank gastrointestinal symptoms.

A key element to the diagnosis of akathisia is awareness of the institution of prescribed medications that have a high incidence of akathisia. These include all the typical antipsychotics. Among atypical antipsychotics, aripiprazole, ziprasidone, and risperidone create more akathisia than other members of this group. Some antidepressants including fluoxetine, bupropion, serotonin–norepinephrine reuptake inhibitors (SNRIs) and tricyclic antidepressants (TCAs) also may cause akathisia. When any of these medications are prescribed for a bipolar condition, it is particularly critical to assess for the presence of akathisia. Patients with akathisia can become sufficiently desperate and attempt drastic solutions to rid themselves of the feeling including attempted or completed suicide.

When akathisia is diagnosed, decreasing the dose or discontinuing the causative medication will usually alleviate the symptomatology. If the offending medication is essential to clinical stability, use of a β-blocker (e.g., propranolol 10–80 mg), an anticholinergic (e.g., benzotropine 1–2 mg) or a benzodiazepine (e.g., alprazolam or lorazepam 0.25–0.5 mg) can often ameliorate the symptoms.

Tremor

Tremor can often be confused by patients and caregivers alike as a symptom of anxiety and may co-occur with elevated mood. While some anxious individuals are tremulous, others with anxiety have minimal or no tremor. Conversely,

TABLE 10.5
Medications used in mental health that can cause tremor

- Lithium
- Selective serotonin reuptake inhibitors and serotonin–norepinephrine reuptake inhibitors
- Stimulants
- Tricyclic antidepressants
- Thyroxine
- Traditional and atypical antipsychotics
- Valproic acid
- Verapamil
- Bupropion

many anxious individuals will experience no tremor whatsoever. Tremors are obvious in writing, grasping objects, eating or serving food, and may be acutely worsened transiently by the ingestion of caffeine. Agents commonly used in psychiatry that can cause tremor are listed in Table 10.5.

When treating patients with elevated mood with these agents and prominent tremor occurs, as in akathisia, discontinuing or decreasing the dose of the offending agent may improve the tremor. If medication cannot be discontinued for clinical stability, the use of a β-blocker (propranolol 10–80 mg) or a benzodiazepine (lorazepam or alprazolam 0.25–0.5 mg) may mitigate tremors. Antitremor remedies are only necessary during waking hours and are generally not needed during sleep. The clinician may give the patient significant latitude on when and how often the antitremor medication is taken. If the patient requires continuous tremor control, the use of a long-acting β-blocker preparation may give satisfactory response.

In evaluating tremor, patients should also be questioned about a positive family history. "Essential" tremor, which tends to be genetically determined, may occur without any causative physical agent, may not respond to the above remedies, and should be evaluated neurologically.

Medication treatments for anxiety in elevated mood

Although the co-occurrence of anxiety disorders with elevated mood is quite common, there have been no randomized placebo-controlled trials looking at the effect of medications on anxiety or specific anxiety disorders in patients with elevated mood or bipolar disorder. Therefore, information and recommendations contained in this section are derived solely from controlled trial evidence of medications on individual anxiety disorders themselves, without the presence of bipolar disorder. Whether the presence of elevated mood and/or bipolar disorder would significantly affect the study outcomes is not known (14). When evaluating the data reviewed here, it is also important to recall that, as with any patient with mood disorder, the potential clinical effect on the patient's mood may have substantial impact on choosing a particular medication or avoiding a particular medication for anxiety. Therefore, each bipolar patient with anxiety as a comorbid symptom should be evaluated on an individual basis for the most effective treatment of anxiety with the least disruption of mood.

Valproic acid

Valproic acid has one small placebo-controlled trial, several case reports, and a number of open-label studies (14–18) that have shown valproate to be useful in the treatment of panic attacks and panic disorder. This response is presumably through its significant positive effect on gamma-aminobutyric acid (GABA) receptors. Although it has not been validated in every study, most open-label trials and case reports of the use of valproic acid in combat-related PTSD reveal positive benefits on sleep disorder, hyperarousal, and intrusive symptoms (19–23). Avoidant symptoms of PTSD are generally less responsive. There are two reports of the use of valproic acid in conjunction with serotonergic medication for the treatment of obsessive-compulsive disorder (24,25). Valproic acid has shown limited efficacy in other anxiety disorders, and particularly in social anxiety.

Carbamazepine

At least three open-label studies have shown carbamazepine to be useful in minimizing the frequency and intensity of PTSD nightmares, flashbacks, and intrusive thoughts (26–28). Carbamazepine has had mixed results in studies of panic disorder and obsessive-compulsive disorder.

Lamotrigine

One small placebo-controlled study indicated a positive response to lamotrigine with PTSD patients, with twice the success rate of placebo (29). There was improvement in re-experiencing phenomena, avoidance, and numbness symptoms. There are no other positive studies for the use of lamotrigine in anxiety disorders.

Atypical antipsychotics

Olanzapine

There have been several positive case series with up to ten patients that showed a distinct reduction in the frequency of panic attacks and anticipatory anxiety when olanzapine was used as monotherapy (30,31). There are a large number of open-label trials and case series that show the beneficial effects of adding olanzapine to selective serotonin reuptake inhibitors (SSRIs) in patients with obsessive-compulsive disorder (32–35). There have also been positive studies of olanzapine, both as monotherapy and as additive treatment in PTSD (36–38). The olanzapine treated groups demonstrated positive response in intrusive PTSD symptoms (flashbacks and nightmares), sleep disturbance, avoidance, and arousal symptoms. There is one small trial of olanzapine in social anxiety disorder with a positive outcome (39), but there are no reports of its use in treating generalized anxiety disorder.

Quetiapine

There is one placebo-controlled study (40) and several open-label reports and case series (41–43) on the use of quetiapine as adjunctive treatment in obsessive-compulsive disorder with modest improvement. There are small open-label trials of quetiapine in PTSD, panic attacks, and social anxiety disorder, all of which showed positive benefit in their respective symptom clusters (44–46).

Risperidone

Three placebo-controlled trials where risperidone was added to SSRIs in obsessive-compulsive disorder that showed positive responses that were further elucidated in several case series (47–49). Risperidone has been found to be useful in reducing irritability, intrusive thoughts, and hyperarousal in PTSD patients in three placebo-controlled trials and various case reports (50–52). No studies of risperidone in generalized anxiety disorder and social anxiety or panic disorder have been reported.

Aripiprazole

Three placebo-controlled studies of aripiprazole as monotherapy or adjunctive therapy with SSRIs in the treatment of residual anxiety and depression in patients with obsessive-compulsive disorder have been published (53–55). No other specific anxiety disorders using aripiprazole have been studied.

Ziprasidone

There have been no reports published of ziprasidone in patients with anxiety disorders.

Antidepressants

It has long been known that virtually every class of antidepressants is efficacious in the treatment of most anxiety disorders (56,57). Many of the SSRIs, SNRIs, and TCAs have FDA-approved indications for a variety of anxiety disorders. Although these agents are clearly useful in patients with bipolar disorder, they are potentially prone to exacerbating mania or precipitating a switch into mania. In treating elevated mood patients with anxiety, therefore, caution should be used to avoid an exacerbation of mania at the expense of anxiety relief.

Other antiepileptics

Topiramate

Topiramate has had efficacy reported in case reports and open-label trials with PTSD (58), social anxiety disorder (59), and as adjunctive treatment for obsessive-compulsive disorder (60). This compound, however, has also been associated with new onset panic attacks and new onset obsessive symptoms. Its use, therefore, in anxiety disorders presents a mixed picture pending further research.

Gabapentin

Gabapentin has shown positive benefit in SSRI-refractory obsessive-compulsive disorder (61) and PTSD (62,63). It has also been useful in patients with refractory panic disorder and social anxiety (64,65).

Pregabalin

Placebo-controlled studies for the treatment of social anxiety and generalized anxiety have shown positive correlations of the use of pregabalin at higher doses (200 mg three times a day) (64,65).

Benzodiazepines

What should not be lost in anxiety treatment with recent trials of mood stabilizers, anticonvulsants, and antidepressants is the role of benzodiazepines. Although this group of compounds clearly has potential downsides, including potential for habituation, withdrawal, abuse, cognitive interference and deficits in coordination and balance, benzodiazepines have been used in the treatment of anxiety for more than four decades (66–69). Easily combinable with virtually all mood medications, adjunctive benzodiazepine therapy may have a significant positive benefit on most anxiety disorders. Because of its somewhat longer half-life and documented (albeit limited) potential for mood stabilization, clonazepam has some benefit over other benzodiazepines in common use. Extended release alprazolam does have some advantage over its shorter half-life, immediate release counterpart. Lorazepam has almost no interaction with other psychotropic and nonpsychotropic medications and has found favor with nonpsychiatric clinicians. In appropriately selected elevated mood patients without a history of substance abuse, the adjunctive use of one of these benzodiazepines may significantly ameliorate mental agitation and other anxious symptoms.

The bottom line

- Anxiety may be an intrinsic part of an elevated mood state or a comorbid symptom.
- Anxiety disorders are the most common comorbidity with bipolar disorders including the following:
  ○ Generalized anxiety disorder
  ○ Panic disorder
  ○ Social anxiety disorder
  ○ PTSD
  ○ Separation anxiety disorder
- Akathisia and tremor can be confused with anxiety in the elevated mood patient.
- Studies evaluating anxiety exclusively in elevated mood patients are scant.
- Antidepressants, antiepileptics, antipsychotics, and benzodiazepines all have a role in the amelioration of anxiety.

REFERENCES

1. Freeman MP, Freeman SA, McElroy SL. The comorbidity of bipolar and anxiety disorders: Prevalence, psychobiology, and treatment issues. *J Affect Disord.* 2002;68:1–23.
2. Boylan KR, Bieling PJ, Marriott M, et al. Impact of comorbid anxiety disorders on outcome in a cohort of patients with bipolar disorder. *J Clin Psychiatry.* 2004;65:1106–1113.
3. Simon NM, Otto MW, Wisniewski SR, et al. Anxiety disorder comorbidity in bipolar patients: Data from the first 500 participants in the Systematic Treatment Enhancement Program for Bipolar Disorder (STEP-BD). *Am J Psychiatry.* 2004;161:2222–2229.
4. Simon NM, Otto MW, Fischmann D, et al. Panic disorder and bipolar disorder: Anxiety sensitivity as a potential mediator of panic during manic states. *J Affect Disord.* 2005;87:101–105.
5. MacKinnon DF, Zandi PP, Cooper J, et al. Comorbid bipolar disorder and panic disorder in families with a high prevalence of bipolar disorder. *Am J Psychiatry.* 2002;159:30–35.
6. Keller MB. Prevalence and impact of comorbid anxiety and bipolar disorder. *J Clin Psychiatry.* 2006;67(Suppl 1):5–7.
7. Jerrell JM, Shugart MA. Community-based care for youths with early and very early onset bipolar i disorder. *Biol Psychiatry.* 1997;42:90–95.
8. Ackerman PT, Newton JE, McPherson B, et al. Prevalence of posttraumatic stress disorder and other psychiatric diagnoses in three groups of abused children (sexual, physical and both). *Child Abuse Negl.* 1998;22:759–774.

9. Wilens TE, Biederman J, Forkner P, et al. Patterns of comorbidity and dysfunction in clinically referred preschool and school-aged children with bipolar disorder. *J Child Adolesc Psychopharmacol.* 2003;13:495–505.

10. Wozniak J, Crawford MH, Biederman J, et al. Antecedents and complications of trauma in boys with ADHD: Findings from a longitudinal study. *J Am Acad Child Adolesc Psychiatry.* 1999;38:48–55.

11. Goldberg JF, Garno JL. Development of posttraumatic stress disorder in adult bipolar patients with histories of severe childhood abuse. *J Psychiatr Res.* 2005;39(6):595–601.

12. Pini S, Abelli M, Mauri M, et al. Clinical correlates and significance of separation anxiety in patients with bipolar disorder. *Bipolar Disord.* 2005;7(4):370–376.

13. Lewinsohn PM, Klein DN, Seeley JR. Bipolar disorders in a community sample of older adolescents: Prevalence, phenomenology, comorbidity, and course. *J Am Acad Child Adolesc Psychiatry.* 1995;34(4):454–463.

14. Keck PE, Strawn JR, McElroy SL. Pharmacologic treatment considerations in co-occuring bipolar and anxiety disorders. *J Clin Psychiatry.* 2006;67(Suppl 1):8–15.

15. Lum M, Fontaine R, Elie R, et al. Divalproex sodium's anti-panic effect in panic disorder: A placbo-controlled study. *Biol Psychiatry.* 1990;27:164A–165A.

16. Primeau F, Fontaine R, Beauclair L, et al. Valproic acid and panic disorder. *Can J Psychiatry.* 1990;35:248–250.

17. Woodman C, Noyes R. Panic disorder: Treatment with valproate. *J Clin Psychiatry.* 1994;55:134–136.

18. Brady KT, Sonne S, Lydiard RB. Valproate treatment of comorbid panic disorder and affective disorders in two alcoholic patients [letter]. *J Clin Psychopharmacol.* 1994;14:81–82.

19. Szymanski HV, Olympia J. Divalproex in post-traumatic stress disorder [letter]. *Am J Psychiatry.* 1991;148:1086–1087.

20. Berigan TR, Holzgang A. Valproate as an alternative in post-traumatic stress disorder: A case report. *Mil Med.* 1995;160:318.

21. Fesler FA. Valproate in combat-related post-traumatic stress disorder. *J Clin Psychiatry.* 1991;52:361–364.

22. Clark RD, Canive J, Calais LA, et al. Divalproex in posttraumatic stress disorder: An open-label trial. *J Trauma Stress.* 1999;12:395–403.

23. Petty F, Davis LL, Nugent AL, et al. Valproate therapy for chronic, combat-induced posttraumatic stress disorder. *J Clin Psychopharmacol.* 2002;22:100–102.

24. Van Ameringen M, Mancini C, Pipe B, et al. Antiepileptic drugs in the treatment of anxiety disorders: Role in therapy. *Drugs.* 2004;64:2199–2220.

25. Deltito JA. Valproate pretreatment for the difficult-to-treat patient with OCD [letter]. *J Clin Psychiatry.* 1994;55:500.

26. Lipper S, Davidson JRT, Grady TA, et al. Preliminary study of carbamazepine in post-traumatic stress disorder. *Psychosomatics.* 1986;27:849–854.

27. Wolf ME, Alavi A, Mosnaim AD. Posttraumatic stress disorder in Vietnam veterans clinical and EEG findings: Possible therapeutic effects of carbamazepine. *Biol Psychiatry.* 1988;23:642–644.

28. Looff D, Grimely P, Kuller F, et al. Carbamazepine for PTSD [letter]. *J Am Acad Child Adolesc Psychiatry.* 1995;34:703–704.

29. Hertzberg MA, Butterfield MI, Feldman ME, et al. A preliminary study of lamotrigine for the treatment of posttraumatic stress disorder. *Biol Psychiatry.* 1999;45:1226–1229.

30. Etxebeste M, Aragues E, Malo P, et al. Olanzapine and panic attacks [letter]. *Am J Psychiatry.* 2000;157:659–660.
31. Shapira NA, Ward HE, Mandoki M, et al. A double-blind, placebo-controlled trial of olanzapine addition in fluoxetine-refractory obsessive-compulsive disorder. *Bio Psychiatry.* 2004;55:553–555.
32. Francobandiera G. Olanzapine augmentation of serotonin uptake inhibitors in obsessive-compulsive disorder: An open study. *Can J Psychiatry.* 2001;46:356–358.
33. Koran LM, Ringold AL, Elliott MA. Olanzapine augmentation for treatment-resistant obsessive-compulsive disorder. *J Clin Psychiatry.* 2000;61:514–517.
34. Crocq MA, Leclerq P, Guillon MS, et al. Open-label olanzapine in obsessive-compulsive disorder refractory to antidepressant treatment. *Eur Psychiatry.* 2002;17:296–297.
35. Marazziti D, Pallanti S. Effectiveness of olanzapine treatment for severe obsessive-compulsive disorder [letter]. *Am J Psychiatry.* 1999;156:1834–1835.
36. Stein MB, Kline NA, Matloff JL. Adjunctive olanzapine for SSRI-resistant combat-related PTSD: A double-blind, placebo-controlled study. *Am J Psychiatry.* 2002;159:1777–1779.
37. Pivac N, Kozaric-Kovacic D, Muck-Seler D. Olanzapine versus fluphenazine in an open trial with psychotic combat-related post-traumatic stress disorder. *Psychopharmacology.* 2004;175:451–456.
38. Labbate LA, Douglas S. Olanzapine for nightmares and sleep disturbance in posttraumatic stress disorder (PTSD) [letter]. *Can J Psychiatry.* 2000;45:667–668.
39. Barnett SD, Kramer ML, Casat CD, et al. Efficacy of olanzapine in social anxiety disorder: A pilot study. *J Psychopharmacol.* 2002;16:365–368.
40. Denys D, deGues F, van Megan HJGM. A double-blind, randomized, placebo-controlled trial of quetiapine addition in patients with obsessive-compulsive disorder refractory to serotonin reuptake inhibitors. *J Clin Psychiatry.* 2004;65:1040–1048.
41. Atmaca M, Kuloglu M, Tezcan E, et al. Quetiapine augmentation in patients with treatment resistant obsessive-compulsive disorder. *Int Clin Psychopharmacol.* 2002;17:37–40.
42. Mohr N, Vythilingum B, Emsley RA, et al. Quetiapine augmentation of serotonin reuptake inhibitors in obsessive-compulsive disorder. *Int Clin Psychopharmacol.* 2002;17:37–40.
43. Francobandiera G. Quetiapine augmentation of sertraline in obsessive-compulsive disorder [letter]. *J Clin Psychiatry.* 2002;63:1046–1047.
44. Hamner MB, Deitsch SE, Brodrick PS, et al. Quetiapine treatment in patients with posttraumatic stress disorder: An open trial of adjunctive therapy. *J Clin Psychopharmacol.* 2003;23:15–20.
45. Takahashi H, Sugita T, Yoshida K, et al. Effect of quetiapine in the treatment of panic attacks in patients with schizophrenia: 3 case reports. *J Neuropsychiatry Clin Neurosci.* 2004;16:113–115.
46. Schutters SIJ, van Megan HJGM, Westenberg HGM. Efficacy of quetiapine in generalized social anxiety disorder: Results from an open-label study. *J Clin Psychiatry.* 2005;66:540–542.
47. McDougle CJ, Epperson CN, Pelton GH, et al. A double-blind, placebo-controlled study of risperidone addition in serotonin reuptake inhibitor-refractory obsessive-compulsive disorder. *Arch Gen Psychiatry.* 2000;57:794–801.

48. Hollander E, Rossi NB, Sood E, et al. Risperidone augmentation in treatment-resistant obsessive-compulsive disorder: A double-blind, placebo-controlled study. *Int J Neuropsychopharmacol.* 2003;6:397–401.
49. Erzegovesi S, Guglielmo E, Siliprandi F, et al. Low-dose risperidone augmentation of fluvoxamine treatment in obsessive-compulsive disorder: A double-blind, placebo-controlled study. *Eur Neurophsychopharmacol.* 2005;15:69–74.
50. Reich DB, Winternitz S, Hennen J, et al. A preliminary study of risperidone in the treatment of posttraumatic stress disordered related to childhood sexual abuse in women. *J Clin Psychiatry.* 2004;65:1601–1606.
51. Bartzokis G, Lu PH, Turner J, et al. Adjunctive risperidone in the treatment of chronic combat-related posttraumatic stress disorder. *Biol Psychiatry.* 2004;57:474–479.
52. Monnelly EP, Ciraulo DA. Risperidone effects on irritable aggression in posttraumatic stress disorder [letter]. *J Clin Psychopharmacol.* 1999;19:377–378.
53. Connor KM, Payne VM, Gadde KM, et al. The use of aripiprazole in obsessive-compulsive disorder: Preliminary observations in 8 patients. *J Clin Psychiatry.* 2005;66:49–51.
54. Worthington JJ, Kinrys G, Wygant LE, et al. Aripiprazole as an augmentor of selective serotonin reuptake inhibitors in depression and anxiety disorders. *Int Clin Psychopharmacol.* 2005;20:9–11.
55. Adson DE, Kushner MG, Fahnhorst TA. Treatment of residual anxiety symptoms with adjunctive aripiprazole in depressed patients taking selective serotonin reuptake inhibitors. *J Affect Disord.* 2005;86:99–104.
56. Davidson JRT, Connor KM. Treatment of anxiety disorders. In: Nemeroff CB, Schatzberg AF, eds. *Textbook of psychopharmacology*, 3rd ed. Washington, DC: American Psychiatric Press; 2004:913–934.
57. Dominguez RA. Serotonergic antidepressants and their efficacy in obsessive-compulsive disorder. *J Clin Psychiatry.* 1992;53(Suppl 5):56–59.
58. Berlant J, van Kammen DP. Open-label topiramate as primary or adjunctive therapy in chronic civilian posttraumatic stress disorder: A preliminary report. *J Clin Psychiatry.* 2002;64:15–20.
59. Berlant JL. Topiramate in posttraumatic stress disorder: Preliminary clinical observations. *J Clin Psychiatry.* 2001;62(Suppl 17):60–63.
60. Van Ameringen MA, Mancini CL, Pipe B, et al. Adjunctive topiramate in treatment-resistant obsessive-compulsive disorder. In: *New research abstracts of the 157th annual meeting of the American psychiatric association.* New York, May 3, 2004: Abstract NR195:71–72.
61. Cora-Locatelli G, Greenberg BD, Martin J, et al. Gabapentin augmentation for fluoxetine-treated patients with obsessive-compulsive disorder [letter]. *J Clin Psychiatry.* 1998;59:480–481.
62. Hamner MB, Brodrick PS, Labbate LA. Gabapentin in PTSD: A retrospective, clinical series of adjunctive therapy. *Ann Clin Psychiatry.* 2001;13:141–146.
63. Malek-Ahmadi P. Gabapentin and posttraumatic stress disorder. *Ann Pharmacother.* 2003;37:664–666.
64. Pollack MH, Matthews J, Scott EL. Gabapentin as a potential treatment for anxiety disorder [letter]. *Am J Psychiatry.* 1998;155:992–993.
65. Pane AC, Davidson JRT, Jefferson JW, et al. Treatment of social phobia with gabapentin: A placebo-controled study. *J Clin Psychopharmacol.* 1999;19:341–348.

66. Pohl RB, Feltner DE, Fieve RR, et al. Efficacy of pregabalin in the treatment of generalized anxiety disorder: Double-blind, placebo-controlled comparison of BID versus TID dosing. *J Clin Psychopharmacol.* 2005;25:151–158.
67. Pande AC, Feltner DE, Jefferson JW, et al. Efficacy of the novel anxiolytic pregabalin in social anxiety disorder. *J Clin Psychopharmacol.* 2004;24:141–149.
68. Shader RI, Greenblatt DJ. Use of benzodiazepines in anxiety disorders. *N Engl J Med.* 1993;328(19):1398–1405.
69. Uhlenhuth EH, Balter MB, Ban TA, et al. International study of expert judgment on therapeutic use of benzodiazepines and other psychotherapeutic medications: VI. Trends in recommendations for the pharmacotherapy of anxiety disorders, 1992–1997. *Depress Anxiety.* 1999;9(3):107–16.

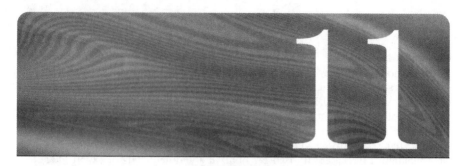

SLEEP AND HYPOMANIA—
THE ABCs OF GETTING YOUR ZZZs

- The reciprocal relationship between mood and sleep
- How much sleep is enough?
- Evaluation of sleep in elevated mood
- Treatment of sleep problems in elevated mood
- Pharmacologic treatment of sleep in elevated mood
- Sleep disorders in patients who abuse substances
- Chronic sleep treatment—good or bad?
- The bottom line

References

The prevalence and consequences of insomnia and poor quality sleep are well known. Worldwide, >60 million adults are affected by sleep disorders (1) and 50% of adults, at some point in their lives, are affected by insomnia (2). Between 10% and 15% of the US population experiences insomnia lasting >6 months (3,4). Insomnia causes significant physiologic morbidity including increased cortisol levels, decreased glucose tolerance, and increased activity of the sympathetic nervous system (5). Long-lasting insomnia can lead to impaired functioning during the waking hours and increased incidence of accidents (6). Within the mood spectrum, persistent insomnia may be a risk factor in developing depression (7). How then do these staggering statistics impact the realm of hypomania and elevated mood?

The reciprocal relationship between mood and sleep

There are at least three connections between disruption of sleep and elevated mood. It has been clinically and experimentally shown that sleep deprivation is associated with the onset of hypomania or mania in patients susceptible to mood disorders (8). When 11 studies were reviewed totaling 631 patients with bipolar disorder (9), sleep disturbance was the most common symptom of mania, reported by more than three quarters of patients, and the sixth most common symptom of bipolar depression, reported by one fourth of the number of patients. Insomnia is also a significant and common problem among patients with bipolar disorder even when they are euthymic. In a recent study (10), ten percent of euthymic patients with bipolar disorder reported a significant sleep disturbance including impaired sleep efficiency, increased anxiety about poor sleep, and decreased daytime activity levels due to lack of sleep. Lastly, it has been suggested that the disruption of the sleep–wake cycle may be a causative factor in the development of bipolar disorder, postulating that these patients have a genetic diathesis for circadian rhythm instability. These authors propose (11,12) that psychosocial stressors may cause disrupted routine and sleep, which consequently disrupts already vulnerable circadian rhythms and may trigger a mood episode. Sleep quality is one of the most objective measures of improvement or deterioration in bipolar disorder and may serve as either a signal, or a trigger of manic, or hypomanic episodes (13,14). Lack of sleep may cause a switch from depression to mania in as many as 6% of vulnerable patients (15). *Therefore, insomnia and disruptive sleep are a consequence of a mood episode, may serve as a signal of an oncoming mood episode, or be a cause of an elevated mood episode. Disrupted sleep and circadian rhythms may also have a causative role in the development of bipolar disorder itself.* It is critical, therefore, for the clinician to monitor sleep–wake cycles and intervene quickly if sleep is disrupted.

How much sleep is enough?

The notion that everyone requires 8 hours of sleep is a myth, and is seldom true for even non–mood disordered patients. In patients with elevated mood, however, the length of sleep necessary for optimum functioning is further complicated by the fact that patients with bipolar disorder, even when relatively euthymic, are often short sleepers. Hyperthymic individuals who function at adequate or even superior levels may require only 4 to 5 hours of sleep over long periods of time. In these individuals, short sleep patterns do not necessarily indicate pathology. As with many areas of elevated mood, assessment of the patient's functioning is the key issue. If a patient has been stable on a short sleep pattern for many months or even years and is functioning well, the pattern need not be changed nor seen as an element of pathology. It is of significance, however, if there is a *recent change in sleep pattern*. The fact that a mood disordered patient who has traditionally slept 6 to 7 hours but begins to sleep 3 to 4 hours per night is a red flag warning, and is a potential sign of an incipient mood change. When necessary, input from other sources such as the patient's spouse or bed partner may be necessary to adequately assess the quality and quantity of the patient's sleep.

Evaluation of sleep in elevated mood

Because of the reciprocal relationship between sleep and mood fluctuations, one may assume that all disordered sleep is referable to the patient's hypomania or mania. Especially during an initial evaluation or early in treatment however, this assumption should not be made until a thorough evaluation of other causes of sleep disturbance is made. Short-term or transient insomnia in a hypomanic patient can also be due to multiple factors such as those listed in Table 11.1.

When evaluating a mood disordered patient with a significant sleep problem, the evaluation should consist of a clinical history, a sleep history, a physical examination, and, when necessary, laboratory assessments. The clinical history should focus on the duration of the sleeping problem.

- How long has the patient had difficulty with sleep?
- When in the night does the problem occur?
- Is there
  - ◦ difficulty falling asleep?
  - ◦ awakening in the middle of the night (sleep continuity disturbance)?
  - ◦ early morning awakening?

The sleep history should obtain information about the lifestyle and sleep environment including cigarette smoking, alcohol and caffeine intake, levels of exercise, and when bedtimes and arising occur. It may be helpful to use a standardized questionnaire such as the Pittsburgh Sleep Quality Index (PSQI) to document these issues (Table 11.2).

A physical examination should focus on ruling out medical conditions and the treatments that are known to cause insomnia including the factors in Table 11.3.

The patient should be screened for the use of various medications and other substances that are known to cause insomnia as shown in Table 11.4.

A physical examination should also include a neurologic examination, assessment for signs of vascular disease, or peripheral neuropathy, assessment of the upper airway and a general examination of cardiac and pulmonary

TABLE 11.1

Factors causing short-term or transient insomnia in hypomanic patients

- Emotional distress or bereavement
- Initiation or discontinuation of pharmaceuticals
- Use/abuse/withdrawal of alcohol or recreational drugs
- Recent onset of a physical or painful illness
- Work shift changes
- Jet lag

TABLE 11.2
Pittsburgh sleep quality index

Pittsburgh Sleep Quality Index (PSQI)

The following questions related to the patient's usual sleep habits during the **past month only**. Answers should indicate the most accurate reply for the **majority** of days and nights in the past month. Answer all questions.

During the past month:

1. What time have you usually gone to bed? _____
2. How long has it taken you to fall asleep each night? _____ (in minutes)
3. What time have you usually gotten up in the morning? _____
4. How many hours of **actual sleep** did you get at night? This may be different than the number of hours you spend in bed) _____ (in hours)
5. How often have you had trouble sleeping because you. . .

Place the number in the parentheses in the box that matches your best answer	Not during the past month (0)	Less than once a week (1)	Once or twice a week (2)	Three or more times a week (3)
a. Could not go to sleep within 30 minutes				
b. Woke up in the middle of the night or early morning				
c. Had to get up to use the bathroom				
d. Could not breathe comfortably				
e. Cough or snore loudly				
f. Felt too cold				
g. Felt too hot				
h. Had bad dreams				
i. Had pain				
j. Other reason(s), please describe how often you have had trouble sleeping because of this reason(s):				

During the past month:
Very good (0), fairly good (1), Fairly bad (2), Very bad (3)

6. How would you rate your sleep overall? _____

(*continued overleaf*)

TABLE 11.2

(*continued*)

Not during the past month (0), less than once a week (1),
Once or twice a week (2), Three or more times a week (3)

7. How often have you taken medicine (prescribed or "over the counter") to help you sleep? _____

8. How often have you had trouble staying awake while driving, eating meals, or engaging in social activity? _____

No problem at all (0), Only a very slight problem (1),
Somewhat of a problem (2), a big problem (3)

9. How much of a problem has it been for you to keep up enough enthusiasm to get things done? _____

10. Do you have a bed partner or roommate? _____Yes _____ No

If you have a bed partner or roommate ask them how often in the past month you have had...

Not during the past month (0), less than once a week (1),
Once or twice a week (2), three or more times a week (3)

a. Loud snoring _____
b. Long pauses between breaths while you sleep _____
c. Legs twitching or jerking while you sleep _____
d. Episodes of disorientation or confusion during sleep _____
e. Other restlessness while you sleep, please describe _____. How often? _____

Scoring

Each component has a score of 0 to 3, with 0 indicating no difficulty and 3 indicating severe difficulty. The seven components are combined to give one global score of 0 to 21, with 0 indicating no difficulty and 21 indicating severe difficulties in all areas.

Component 1—Subjective Sleep Quality	**Component Score** _____

Component score = question 6 score

Component 2—Sleep Latency	**Component Score** _____

1. If question 2 score is ...
   ≤15 minutes; component score = 0
   16–30 minutes; component score = 1
   31–60 minutes; composite score = 2
   >60 minutes; composite score = 3

2. Question 5a score

3. Sum of question 2 score + question 5a score is ...
   If 0, then component score = 0
   If 1–2, the component score = 1
   If 3–4, then component score = 2
   If 5–6, then component score = 3

TABLE 11.2

(continued)

Component 3—Sleep Duration	Component Score _____

For question number 4:
   If >7, then component score = 0
   If 6–7, then component score = 1
   If 5–6, then component score = 2
   If <5, then component score = 3	

Component 4—Habitual Sleep Efficiency (HSE)	Component Score _____

HSE% = (# hours asleep—# hours in bed) × 100
   If >85%, then component score = 0
   If 75–84%, then component score = 1
   If 65–74%, then component score = 2
   If <65%, then component score = 3	

Component 5—Sleep Disturbance	Component Score _____

Sum of score for question 5b through 5j
   If 0, then component score = 0
   If 1–9, then component score = 1
   If 10–18, then component score = 2
   If 19–27, then component score = 3	

Component 6—Use of Sleep Medication	Component Score _____
Component score = question 7 score	

Component 7—Daytime Dysfunction	Component Score _____

Sum of question 8 score + question 9 score
   If 0, then component score = 0
   If 1–2, then component score = 1
   If 3–4, then component score = 2
   If 5–6, then component score = 3	

Global Score	**Global PSQI Score** _____
Add the 7 components together	

Adapted from Buysse DJ, Reynolds CF III, Mont TH, et al. The pittsburgh sleep quality index: A new instrument for psychiatric research and practice. *Psychiatry Res* 1989;28(2):193–213.

function (16). If there is suspicion of a sleep-related breathing disorder, periodic leg movements, or nocturnal seizure disorder, polysomnography, a nocturnal electroencephalograph (EEG), or electromyography (EMG) may be helpful. These tests, however, are not routinely performed in the patient with elevated mood unless there are signs of these disorders. As with most patients with elevated mood who are to be placed on medication, a battery of laboratory screening tests including routine electrolytes, chemistries, blood

TABLE 11.3
Medical illnesses known to cause insomnia

- Hypertension
- Hyperthyroidism
- Chronic pain
- Asthma
- Rheumatoid arthritis
- Cardiac obstructive pulmonary disease
- Cardiac ischemia
- Fibrosis
- Menopausal symptoms
- Gastroesophageal reflux
- Irritable bowel syndrome
- Chronic renal failure
- Liver failure

urea nitrogen (BUN), creatine, liver function, thyroid-stimulating hormone (TSH), and complete blood count (CBC) should be obtained.

Treatment of sleep problems in elevated mood

Regardless of what else is done to specifically treat the patient's elevated mood, sleep should be given a top priority. Sleep treatment is separated into non-pharmacologic and pharmacologic approaches. Non-pharmacologic treatments include the following sleep hygiene recommendations that should be given to all patients with insomnia:

- A regular activity schedule with approximately the same bedtime and morning arising time each day should be followed. Patient should be counseled against "sleeping in" on weekends or marked variations in bedtime.
- Avoid naps during the day.
- Heavy meals should be avoided before sleep, although a light snack may be useful at bedtime (particularly for geriatric patients with insomnia).
- Regular exercise should be done three to four times per week, although it is best not performed after dinner because adrenaline stimulation may exacerbate sleep difficulties. Inform the patient that any exercise regime that aids sleep will take up to 6 weeks to have a beneficial sleep effect.
- Control bedroom temperature and surroundings. Most individuals do not sleep well in rooms that are excessively hot, cold, noisy, or brightly lit. If

TABLE 11.4

Medications and other substances known to cause sleep disturbance

Medications
- Alpha-Adrenergic agonists
- Amphetamines
- Quinolone antibiotics
- Anticonvulsants
- Antidepressants
- Antihypertensives
- Antineoplastic agents
- Glucocorticoids
- Hypnotic agents
- Levadopa
- Niacin
- Oral contraceptives
- Psychostimulants
- Sympathomimetics
- Theophylline
- Thyroid preparations

Other substances
- Caffeine
- Cocaine
- Nicotine
- Alcohol

Adapted from Pagel JF, Parnes BL. Medications for the treatment of sleep disorders: An overview. Prim care companion. *J Clin Psychiatry.* 2001;3:188–125 (17).

necessary, advise the use of earplugs, sleep masks, white-noise machines or fans to maintain comfortable, consistent bedroom conditions.
- Encourage relaxing activities and a "ritual wind down" in the hour before going to bed. This may involve reading, television, relaxation exercises, or yoga. At times, progressive relaxation training is useful (see Chapter 6).
- Avoid stimulating or emotionally charged issues (e.g., bothersome work issues, excessively arousing reading, or emotionally laden discussions) before going to bed.
- Avoid caffeine after the noontime meal.
- Avoid alcohol after dinner.
- Advise that the bed be used only for sleeping or sexual activity, and not as a place for watching television, eating, or other activities.
- If patients have not fallen asleep within 30 minutes after going to bed, advise getting up and engaging in a pleasant, relaxing activity such as reading, listening to music, or watching television until becoming drowsy. Only then, should the patient return to bed. Advise against staying in bed, tossing, turning, and looking at the clock.

- Similarly, if patients awaken in the middle of the night and have not fallen back to sleep within 30 minutes, advise getting up and following the suggestions in the preceding text until drowsy.

Pharmacologic treatment of sleep in elevated mood

If there is no history of substance abuse or other contraindications, the clinician should be liberal with the use of sleep medication in patients with elevated mood. Because disordered sleep can precipitate manic or hypomanic episodes, the patient should be instructed to contact the clinician if there are more than two nights of significantly disturbed sleep. At such times, the clinician should evaluate the problem, and select both nonpharmacologic and possible medication interventions. Medications for sleep in the patient with elevated mood can include those that have mood effects and those that are primarily hypnotics.

There are many medications with sedative properties that are used in the stabilization of mood and treatment of hypomania and depression. When appropriate, the addition of these medications can have dual purposes. Antimanic agents including lithium carbonate, carbamazepine, valproic acid, atypical antipsychotics (especially olanzapine, risperidone, and quetiapine), traditional neuroleptics, lamotrigine, and oxcarbazepine may all have some sedative effect. With the exception of quetiapine, which is frequently used as a nonhabituating sedative in patients with bipolar disorder, most of the agents mentioned earlier would be used for mood stabilization or antimanic activity and not as a primary hypnotic. Antidepressants such as trazodone, nefazodone, and mirtazapine are frequently prescribed for patients with unipolar depression in need of bedtime sedation. The use of these medications in the patient with elevated mood, however, should be evaluated carefully. Because they are antidepressants, they may disrupt the stability of a mood patient. Patients with bipolar depression in whom a decision was made to treat with antidepressant medications and sleep disorder was part of the depression are exceptions to this general principle. In these patients, the use of a sedative antidepressant could successfully treat both elements of the condition with one medication.

Medications used for their hypnotic properties alone and which do not have prominent mood effects include over-the-counter and herbal sleeping aids as well as sedative hypnotics that can be benzodiazepines or non-benzodiazepines. Although some elevated mood patients may respond to over-the-counter sleep aids, in general, a sleep disturbance associated with hypomania seldom responds to these preparations. Some of these sleep aids are listed in Table 11.5.

The sleep promoting effect of over-the-counter medications has been only minimally studied and their proven efficacy is limited. Herbal preparations have not been studied with rigorous scientific methodology and their use and efficacy is limited in this patient population.

TABLE 11.5
Over-the-counter and herbal preparations for sleep

- Diphenhydramine (Benadryl)
- Diphenhydramine (includes Tylenol PM)
- Melatonin
- Valerian root

Benzodiazepine hypnotics have been used for several decades by primary care and mental health clinicians to treat various sleep disorders, and their usage has been high. The commonly used benzodiazepines are shown in Table 11.6.

Although moderately to significantly effective as hypnotics, these medications have complications. Medication abuse, dependence, discontinuation syndrome, and excessive sedative effects during the day are potential difficulties. Extraordinary care should be exercised when prescribing these medications for patients with a history of substance abuse. When indicated, choice of benzodiazepine is based on individual response, clinician preference and half-life. Longer half-life preparations (diazepam and flurazepam) are generally avoided because their sedative "hang over" effects are often problematic. Intermediate half-life products (temazepam and clonazepam) are more desirable, particularly if sleep continuity disturbance is a problem. Short half-life products (alprazolam and triazolam) are generally useful for patients who have specific difficulty in sleep initiation, but can remain asleep for an adequate period once sleep onset is achieved. Such short half-life products are generally not useful in patients who have middle-of-the-night insomnia.

TABLE 11.6
Benzodiazepine hypnotics

- Alprazolam (Xanax)
- Clonazepam (Klonopin)
- Estazolam (ProSom)
- Diazepam (Valium)
- Flurazepam (Dalmane)
- Lorazepam (Ativan)
- Temazepam (Restoril)
- Triazolam (Halcion)

TABLE 11.7
Non-benzodiazepine receptor agonists

- Zolpidem (Ambien, Ambien CR)
- Zaleplon (Sonata)
- Eszopiclone (Lunesta)

Non-benzodiazepine sedative hypnotics have become popular with clinicians over the past decade. These include the medications listed in Table 11.7.

These products have shown significant advantages over benzodiazepines including lower habit-forming potential, less disruption of normal sleep architecture, fewer medication interactions, and minimal rebound insomnia. Eszopiclone and zolpidem controlled release, have demonstrated safety of usage and lack of tolerance when used over 6 months and 3 months, respectively, adding to the data that, when necessary, long-term use of these newer hypnotics may be safe and effective.

Sodium oxybate (Xyrem) is another possible hypnotic for sleep-disordered patients. Its active ingredient is GHB (gamma hydroxybutyrate) that was initially marketed for cataplexy. Sodium oxybate, an indigenous metabolite of gamma aminobutyric acid (GABA), is a neuromodulator of GABA, dopamine, serotonin and endogenous opioids. Binding to the GABA-B receptor, it has hypnotic effect and a sustained decrease in daytime sleepiness for up to 12 months. Sodium oxybate consolidates nighttime sleep, increases stage 3 and 4 sleep with decreased nighttime awakenings and shows no evidence of tolerance with long-term use. It does have the downside of requiring a middle-of-the-night second dosage because of its very short half-life.

Sleep disorders in patients who abuse substances

Elevated mood patients with a history of substance abuse create a clinical challenge, because the use of benzodiazepines and perhaps non-benzodiazepine hypnotics, such as zolpidem, zaleplon and eszopiclone may be subject to abuse by these patients. The conundrum is that disordered sleep can predispose to manic, hypomanic, and depressive episodes, yet the clinician must be wary of a medication regimen that may lead to further abuse.

In general, nonhabituating agents should be used as first-line treatment for substance abusing patients. These include agents listed in Table 11.8.

The medications, which have mood effects, antidepressant action or antipsychotic treatment, also have sedation as a common side effect. In addition to potentially affecting mood positively, these sedative effects can be extremely useful for sleep maintenance in patients with history of substance abuse. The pros and cons of the use of mood stabilizers, antidepressants, and

TABLE 11.8
Nonhabituating sedative/hypnotic agents

- Mood stabilizers including the following:
  - Lithium
  - Carbamazepine
  - Valproic acid

- Atypical antipsychotics
  - Olanzapine
  - Quetiapine
  - Risperidone

- Anticonvulsant agents including the following:
  - Topiramate
  - Lamotrigine
  - Gabapentin

- Sedative antidepressants (when not otherwise contraindicated)
  - Trazodone
  - Nefazodone
  - Mirtazapine

- Miscellaneous agents
  - Sodium oxybate
  - Over-the-counter sleep preparations
  - Pregabalin
  - Ramelteon

atypical antipsychotics have been discussed previously in this chapter. Other nonhabituating medications include the following:

- Alpha-2-delta antagonists including gabapentin (Neurontin) and pregabalin (Lyrica) which may, in some patients, have a sedative effect and are non–habit forming. These agents also reduce anxiety and pain and may be useful treatment agents for selected hypomanic individuals.
- Ramelteon (Rozerem), a melatonin receptor agonist approved by the U.S. Food and Drug Administration (FDA) for treatment of insomnia. Ramelteon shows no evidence of habituation or tolerance over extended usage. It might be used in a patient with a history of substance abuse or who is particularly concerned about the potential for tolerance developing from chronic use of a hypnotic agent.

Although not generally advisable, some patients with a history of substance abuse who are dependable, responsible, and are not currently abusing substances, may be treated with benzodiazepines under careful supervision and follow-up from the clinician. If this practice is undertaken, clear clinical documentation of the rationale for this treatment should be noted in the patient's chart. Additionally, the patient must be warned that if there are signs of abuse or increasing utilization of the medication, the medication will be discontinued.

Chronic sleep treatment—good or bad?

Patients with chronically elevated mood or frequent hypomanic exacerbations triggered by sleep loss raise the issue of possible long-term administration of sedative hypnotic agents. Although not a desirable mode of treatment for most insomnia patients, the risks of hypomania/mania in patients with bipolar disorder may favor the long-term prescription of sedative hypnotics, when necessary. In general, it is advisable to utilize mood stabilizing sedative compounds such as those listed in Table 11.8 as first-line treatments for sleep problems in this population. However, if substance abuse is not present currently or in the patient's history, the use of non-benzodiazepine hypnotics on a long-term basis may be good treatment. In the context of overall functioning, such agents provide less risk to patients than becoming hypomanic or manic triggered by sleep loss. Whenever treating chronic insomnia with long-term hypnotics, the clinician should clearly document his or her rationale in the patient's record.

The bottom line

- There is a reciprocal relationship between elevated mood and adequate sleep.
- Insomnia may be a consequence of a mood episode, serve as a signal of an oncoming mood episode, or be a cause of a mood episode.
- All patients with elevated mood and insomnia should receive education on sleep hygiene.
- There are a wide variety of medications that can be useful treatments for elevated mood patients.
- If there is no history of substance abuse, chronic prescription of hypnotics may be less harmful than risking serious mood elevation due to sleep loss.

REFERENCES

1. Karacam I. Pharmacotherapy of insomnia. *Essent Psychopharmacol.* 1996; 1(2):167–181.
2. The Gallup Organization. *Sleep in America: a national survey of US Adults.* National Sleep Foundation; 1995.
3. Breslau N, Roth T, Rosenthal L, et al. Sleep disturbance and psychiatric disorders: A longitudinal epidemiological study of young adults. *Biol Psychiatry.* 1996;39:411–418.
4. Ohayon MM. Epidemiological study on insomnia in the general population. *Sleep.* 1996;19:S7–S15.
5. Spiegel K, Leproult R, Van Cauter E. Impact of sleep debt on metabolic and endocrine function. *Lancet.* 1999;354:1435–1439.

6. Stutts JC, Wilkins JW, Osberg S, et al. Driver risk factors for sleep-related crashes. *Accid Anal Prev.* 2003;35:321–331.
7. Riemann D, Vonderholzer U. Primary insomnia: A risk factor to develop depression. *J Affect Disord.* 2003;76:255–259.
8. Wu JC, Bunney WE. The biological basis of an antidepressant response to sleep deprivation and relapse: Review and hypothesis. *Am J Psychiatry.* 1990;147:14–21.
9. Jackson A, Cavanagh J, Scott J. A systematic review of manic and depressive prodromes. *J Affect Disord.* 2003;74:209–217.
10. Harvey A, Schmidt A, Scarna A, et al. Sleep-related functioning in euthymic patients with bipolar disorder, patients with insomnia and subjects without sleep problems. *Am J Psychiatry.* 2005;162:50–57.
11. Goodwin F, Jamison K. *Manic-depressive illness.* New York: Oxford University Press; 1990.
12. Wehr TA, Sack DA, Rosenthal NE. Sleep reduction as a final common pathway in the genesis of mania. *Am J Psychiatry.* 1987;144:201–204; correction, 144:542.
13. Leibenluft E, Albert PS, Rosenthal NE, et al. Relationship between sleep and mood in patients with rapid-cycling bipolar disorder. *Psychiatry Res.* 1996;63:161–168.
14. Wehr TA, Turner EH, Shimada JM, et al. Treatment of rapidly cycling bipolar patient by using extended bed rest and darkness to stabilize the timing and duration of sleep. *Biol Psychiatry.* 1998;43:822–828.
15. Colombo C, Benedetti F, Barbini B, et al. Rate of switch from depression into mania after therapeutic sleep deprivation in bipolar depression. *Psychiatry Res.* 1999;86:267–270.
16. Buysse DJ, Reynolds CF III, Mont TH, et al. The pittsburgh sleep quality index: A new instrument for psychiatric research and practice. *Psychiatry Res* 1989;28(2):193–213.
17. Pagel JF, Parnes BL. Medications for the treatment of sleep disorders: An overview. Prim care companion. *J Clin Psychiatry.* 2001;3:118–125.

MEDICAL CONDITIONS AND ELEVATED MOOD

- Primary versus secondary mania
- Corticosteroid-induced mania
- Brain injury and elevated mood
- Late-onset secondary mania
- Medical illnesses with late-onset elevated mood

- Differentiating late-onset bipolar disorder from agitated dementia
- Treatment of secondary mania
- Medical comorbidities of elevated mood
- The bottom line
  References

Diagnosable medical conditions have at least two interfaces with elevated mood. The first is when the medical condition is causative for the onset of elevated mood, leading to what has been called *secondary mania*. The second relates to medical comorbidities coexisting with elevated mood, but not necessarily having a causative effect.

Primary versus secondary mania

The elevated mood/hypomania/mania referred to in most of this text has also been labeled *primary mania*. Although the underlying cause of primary mania is usually unknown, in other situations, there appears to be a clearly identified medical cause for the onset of bipolar elevated mood. In this situation, referred to as *secondary mania*, identification and treatment of the medical cause are essential for adequate management of any mood alteration. This section discusses the evaluation, identification, and treatment of secondary mania.

Secondary mania may appear at any age but has a higher late-onset incidence because of medical causes and comorbidities. In an ideal world, every patient with new-onset elevated mood symptoms should be thoroughly evaluated medically and neurologically for identifiable medical causes. This, however, is neither cost effective nor always possible. Younger patients with new-onset elevated mood do require a thorough medical evaluation when they

TABLE 12.1
Possible indications of secondary mania in younger patients

- Manic symptoms interspersed with neurologic signs (e.g., gait, vision, or sensory disturbances)
- Patients with no family history of affective disorder
- Persistent sensitivity to mood stabilizing or antidepressant medications; side effects such as difficulty with balance, speech, or vision
- History of recent head injury

show any of the symptoms listed in Table 12.1. The known physical causes of mania are shown in Table 12.2.

Induction of mania has also been associated with a wide variety of disparate medications. These are shown in Table 12.3.

Corticosteroid-induced mania

Brought into the public eye by Jane Pauley's autobiographic account of corticosteroid-induced mania, this common side effect occurs frequently and bears special mention. A variety of studies over the past 25 years have documented the frequency of mood-related symptoms secondary to the use of corticosteroids (1–4). Depending on the study, mania and hypomania were either more or less prevalent than depression, but in all studies both elevated mood and depression were common side effects. In these studies, mania and hypomania were shown to occur in 28% to 35% of patients who had been treated with steroids for a variety of medical conditions. Mixed mood episodes were also common, ranging from 8% to 12% of those treated with

TABLE 12.2
Medical causes of secondary mania

1. Head injury
2. Stroke (including silent cerebral infarction)
3. Dementia
4. Infection
5. Tumor
6. Other neurologic disorders such as multiple sclerosis
7. Medication-induced elevated mood (see Table 12-3)

TABLE 12.3

Medications associated with the induction of mania

- Amphetamines
- Anticholinergics
- Benztropine
- Corticosteroids
- Cyclosporine
- Baclofen
- Bromocriptine
- Captopril
- Cimetidine
- Disulfiram
- Hydralazine
- Isoniazid
- Levodopa
- Levothyroxine
- Metrizamide
- Opioids
- Procarbazine
- Procyclidine
- Trihexyphenidyl
- Yohimbine

Adapted from Medicines that can cause mood disorders. Cleveland clinic health system 2004 accessed at http://www.cchs.net/health/health-info/2200/2284.asp?index=9287. (5)

corticosteroids (1,2). Because steroids are commonly indicated for a variety of medical conditions, including Addison's disease, asthma, inflammatory bowel disease, multiple sclerosis, organ transplant, rheumatoid arthritis and systemic lupus erythematosus, this medical cause of elevated mood is seen frequently in medical and consultation services.

A review of steroid-induced mania by Michael Cerullo (4) has studied the characteristics of this disorder. Typically, psychiatric symptoms emerge from 3 to 11 days after steroid therapy is begun and, when present, mania may persist for 3 weeks after steroids are discontinued. The incidence of psychiatric side effects is higher as the daily dose of steroid is increased with

- 1.3% incidence on <40 mg a day,
- 4.6% on 40 to 80 mg a day,
- 18.4% in those individuals taking >80 mg a day (6).

TABLE 12.4

Mood stabilizers with evidence of benefit in treating corticosteroid-induced mania

- Preventing psychiatric effects in patients requiring long-term corticosteroids
  - Lithium at 0.8 to 1.2 mEq/L

- Preventing recurrence of manic symptoms in patients requiring additional steroid pulses
  - Carbamazepine at 8–12 μg/mL
  - Gabapentin 300 mg t.i.d.

- Treating steroid-induced manic symptoms
  - Olanzapine 2.5–30 mg/day
  - Lithium 0.7 mEq/L
  - Quetiapine 25–50 mg/day
  - Carbamazepine at 8–12 μg/mL
  - Haloperidol 2–20 mg/day

Adapted from Cerullo MA. Corticosteroid-induced mania: Prepare for the unpredictable. *Current Psychiatry.* 2006;5(6):43–58.

Psychiatric symptoms do not consistently appear with each exposure to steroids. Therefore, a history of previous exposure without psychiatric sequelae does not confer protection against such an occurrence during a subsequent exposure (1).

Although no double-blind, placebo-controlled studies have specifically examined the prevention or treatment of steroid-induced mania, patient reports and uncontrolled trials suggest that a variety of psychotropic agents may be beneficial in treating steroid-induced psychiatric symptoms (shown in Table 12.4).

Brain injury and elevated mood

There have been isolated case reports of hypomania, mania, or bipolar disorder with onset after traumatic brain injury (TBI). Most of these reports are on studies with one or two patients. One large-scale review, however, was performed by Jorge et al. (7). This comprehensive study reviewed a consecutive series of 66 patients with closed head injury who were followed at 3-, 6-, and 12-month intervals following the injury. Semistructured psychiatric interviews were conducted and activities of daily living, intellectual and social functioning were evaluated. Six patients (9%) met the criteria for mania at some point during follow-up. This secondary mania was not found to be associated with the severity of brain injury, degree of physical or cognitive impairment, level of social function, or previous family or personal history of psychiatric disorder. The duration of mania lasted for approximately 6 months; although methods of treatment that could affect this statistic were not specified in the report. This frequency of mania is suggested by the authors to be significantly greater than that seen in other brain-injured populations (e.g., patients with stroke).

A smaller series (8) of eight patients looked at brain loci through neuroimaging for possible correlation between mania onset and the location of the TBI. None of the series showed a consistent pattern of TBI location with the onset of secondary mania, and to-date, it is unclear whether location is a crucial factor in the development of secondary mania from TBI. When treatment was indicated for the secondary mania in this group, the most successful outcome involved the use of anticonvulsants, most notably sodium valproate.

Late-onset secondary mania

Although elevated mood with a medical cause can occur at any age, it is particularly common in later life. The so-called *late-onset* hypomania/mania, that is, mania that occurs after the age of 50, is a form of mania that requires special consideration both in diagnosis and treatment. Late-onset elevated mood may have a clinical presentation among those identified in Table 12.5.

Compared to younger individuals, late-onset mania tends to be more debilitating with lower global assessment scale scores (9) and increased cognitive impairment (10). Mania, however, represents one of the few potentially reversible causes of what appears to be cognitive decline in later life. Symptoms of mania in late life include unusually elevated or irritable mood lasting for at least 1 week along with typical manic symptoms including decreased need for sleep, increased talkativeness, flight of ideas, grandiosity, distractibility, and psychomotor agitation. The intensity of symptoms in older patients may be attenuated as compared to younger patients.

Although primary bipolar disorder can first emerge after age 50 without a previous psychiatric history or family history of bipolar disorder (11–13), late-onset elevated mood is more commonly caused by neurologic, pharmacologic or metabolic factors (14,15). Tohen and et al. performed a retrospective study of 50 patients with mania present after age 65. First-onset mania occurred in

TABLE 12.5
Symptomatic patterns in late onset of elevated mood

- Elevated mood with a medical cause (see Table 12.2)
- Long-standing episodes of depression with emergence of a hypomanic/manic episode in late life
- Pharmacologically induced elevated mood
- Late-onset primary bipolar disorder (i.e., no other medical causes)

approximately one fourth of the patients and three fourths of these patients had a comorbid neurologic disorder (15). Because of the increased risk in older adults from medical comorbidities and neurologic disorders, as well as increased sensitivity to medications, *it is important that any late-onset episode of elevated mood be evaluated with a thorough medical and neurologic work-up including neuroimaging.* The clinician should consider late-onset primary bipolar disorder as a diagnosis of exclusion, made only after other medical causes and comorbidities are ruled out.

Medical illnesses with late-onset elevated mood

Although all of the conditions in Table 12.2 have been causally related to the emergence of late-onset bipolar disorder, there are other medical conditions with significantly high incidence of comorbidity in the late-onset bipolar group. These are shown in Table 12.6.

Regardless of age, the association between bipolar disorder and epilepsy bears special note. A recent demographic sample from over 600,000 U.S. households showed that bipolar symptoms were 6.6 times more likely to appear in those with epilepsy than a control group (18). In the same study, 26.3% of the subjects with epilepsy had been diagnosed with unipolar depression. Because bipolar disorder is so common in this population, clinicians should carefully ask epilepsy patients about the presence of elevated mood symptoms when evaluating depression. Secondly, because hypomanic or manic symptoms can be precipitated by antidepressants, clinicians should be cautious in their use when treating what appears to be unipolar depression in this population. Lastly, epileptic patients who have comorbidity of affective

TABLE 12.6
Medical comorbidities with late-onset bipolar disorder

- Epilepsy
- Substance abuse
- Migraine headaches
- Endocrine abnormalities, particularly thyroid disorders including hyper- and hypothyroidism
- Obesity
- Type 2 diabetes
- Cardiovascular disease
- Tourette's syndrome
- Multiple sclerosis

(16,17)

symptoms should preferentially be treated with anticonvulsants that have some mood stabilizing properties (e.g., divalproex sodium, carbamazepine, or lamotrigine) rather than anticonvulsants lacking mood stabilization properties in this area (e.g., dilantin, gabapentin, or topiramate).

Substance abuse is common in the elderly population and can also be a comorbidity with elevated mood (see Chapter 14). Substance abuse can account for impulsivity, aggression, and other symptoms that may appear to be hypomanic in origin (11). Because older adults may be more sensitive to effects of alcohol and other drugs such as cocaine, methamphetamine, and amphetamine, substance use should always be considered in evaluating this population. When the clinician's index of suspicion of substance use is raised in the elevated mood patient, a liver panel and serum drug screen is indicated.

Medications associated with the precipitation of late-onset bipolar disorder include those listed in Table 12.7. This smaller list is in contrast to the longer list in Table 12.3 that lists medication associated with bipolar disorder.

Differentiating late-onset bipolar disorder from agitated dementia

As noted in the preceding text, patients with late-onset primary bipolar disorder may show cognitive impairment, which has the potential for partial reversibility. Therefore, it is important to distinguish this cause of cognitive impairment from a dementia that may be less amenable to treatment.

TABLE 12.7

Medications associated with late-onset mania

- Antidepressants
  - Tricyclic antidepressants
  - Serotonin-specific reuptake inhibitors
  - Serotonin–norepinephrine reuptake inhibitors

- Atypical antipsychotics
  - Olanzapine
  - Risperidone
  - Quetiapine
  - Ziprasidone

- Antibiotics
  - Macrolides
  - Clarithromycin

- Corticosteroids
- St. John's Wort

Brooks JO, Hoblyn JC. Secondary mania in older adults. *Am J Psychiatry.* 2005;162(11):20–35.

In dementia, cognitive changes typically occur early in the course of the illness and seldom have affective components. These changes gradually progress over many months. Affective symptoms often appear in dementia patients only after several years. The treatment of these affective symptoms seldom diminishes the severity of the cognitive changes. Agitation and restlessness that begin in the late afternoon and early evening are also more characteristic of dementia than mania. By contrast, hypomania or mania tends to have a relatively abrupt onset of affective symptoms. Any cognitive impairment associated with such mania is also abrupt in onset and is more likely to recover when the elevated mood is treated.

Acute delirium and its associated cognitive changes may also present with agitation that can at times be confused with elevated mood. In general, delirium shows a waxing and waning pattern of alteration in consciousness that accompanies cognitive changes. Therefore, longitudinal observations of the patient are important to distinguish this cardinal feature of delirium from the steadier affective symptomatology of elevated mood associated with mania.

Treatment of secondary mania

In general, the treatment of secondary mania is similar to the treatment of primary mania, but there are additional considerations. When the medical cause of secondary mania is elucidated and treatment is initiated, hypomanic/manic symptoms may quickly resolve. For example, if a benign brain tumor is diagnosed and removed, mood stabilizing medication may be necessary only until the patient recovers from surgery. At this point, medication may gradually be decreased and ultimately discontinued without re-emergence of elevated mood symptoms. Likewise, elevated mood associated with thyroid abnormalities, neurologic infections and pharmacologic induction can have relatively benign outcomes, and will not require chronic treatment. Alternatively, when the medical cause is not treatable or only partially so, treatment of the elevated mood symptoms may be complex and these patients may present treatment challenges. Patients with elevated mood associated with cerebrovascular accidents, multiple sclerosis, Tourette's syndrome or diabetes mellitus may require continued treatment for elevated mood despite appropriate treatment measures for the underlying medical condition.

There is no single ideal treatment for late-onset secondary mania. Regardless of the agent chosen, medication treatment of secondary mania must be judged on an individual basis. The clinician must take into account medical comorbidities and the specific side effect profile of possible medications when selecting the best agent or combination of agents to be used. Many of the studies on which the following recommendations are made were conducted in elderly patients with secondary mania. It is assumed (without specific evidence, however) that the recommendations would also apply to younger secondary mania patients. The relative merits of mood stabilizing medications used in secondary mania are as follows:

Sodium valproate. Sodium valproate, whether in its generic or branded preparations, is generally acknowledged as the most useful treatment for secondary mania (16,19). It shows effectiveness in modulating elevated mood and providing some control of agitated behavior. It also provides anticonvulsive effectiveness when needed (e.g., in the presence of epilepsy or tumor). Common side effects of valproate may, however, create some difficulty for certain patients. These include sedation, weight gain, gastrointestinal upset, tremor, and decreased platelets. Hepatotoxicity and pancreatitis are serious side effects, but occur rarely.

Carbamazepine. Carbamazepine, whether in the generic or recently branded preparation (Equetro), is effective in controlling secondary elevated mood. Sedation, visual and gait abnormalities, and decreased numbers of white blood cells, however, can create problems. Also, carbamazepine has multiple drug interactions that may affect the serum levels of medications commonly used in the elderly population including other anticonvulsants, warfarin, cardiovascular agents, and digoxin.

Lithium carbonate. Although clearly effective for elevated mood in general, lithium may be a problematic medication in the elderly. Side effects of polydipsia, polyuria, decreased thyroid function, and alterations of salt and fluid balance can create complications in fragile seniors. Elderly patients may also be more vulnerable to adverse side effects from mild to moderate lithium toxicity.

Antipsychotics. Antipsychotics have long been used to control either primary or secondary manic behavior. Over the past decade, atypical antipsychotics have been used preferentially because of the lack of extrapyramidal side effects and minimal potential for irreversible tardive dyskinesia. Recently, however, these agents have been cited for an increase in mortality rates associated with their use in elderly patients who have dementia. The current expert consensus guidelines for the use of antipsychotic agents in older patients suggest that antipsychotics be avoided for mild mania, which presumably would include all those with hypomania. Antipsychotics, however, are considered adjunctive treatment with primary mood stabilizers for psychotic mania or severely uncontrolled nonpsychotic mania (20).

Benzodiazepines. Although effective for the acute agitation associated with secondary mania, benzodiazepines present particular concerns in the elderly population. With an associated fall rate as high as 40%, as well as problems with coordination, balance, cognition, and oversedation, long-acting benzodiazepines are particularly problematic. Despite the fact that benzodiazepines are a target of oversight by the Federal government in long-term care facilities, small doses of short to medium half-life agents such as lorazepam or clonazepam might be reasonable choices for acute agitation (16,19).

Other anticonvulsants. Other anticonvulsants that have been purported to have mood stabilization properties run the gamut from those
that have strong evidence for efficacy (e.g., lamotrigine) to those that
have relatively weak or nonexistent research to support mood stabilization efficacy (e.g., topiramate, gabapentin, oxcarbazepine). None
of these latter agents have been studied specifically in patients with
secondary mania or late-onset bipolar disorder. Conversely, lamotrigine clearly has the best evidence for mood stabilization and efficacy in
bipolar depression and, therefore, is a more likely candidate for usage.

Medical comorbidities of elevated mood

Having looked at medical illnesses that have a causative role in mania,
we now focus on medical conditions that show frequent comorbidity with
elevated mood, but that do not have apparent causative effect. It has long
been known that medical conditions can be quite common in individuals
with major mental illnesses and that the presence of mental illness increases
morbidity and mortality from the medical conditions. Retrospective analyses
of patients with mental illness have shown an increased risk of death from
cardiovascular and cerebrovascular disorders. Diabetes and obesity have also
been correlated with bipolar I disorder (21,22).

A recent study looked at the prevalence of specific medical comorbidities
in 174 patients with bipolar I disorder (Table 12.8, [22]). Thompson, Kupfer
et al. showed that a variety of medical conditions were common in this cohort
of patients with bipolar I disorder.

This study also confirmed previous evidence that the presence of medical
comorbidities in an individual with bipolar I disorder is correlated with poor
prognosis outcome for the bipolar disorder. These individuals had a longer
total duration of lifetime depressive episodes, longer total duration of total
lifetime inpatient depressive episodes, and higher baseline Hamilton Rating
Scale for Depression (HAM-D) scores. The authors speculate that these
medical illnesses could be influencing the outcome of the mood disorder
through several factors including the following:

- A negative impact on quality of life
- A disruption of circadian rhythms causing mood destabilization
- The degree of suicidality

Although there was an association between medical comorbidities and
depression, there was lack of statistical significance between increased medical burden and mania. It is speculated by the authors that the size of the
patient sample might not have been large enough to elucidate such a possible
connection.

TABLE 12.8

Active medical comorbidities in 174 patients with bipolar I disorder

Category	Number of active comorbidities
• Asthma/respiratory	41
• Bone/joints/muscles	56
• Cardiovascular	32
• Diabetes	2
• Gastrointestinal	59
• Genital/urinary	43
• Headache/migraine	42
• Obesity	58
• Skin	23
• Thyroid dysfunction	22
• Others	43

Adapted from Thompson WK, Kupfer DJ, Fagiolini A, et al. Prevalence and clinical correlates of medical co-morbidities in patients with Bipolar I Disorder: Analysis of acute-phase data from a randomized controlled trial. *J Clin Psychiatry.* 2006;67. (23)

The bottom line

- Certain medical conditions that can cause secondary mania include head injury, stroke, dementia, infection, or tumor.
- Epilepsy, migraine headaches, hyper- and hypothyroidism, type 2 diabetes and Tourette's syndrome are associated with late-onset bipolar disorder.
- Late-onset elevated mood patients (>50 years old) should be evaluated thoroughly for possible medical causes.
- The use of sodium valproate has gained wide acceptance in treating secondary mania.

REFERENCES

1. Lewis DA, Smith RE. Steroid-induced psychiatric syndromes. A report of 14 cases and a review of the literature. *J Affect Disord.* 1983;5:319–332.
2. Sirois F. Steroid psychosis: A review. *Gen Hosp Psychiatry.* 2003;25:27–33.
3. Nabar D, Sand P, Heigl B. Psychopathological and neuropsychological effects of 8-days' corticosteroid treatment. A prospective study. *Psychoneuroendocrinology.* 1996;21:25–31.

4. Cerullo MA. Corticosteroid-induced mania: Prepare for the unpredictable. *Curr Psychiatry*. 2006;5(6):43–58.
5. Medicines that can cause mood disorders. Cleveland clinic health system 2004 accessed at http://www.cchs.net/health/health-info/2200/2284.asp?index=9287.
6. The Boston Collaborative Drug Surveillance Program. Acute adverse reactions to prednisone in relation to dosage. *Clin Pharmacol Ther*. 1972;13:694–698.
7. Jorge RE, Robinson RG, Starkstein SE, et al. Secondary mania following traumatic brain injury. *Am J Psychiatry*. 1993;150(6):916–921.
8. Starkstein SE, Mayberg HS, Berthier ML, et al. Mania after brain injury: Neuroradiological and metabolic findings. *Ann Neurol*. 1990;27(6):652–659.
9. Young RC, Klerman GL. Mania in late life: Focus on age at onset. *Am J Psychiatry*. 1992;149:867–876.
10. Mirchandani IC, Young RC. Management of mania in the elderly: An update. *Ann Clin Psychiatry*. 1993;5:67–77.
11. Depp CA, Jin H, Mohamed S, et al. Bipolar Disorder in middle-aged and elderly adults: Is age of onset important. *J Nerv Ment Dis*. 2004;192:796–799.
12. Depp CA, Jeste DV. Bipolar Disorder in older adults: A critical review. *Bipolar Disord*. 2004;6:343–367.
13. Moorhead SR, Young AH. Evidence for a late onset Bipolar I Disorder sub-group from 50 years. *J Affect Disord*. 2003;73:271–277.
14. Krauthammer C, Klerman GL. Secondary mania: Manic syndromes associated with antecedent physical illness or drugs. *Arch Gen Psychiatry*. 1978;35:1333–1339.
15. Tohen M, Shulman Kl, Satlin A. First-episode mania in late life. *Am J Psychiatry Res*. 1975;12:189–198.
16. Brooks JO, Hoblyn JC. Secondary mania in older adults. *Am J Psychiatry*. 2005;162(11):1333–1339.
17. McElroy SL.Diagnosing and treating comorbid (complicated) Bipolar Disorder. *J Clin Psychiatry*. 2004;65(Suppl 15):35–44.
18. Ettinger AB, Reed ML, Goldberg JF, et al. Prevalence of Bipolar symptoms in epilepsy vs other chronic health disorders. *Neurology*. 2005;65:535–540.
19. Snader TC. Current treatment options for Bipolar Disorder in the older patient. The University of Florida CME, peerview institute for medical education accessed at www.peerviewpress.com/r/inR106.
20. Alexopoulos GS, Streim JE, Carpenter D. Expert consensus guidelines for using antipsychotic agents in older patients. *J Clin Psychiatry*. 2004;65(Suppl 2):5–99.
21. Cassidy F, Ahearn E, Carroll B. Elevated frequency of diabetes mellitus in hospitalized manic-depressive patients. *Am J Psychiatry*. 1999;156:1417–1420.
22. Fagiolini A, Frank E, Houck PR, et al. Prevalence of obesity and weight change during treatment in patients with Bipolar I Disorder. *J Clin Psychiatry*. 2002;63:528–533.
23. Thompson WK, Kupfer DJ, Fagiolini A, et al. Prevalence and clinical correlates of medical co-morbidities in patients with Bipolar I Disorder: Analysis of acute-phase data from a randomized controlled trial. *J Clin Psychiatry*. 2006;67:783–788.

13

ELEVATED MOOD
AND SUBSTANCE ABUSE

- Why do elevated mood patients drink?
- Effects of alcohol on mood-stabilizing medication
- Recreational drugs and elevated mood
- The bottom line
  References

The frequent comorbidity of substance abuse with bipolar disorder has long been known (1–3). Data from the National Epidemiological Survey on Alcohol-Related Conditions (NESARC) show that bipolar disorder has the strongest association with alcohol use disorders (AUDs) of any mood or anxiety disorder (2). Both clinical and community populations show that alcohol is the most commonly abused medication for both bipolar I and bipolar II disorders (2,3). Bipolar I patients with current alcohol use have been differentiated from patients with other bipolar disorders in that they show increased numbers of manic symptoms, increased impulsivity and increased high-risk of violent behavior (4,5). Hypomania and bipolar II disorder also put a patient at high risk for alcohol abuse and dependence. A 20-year longitudinal study comparing over 600 subjects with bipolar II disorder to those who did not develop mood disorders, revealed that those with bipolar II disorder had a 4.6-fold increased likelihood of developing alcohol abuse and a 2.2-fold increased likelihood to become alcohol dependent.

Not only is the co-occurrence of AUDs and bipolar disorders very common, but the use of alcohol also worsens the prognosis for bipolar disorder on virtually all parameters, as shown in Table 13.1.

Interestingly, although in the general population the risk of alcohol use and abuse is higher for men, Frye, Altshuler et al. showed that in patients with bipolar disorder, the risk of alcoholism was greater for women (odds ratio = 7.35) than for men (odds ratio = 2.77) (6). Women are also physically more vulnerable to the effects of alcohol than men. Women who abuse alcohol show increased liver and brain damage, increased negative effects

TABLE 13.1
Deleterious effects of alcohol use on bipolar disorder

The presence of an alcohol use disorder worsens the prognosis for bipolar disorder by

- delaying recovery from an acute episode
- increasing recurrence
- increasing frequency of hospitalization
- increasing interepisode symptomatology, leading to poorer symptomatic and functional recovery
- decreasing adherence and compliance to treatment regimens
- increasing the development of mixed states
- increasing suicidal ideation and attempts

Adapted from references (1–4)

on cognition, increased rates of hepatitis C, human immunodeficiency virus (HIV)/acquired immunodeficiency syndrome (AIDS), and breast cancer, as compared to those who do not abuse alcohol and as compared to men. Women with comorbid bipolar disorder and alcoholism are more prone to victimization, violence, and sexual abuse. These comorbid women also have nine times the rate of polysubstance abuse, three times the rate of social anxiety disorder, and four times the rate of depressive episodes as compared to women with bipolar disorder without alcoholism. They are also less likely to receive treatment for alcoholism than men with bipolar disorder (4,6).

Why do elevated mood patients drink?

It has been commonly accepted that patients with elevated mood drink to "self-medicate" and therefore, "treat" unpleasant affective symptoms through alcohol use. This concept would predict that alcohol use should increase during affective episodes and that affective symptoms should improve during periods of alcohol use. There is, however, little evidence to support this hypothesis and most evidence indicates that substance use makes mood symptoms worse (7). Although it is certainly possible that some patients with bipolar disorder drink to decrease the perceived negative effects of either elevated mood or depression, there are other possibilities. Some patients may drink to initiate or enhance euphoric feelings. Other authors have speculated that the poor judgment, impulsivity, and excessive involvement in pleasurable activities associated with bipolar disorder may predispose an individual to an alcohol use disorder (8). Citing the neurobiologic similarities in neural transmitter symptoms and adaptation in signaling pathways common to both disorders, some suggest that substance abuse "unmasks" a bipolar disorder in a vulnerable individual (9). Because the ultimate causal connection between bipolar disorder and alcohol abuse remains unclear, this relationship is complex and bidirectional (8).

Effects of alcohol on mood-stabilizing medication

It is well known that individuals with bipolar disorder who drink have a poor response to lithium therapy. Patients with an AUD are likely to be less compliant with a medication regimen, regardless of which mood-stabilizing medication they use. Poor compliance leads to increased relapse and a poor overall prognosis.

There is some evidence for the use of valproic acid in this clinical group. When valproate was added to the regimen of 59 subjects who continued their usual clinical care (lithium carbonate and psychosocial treatments for alcohol dependence), valproate appeared to decrease the amount of heavy drinking in this cohort. Compared with placebo, there were significantly fewer drinking days reported in the valproate group (10).

This advantage for valproate may not apply to rapid cycling bipolar disorder as investigated by Calabrese et al. (11). In a study of 254 patients with either bipolar I or bipolar II disorder who were treated with either lithium or valproate and followed up for 20 months, there were no significant differences in rates of relapse into mood episodes. Most patients on either monotherapy experienced a mood relapse with a preponderance of depressive relapses as compared to manic relapses, regardless of treatment. On the basis of this information, the authors opine that rapid cycling, in and by itself, appears to be a predictor of nonresponse with any treatment.

Beyond knowing that substance use worsens the prognosis for bipolar disorder, one study that specifically studied recovery from substance use, investigating whether it had a *positive* effect on the outcome of bipolar disorder (12,13). Those patients who did obtain a sustained remission from substance use fared better than patients with current substance use, but not as well as those who had never had a substance abuse problem.

Although common knowledge suggests that heavy use of alcohol would negatively affect the prognosis of a bipolar disorder, a recent study suggests that even modest drinking may worsen measures of illness severity in both men and women (14). In this study, the mean weekly alcoholic beverage consumption was minimal among both men and women (3.8 drinks per week and 1.2 drinks per week, respectively). Spirit consumption among men was strongly associated with more lifetime manic episodes and emergency room visits. Women showed increased lifetime episodes of depression and hypomania associated alcohol consumption. Although this finding remains to be confirmed, this study suggests that the usual recommendations to psychiatric patients (i.e., modest, low level alcohol use may be safe) may not apply to bipolar disorder, and that clinicians should advise abstinence for all patients with elevated mood.

Recreational drugs and elevated mood

Although somewhat less studied than alcohol abuse, recreational or street drug abuse is also relatively common in patients with bipolar disorder. The NESARC study cited in the preceding text also showed that the prevalence for drug use in mania was 37.5% and in hypomania was 25.2% (15).

Although, as in other studies, alcohol was the most commonly abused substance, other drugs of abuse were commonly misused by patients with bipolar disorder, including

- marijuana (16%),
- cocaine (9%),
- stimulants (9%),
- sedatives (8%),
- opiates (7%) (16).

Although there have been few specific studies evaluating the effects of treatment on bipolar disorder with comorbid recreational drug abuse, there are several studies worthy of note. Geller et al. (17) studied 25 adolescent patients who had been diagnosed with bipolar disorder and secondary substance abuse, including marijuana, inhalants, or multiple drugs. Treated with lithium carbonate, the patients showed improvement in both symptoms of bipolar disorder (as measured by ability to function in family, school, and social settings) and lessened drug usage (drug-positive urine samples dropped from 40% to 10%).

Lamotrigine was shown to be effective for bipolar disorder and comorbid cocaine dependence by Brown et al. (18) in two separate studies. The first involved 340 patients with comorbid bipolar disorder and cocaine dependence and the second involved an additional 32 cocaine-dependent patients. Although open-label and uncontrolled, the studies revealed that lamotrigine-treated patients showed significantly decreased drug craving and drug use as well as improvement in mood.

The bottom line

- Substance use and substance use disorders are very common comorbidities with bipolar disorder.
- In the bipolar population, alcohol is the most frequently abused substance but marijuana, cocaine, stimulants, sedatives, and opiates are also abused.
- Substance abuse, even when modest may worsen the treatment outcome and prognosis for bipolar disorder.
- There is limited evidence that mood-stabilizing medication may improve the clinical condition of comorbid patients for bipolar disorder and substance abuse—lamotrigine (cocaine), valproic acid (alcohol), and lithium (multiple substances).

REFERENCES

1. Cassidy F, Ahearn EP, Carroll BJ. Substance abuse in Bipolar Disorder. *Bipolar Disord.* 2001;3:181–188.
2. Grant BF, Stinson FS, Dawson DA, et al. Prevalence and co-occurrence of substance use disorders and independent mood and anxiety disorders: Results from the National Epidemiologic Survey on Alcohol and Related Conditions. *Arch Gen Psychiatry.* 2004;61:807–816.
3. Chengappa KNR, Levine J, Gershow S, et al. Lifetime prevalence of substance or alcohol abuse and dependence among subjects with Bipolar I and II disorders in a voluntary registry. *Bipolar Disord.* 2000;2:191–195.
4. Salloum IM, Thase ME. Impact of substance abuse on the course and treatment of Bipolar Disorder. *Bipolar Disord.* 2000;2:269–280.
5. Merikangas KR. Substance abuse and bipolar disorder presented at *The 6th International Conference on Bipolar Disorder.* Pittsburgh PA: June 2005.
6. Frye MA, Altshuler LL, McElroy SL, et al. Gender differences in prevalence, risk and clinical correlates of alcoholism comorbidity in Bipolar Disorder. *Am J Psychiatry.* 2003;160:883–889.
7. Verduin ML, Tolliver BK, Brady KT. Substance abuse and Bipolar Disorder. *Medsc Psychiatr Ment Health.* Posted December 2005.
8. Strakowski SM, Sax KW, McElroy SL, et al. Course of psychiatric and substance abuse syndromes co-occurring with Bipolar Disorder after a first psychiatric hospitalization. *J Clin Psychiatry.* 1998;59:465–471.
9. Markou A, Kosten TR, Koob GF. Neurobiological similarities in depression and drug dependence: A self-medication hypothesis. *Neuropsychopharmacology.* 1998;18:135–174.
10. Salloum IM, Cornelius JR, Daley DC, et al. Efficacy of valproate maintenance in patients with Bipolar Disorder and alcoholism: A double-blind placebo-controlled study. *Arch Gen Psychiatry.* 2005;62:37–45.
11. Calabrese JR, Shelton MD, Rapport DJ, et al. A 20-month, double-blind, maintenance trial of lithium versus divalproex in rapid-cycling Bipolar Disorder. *Am J Psychiatry.* 2005;162:2152–2161.
12. Weiss RD, Ostacher MJ, Otto MW, et al. Does recovery from substance use disorder matter in patients with Bipolar Disorder. *J Clin Psychiatry.* 2005;66:730–735.
13. Weiss RD, Ostacher MJ, Otto MW, et al. Does recovery from substance use disorder matter in patients with Bipolar Disorder? *J Clin Psychiatry.* 2005;66:730–735.
14. Goldstein BI, Velyvis VP, Parihk SV. The association between moderate alcohol use and illness severity in Bipolar Disorder: A preliminary report. *J Clin Psychiatry.* 2006;67:102–106.
15. Conway KP, Compton W, Stinson FS, et al. Lifetime comorbidity of DSM-IV mood and anxiety disorders and specific drug use disorders: Results from the national epidemiologic survey on alcohol and relation conditions. *J Clin Psychiatry.* 2006;67:247–257.
16. McElroy SL, Altshuler LL, Suppes T, et al. Axis I psychiatric comorbidity and its relationship to historical illness variables in 288 patients with Bipolar Disorder. *Am J Psychiatry.* 2001;158:420–426.

17. Geller B, Cooper TB, Sun K, et al. Double-blind and placebo-controlled study of lithium for adolescent Bipolar Disorders with secondary substance dependency. *J Am Acad Child Adolesc Psychiatry.* 1998;37(2):171–178.
18. Brown ES, Perantie DC, Dhanani N, et al. Lamotrigine for Bipolar Disorder and comorbid cocaine dependence: A replication and extension study. *J Affect Disord.* 2006;93(1-3):219–222.

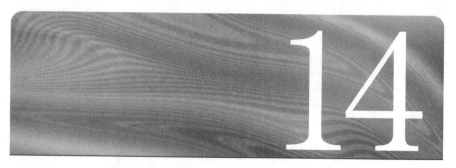

PREGNANCY AND ELEVATED MOOD

C aring for an elevated mood patient who wishes to become pregnant or becomes pregnant requires skill, tact, and an ability to work cooperatively with the woman and her partner. There are four distinct stages to this treatment, each of which has separate principles and guidelines.

- Treating the potentially pregnant woman during the planning and prepregnancy period
- Treating elevated mood during pregnancy
- Peripartum period issues
- Postpartum and lactation

Clinical principles

There is a paucity of information that specifically relates to hypomania in prepregnant and pregnant women. Therefore, we must extrapolate treatment principles on the basis of information derived from investigation of bipolar disorder. Hyperthymic and mildly hypomanic women may not present to a mental health professional for evaluation or treatment at all. These patients, when they present to their maternal health care professional, may show minimal, if any, signs of psychiatric pathology. It would be easy for a health-care professional to mistake mildly elevated mood for the joy and pleasure of anticipating or being pregnant. Therefore, the principles discussed in the rest of this section are for the more easily identifiable hypomanic patients or those women who develop full-fledged mania.

"Traditional wisdom" has suggested that pregnancy may provide protection against bipolar relapse. However, more recent studies suggest otherwise (1–3). When a cohort of women with predominately bipolar I disorder who were studied as part of the National Institute of Mental Health (NIMH) Genetics Initiative became pregnant, half of them described severe emotional disturbances in relation to childbearing (4). Viguera et al. (2) found that the rate of recurrence of bipolar I and bipolar II disorders were approximately equal in pregnant and nonpregnant women. When these patients with bipolar disorder from the Massachusetts General Hospital Perinatal and Reproductive Psychiatry program were followed up over the course of their pregnancy, the overall recurrence risk for a mood episode in this sample was 66%, including 58% showing major depression, 16% showing mania, 13% showing hypomania, and 13% showing mixed states. Therefore, one fourth the number of these patients showed hypomania or a mixed affective state and approximately one sixth of them showed mania. These studies contradict previously held beliefs and indicate that *the risk of elevated mood and depression is significant during pregnancy.*

In the pregnant patient with minimal elevation of mood, consideration should be given to providing a limited treatment of close observation and follow-up. If treatment is necessary, in general, the psychotherapeutic strategies as outlined in Chapter 6 are first-line and preferable to medication. Those with mild symptomatology may respond to cognitive behavioral therapy (CBT), interpersonal psychotherapeutic strategies, psychoeducation, and lifestyle hygiene recommendations. Although it may be theoretically desirable for women with bipolar disorder to remain medication-free during pregnancy, this may not, however, be possible and maintenance treatment during pregnancy may be necessary. Even those patients who initially decide to discontinue medication during pregnancy may relapse with such significant symptomatology that the reintroduction of medication is indicated.

When medication is considered, it is the role of the clinician to do the following:

- Provide up-to-date and balanced information to the patient about possible risks of medication and/or the possible complications of untreated mood illness.
- Assist the woman to make the best decision for herself, always being cognizant that the final decision rests with the patient.

- Once a decision is reached, verbally support the final choice of the patient and her partner.

  If medication is being prescribed during the pregnancy, the following clinical guidelines should be adhered to.

- The lowest possible dose that treats the symptoms satisfactorily should be used. Consider intermittent dosing if feasible, but do not hesitate to increase medication dosages to full therapeutic range if necessary for adequate symptom control.
- Once a patient decides to use or restart medication, the clinician should be positive, encouraging, and supportive even if there are known risks to this course of action.
- If elevated mood symptoms worsen to the point of full mania, especially with psychotic symptoms, the clinician should make a strong case for starting or continuing medication. In general, the risk to mother and fetus is small from medication treatment as compared to the effects of a major manic episode. Hospitalization or electroconvulsive therapy (ECT) may also be considered.
- For the patient who has elevated mood escalating to confusion or disorganized thinking, or when manic delusions are present, the care giver should include input from the partner or caretakers to both assess the extent of symptomatology and behavioral risks during pregnancy. For patients who are declared legally incompetent, involve a guardian in any decision to start or restart medication.
- If possible, use monotherapy and avoid polypharmacy.
- In general, it is best to return to a medication that was therapeutically effective and tolerated before pregnancy. Pregnancy is not the time to be experimenting with a new medication regimen unless earlier medications were ineffective. Exceptions to this principle would be during the first trimester with carbamazepine or valproic acid (see the subsequent text), which are pregnancy Class D medication. Other alternatives should be considered at least for the first trimester.

Preplanning with fertile women who have elevated mood

Patients seen for the treatment of elevated mood who are fertile and potentially pregnant require a discussion regarding the benefits of a planned pregnancy. If medication is to be started or has been ongoing, use of birth control should be discussed with all female patients of childbearing age and documented in the chart. For any woman of childbearing age where there are symptoms suggestive of pregnancy or the possibility of pregnancy cannot be ruled out with certainty, a pregnancy test should be obtained before the patient begins medication.

Some patients may present to a clinician in the midst of a major elevated mood episode, expressing their interest in becoming pregnant. The clinician should advise the patient to delay conception until her mental health episode is stabilized. Such a suggestion may displease a hypomanic woman. Providing an approximate time frame for a safe conception is useful in hopes that the patient will be more stable and able to make appropriate decisions about medication and pregnancy.

When an elevated mood patient becomes pregnant

Recommended steps for the clinician treating a patient with elevated mood who suspects or documents a pregnancy are as follows:

- Document when the clinician was informed of the possibility of pregnancy, when it was confirmed by test and the estimated time of delivery.
- Document any other medications taken at the time of conception over and above any psychotropics being prescribed by the clinician.
- Document any history of ongoing alcohol or drug abuse.
- If necessary, order a pregnancy test for confirmation.
- If necessary, assist the patient in finding an obstetrical care provider and prenatal care.
- Unless there is a previously agreed-upon plan, the treater should immediately schedule an appointment to discuss the medication treatment plan during the pregnancy.
- Involve the patient's partner in education and decisions about medication.
- If the patient wishes to be medication-free, it is generally better to stop medications quickly rather than utilize a prolonged taper, even if this might be the preferred schedule during nonpregnant circumstances. Pregnant women who strongly wish to be off medication will generally appreciate this short interval to a medication-free state.
- If medication is to be continued, it should be decreased to the lowest dose that provides reasonable symptom control.
- Avoid polypharmacy. If the patient has been maintained on a combination of medication, monotherapy should be considered.
- If the pregnancy is unplanned, the clinician can serve as an objective sounding board to assist the patient in evaluating whether to keep or terminate the pregnancy.
- When possible, avoid medication in the first trimester when the teratogenic effect of medication is at its highest.
- Maintain flexibility in the use of medication and/or other treatment, pending any change in clinical circumstances. Some patients may benefit from reinstituting medication in the second or third trimester when the risk of teratogenicity is less.
- Monitor the patient directly in face-to-face evaluation more frequently. If the patient sees a psychotherapist in split treatment, maintain close contact with this therapist.

- Consider nonpharmacologic interventions including CBT, individual or group therapy, or light therapy for depression.
- Evaluate life stressors. When necessary, recommend psychotherapy to address job, family, and relationship issues.
- If the patient is experiencing severe symptoms of elevated mood or depression, make a strong case for starting or continuing medication. In general, the risk of medication side effects to mother and fetus are small in comparison to the sequelae of a major mood episode. Maternal stress and distress, anxiety and depression have also been clinically associated with a wide variety of abnormalities in newborns including lower birth weight (3,4).
- Once it is decided to use medication during the pregnancy, be positive, encouraging and supportive toward the patient's decision even if there are some known risks.
- In general, use medications that were successful and well tolerated earlier. Pregnancy is not a time to be experimenting with a new medication regimen.
- Consider hospitalization and/or the use of ECT as an alternative for severe mood symptoms. For manic individuals with psychotic symptoms, involve the partner or caretakers in any decision about treatment and medication. For patients declared legally incompetent, involve the guardian.
- Unless the patient is declared incompetent or incapacitated (this is unlikely in hypomania), the clinician cannot make unilateral decisions for the patient regarding use of medication during pregnancy.

Peripartum and postpartum

As the delivery date approaches, the clinician and patient should discuss plans for the last several weeks of the pregnancy and the immediate postpartum period. Mood stabilizers and antidepressants may be tapered and discontinued in the 7 to 10 days before delivery to prevent neonatal withdrawal, particularly with short half-life antidepressants such as paroxetine, venlafaxine, or benzodiazepines. Tapering of medication may become a moot point in the patient who has a spontaneous early labor.

The immediate postpartum period has long been known for exacerbation of mood disorders. Postpartum depression is common. Postpartum psychosis, although infrequent, is potentially catastrophic. Patients with a history of bipolar disorder are at special risk for worsening of their mood disorder during the postpartum period (5,6). This occurs with enough frequency that postpartum worsening of a mood disorder is one signal supporting a diagnosis of bipolar disorder. Studies with American and international populations of women have shown that women who are at risk for postpartum depression can be identified as early as the third postpartum day (7–10). Instruments such as Maternity Blues Scale and the Edinburgh Postnatal Depression Scale are useful tools for this early detection.

The most recent research on postpartum psychosis (11) confirms the risk. Blackmoor et al. studied 129 white women with lifetime diagnoses of bipolar or schizoaffective disorder of the bipolar type who had suffered at least one manic or affective psychotic episode within 4 weeks after childbirth. Ninety-seven percent of these psychotic episodes had the onset within the first 2 weeks after delivery. Comparison of these findings with 75 unaffected deliveries showed that 82% of these high-risk women had psychotic episodes after their first deliveries. The only other risk factor that could be confirmed in this study was self-reported complications with labor and delivery that also increased postpartum psychosis. This study confirms the necessity of evaluating all pregnant women for history of previous psychiatric disorder. Women with a prior history of bipolar or psychotic disorder should be monitored very carefully during the first several weeks following delivery. Any evidence of severe mood disorder and/or psychotic symptomatology bears immediate action.

Because of this high risk, most, if not all, patients with bipolar disorder should receive a recommendation to rapidly reinstitute mood-stabilizing and possibly antidepressant medication shortly after delivery unless a definitive decision by the mother has been reached to not restart medications. On the basis of current data, the clinician should make a strong recommendation to medicate in this critically vulnerable period.

Breast-feeding

Prospective evidence-based data on the use of psychotropics during breast-feeding is virtually absent, so the evidence for the recommendations in this text comes solely from isolated case examples and on retrospective review of data. Women and their partners, therefore, must be advised that recommendations have little documented supporting evidence. This being said, from the information that we do have, it appears that psychotropic medications in general do not *seem* to have long-term effects on the infant. Adverse effects seen in infants are generally reversible side effects rather than long-term brain toxicity (12). Mothers should, however, be informed that virtually all psychotropic medications taken during breast-feeding do appear in breast milk in varying concentrations. In general, these concentrations are small but the long-term effect of this small amount of medication is uncertain. The following principles and strategies are useful for the patient with elevated mood who will be medicated while breast-feeding.

- Many mothers have a strong predisposition to breast-feed despite any medication risk. Beyond the opportunity for mother–child bonding, there is clear evidence that breast-fed infants may have lower rates of various medical problems (13,14).
- Although the exact incidence is not known, risk to infants from mood stabilizers and antidepressant exposure during breast-feeding appears low.

The risks of harm and neglect to the infant from a mother who is profoundly manic, psychotic and/or depressed can be significant and, at times, catastrophic. In any patient with serious mood symptoms, the treatment should favor the maintenance of the mother's mental health, which is likely to include psychotropic medication.

- Maintain the lowest possible medication dose that controls the patient's symptoms. Premature infants have less well-developed hepatic and kidney function and, therefore, this information should be taken into account before a mother on medication decides to breast-feed.
- It may be useful to suggest weaning an infant sooner than the mother might otherwise do, to reduce the infant's exposure to psychotropic medication.
- Ensure that the condition of the baby is carefully monitored by both the mother and the pediatrician.
- As with pregnancy, the breast-feeding period is not a time for new, untried medication unless all previous medications have been unsuccessful or poorly tolerated.

Specific medications

Having described the clinical principles and overarching clinical guidelines for dealing with the pregnant patient who evidences elevated mood, we turn our attention to specific medications and medication groups that are commonly used to treat elevated mood in the pregnancy.

Lithium

Since lithium came into common use in the late 1960s and early 1970s, there has been concern about an association between first-trimester lithium exposure and congenital malformations. This was particularly of concern with Ebstein's anomaly (a malformation with downward displacement of the tricuspid valve into the right ventricle, causing backward leakage and weakening of the ventricular outflow to the lungs). An early voluntary physician-reported database cited a 400-fold higher rate of Ebstein's anomaly in infants exposed to lithium (15). Recent estimates (16–18) show an incidence of between 1 and 2 per 1,000 babies born to mothers on lithium. Because the overall incidence of this anomaly in the general population is approximately 1 in 20,000, this yields a rate 20 to 40 times higher than the general population. The absolute risk, however, remains small. Cardiac fetal ultrasound evaluation performed at 16 to 19 weeks of pregnancy can reveal the presence of Ebstein's anomaly. This may be a useful diagnostic tool to patients who have had first-trimester lithium exposure to aid in decisions regarding pregnancy continuation.

Regarding neurobehavioral teratogenicity, a follow-up study of children in the register of lithium babies, where 60 children were exposed to lithium either during the first trimester or throughout pregnancy, did not show behavioral differences when compared to their nonexposed siblings (19). The so-called "floppy baby" syndrome, characterized by cyanosis and lowered muscle tone as possible sequelae of infant lithium exposure, can be minimized by close monitoring of lithium levels during the mother's labor (20,21).

Consistent lithium levels may be maintained throughout pregnancy by more frequent dosing (three to four times a day), thereby avoiding peaks of lithium concentration. This may or may not be of significant benefit to the fetus (22,23). Over the course of pregnancy renal lithium excretion increases, requiring an increase in dose over the course of the first 8.5 months. Frequent monitoring should be undertaken, particularly in circumstances that might cause increased lithium levels such as vomiting or febrile illnesses.

In the several weeks before delivery, the dosage of lithium should be significantly decreased because increased serum levels and toxicity may result from the dramatically decreased blood and fluid volumes immediately following childbirth. During delivery and in the immediate postpartum period, close monitoring of serum lithium levels and clinical symptoms must be undertaken to avoid relapse. Adequate hydration should be maintained and IV fluids may be necessary for patients who experience a prolonged labor.

Measurements of the ratio of lithium concentrations in umbilical blood to maternal cord blood shows uniformity across a wide range of maternal concentrations. Because neuromuscular complications lower APGAR (**A**ctivity, **P**ulse, **G**rimace, **A**ppearance, and **R**espiration) scores, longer hospital stays are seen in infants with higher lithium concentrations at delivery (>0.64 mEq/L). Lithium therapy should be withheld totally for 24 to 48 hours before delivery. This results in a reduction in maternal lithium concentration of 0.28 mEq per L (24).

Anticonvulsants

As has been described, a variety of anticonvulsants including valproic acid, carbamazepine, and lamotrigine have been mainstays in the treatment of elevated mood and bipolar disorder. The use of these medications as primary anticonvulsants has provided significant data to aid in the decision making regarding their use for stabilizing mood during pregnancy.

Valproic acid

Valproic acid monotherapy is a known human teratogen and is associated with neural tube defect rates between 5% and 9%. This risk is dose related to its use between day 17 and 30, postconception (25–27). Valproic acid has been associated with a two-fold increase in the rate of fetal malformations including spina bifida, cranial facial anomalies, growth retardation, and cardiac defects (27,28). In general, the combination of valproic acid with carbamazepine should be avoided in the first trimester, particularly if there is a family history of neural tube defects. Combined therapy has shown a higher teratogenetic risk than monotherapy (29,30). Stillbirth and miscarriages are also higher in those treated with anticonvulsants (14%) as compared to unmedicated epileptic women (4%) (31).

Valproate has also been associated with the "fetal valproate syndrome" and neonatal complications including decreased heart rate and withdrawal symptoms of jitteriness, abnormal muscle tone, and irritability (25,27). In general, it is best that women treated with valproic acid be changed to another mood stabilizer before conception. The large percentage of unplanned pregnancies in women with elevated mood, however, means that many do not discover they are pregnant until the deleterious effects of valproate exposure have already occurred. Some incidence of neural tube defects may be decreased by the use of folic acid 4 to 5 mg per day before and during the pregnancy or at least through the first trimester (28). Fertile women on valproic acid should be considered for routine folic acid maintenance. The mother's weight during pregnancy should be monitored because exceptionally high weight gains have been associated with risk for neural tube defects (29,30). Should such weight gain occur, the clinician should assist the patient in dietary consultation. For these reasons, valproate is not a good choice of mood medications in this patient population unless clinically necessary.

Carbamazepine

Carbamazepine, also a human teratogen, has been shown to be associated with an 11% risk of cranial facial defects, a 26% incidence of fingernail hypoplasia, a 20% increase in developmental delay, as well as a 0.5% to 1% rate of neural tube defects (31,32). Carbamazepine has also been associated with decreased birth weight, hyperbilirubinemia, and transient hepatic toxicity. Cognitive dysfunction, however, has not been detected in controlled studies (33). Carbamazepine has also been shown to cause a risk of neonatal hemorrhage due to vitamin K deficiency. This risk can be reduced be giving 20 mg of vitamin K daily during the last 1 to 2 months before delivery in those women taking carbamazepine as well as 1 mg intramuscularly to the neonate after delivery (30,34).

Because of these risks, carbamazepine is a poor choice during the period leading to conception and during the first trimester unless other alternatives fail or are even less desirable.

Lamotrigine

In contrast to the elevated rates associated with use of carbamazepine and valproate, lamotrigine has shown a rate of major malformations similar to that in the general population with the exception of a possible increase in oral clefts. This data is from the Lamotrigine Pregnancy registry maintained by the manufacturer (35,36). The single follow-up study of 23 lamotrigine-exposed infants showed no neurobehavioral teratogenicity at 1 year of age (36). An added consideration with lamotrigine is that the clearance of this compound is *increased* over the course of the pregnancy, leading to a *decrease* in serum concentration. The serum level rapidly returns to preconception levels after delivery. Therefore, if the oral dosage has been increased over the course of the pregnancy for control of symptoms, the patient's condition should be carefully monitored in the immediate postpartum period. A dosage decrease after delivery may be necessary.

Other anticonvulsants including topiramate and zonisamide have minimal pregnancy-related and neonatal-related data on which to base any recommendations; they should be used only when there is a clear positive benefit ratio in a given patient.

Benzodiazepines

Although early reports suggested a relationship between oral cleft development and the use of benzodiazepines during pregnancy (37), follow-up evaluations did not support this association (38,39). However, a recent, more detailed analysis did demonstrate a relationship between benzodiazepine exposure and cleft lip and palate at the rate of approximately 11 per 10,000 births, which is higher than the risk rate in the general population of 6 per 10,000. Therefore, although the rate for this abnormality is increased, it is still rare. Some authorities have suggested the use of level 2 ultrasonography for those in whom there has been first-trimester exposure (40). This low incidence may be further reduced by using high-potency benzodiazepine agents such as clonazepam or lorazepam. No complications of intrauterine growth have been noted with these two compounds. Neonatal toxicity was not found in a small study of infants of mothers who had taken clonazepam (0.5 to 3.5 mg per day) in treatment for panic disorder. The use of benzodiazepines near term has, however, been associated with lower APGAR scores, muscular hypertonia, and failure to feed. Mothers who chronically use benzodiazepines may deliver infants who show withdrawal symptoms including tremor, irritability, hypertonicity, diarrhea, and vomiting (41).

First-generation antipsychotics

Although utilized in much smaller numbers than in the past, first-generation (typical) antipsychotics are still used as treatment for patients who do not respond to second-generation antipsychotics or mood stabilizers. Because these agents were used to treat hyperemesis gravidarum in low doses in the 1950s, there is considerable data on the use of phenothiazines, particularly chlorpromazine, in the pregnant population. A large scale study of >50,000 mother–child pairs revealed 142 women who had first-trimester exposures to chlorpromazine. In this study, there was no elevation in the rate of physical malformations. The study also suggested that other first-generation antipsychotics such as perphenazine, trifluoperazine, and prochlorperazine were similarly not associated with higher respective rates of malformation (42). Some experts suggest that first-generation antipsychotic agents are safer than traditional mood stabilizers such as lithium, valproic acid, and carbamazepine and, are therefore preferable in the treatment of acute mania or severe hypomania during pregnancy (43).

McKenna and other researchers in Canada and Israel assessed the outcomes of pregnancies in women who took one of four second-generation antipsychotics during their first trimester (olanzapine, quetiapine, risperidone and clozapine) (44). In this first prospective comparative study using drugs of this class, the only statistically significant difference between the pregnancies of patients who took antipsychotics and matched controls was in the rates of low birth weight (10% to 2%) respectively and the frequency of therapeutic abortions. There were 110 live births to the 151 women studied, with only one major malformation. A separate study of atypical antipsychotics during pregnancy showed a congenital malformation rate of less than half the baseline rates in the general population. Rates of other perinatal complications were within normal historical control rates (43). Therefore, with the data available to date, this class of medication does not appear to confer added teratogenic risk and may be a useful class of treatment for elevated mood.

Antidepressants

Selective serotonin reuptake inhibitors (SSRIs) and other second-generation antidepressants have not been associated with major fetal abnormalities when taken by women during pregnancy (45–47). However, a recent set of reports has indicated that neonatal withdrawal reactions including irritability, tremor, abnormal crying, and convulsions have occurred in newborns of mothers who have taken SSRIs during pregnancy (48). This resulted in a U.S. Food and Drug Administration (FDA) class labeling change and suggests tapering the dose of an antidepressant in the third trimester. The authors suggest that paroxetine may be the most egregious agent causing both potentially acute toxicity in the infant and withdrawal symptoms, possibly related to its potent affinity for the serotonin transport, its strong anticholinergic activity, its short half-life, and its lack of active metabolites. A review by Sanz et al. looked at a World Health Organization database and located 102 cases of neonatal convulsions or withdrawal in association with maternal SSRI use during pregnancy (48). Most of these cases involved paroxetine at doses between 10 and 50 mg a day. A smaller number of other SSRIs were implicated as well. On the basis of this data, the investigators suggested that late pregnancy use of SSRIs, particularly paroxetine, raised the risk of neonatal convulsions and withdrawal syndrome. The pregnancy category of paroxetine has been changed from category C to category D.

Another antidepressant of concern that is already associated with potentially intense withdrawal reactions in adult patients is the serotonin–norepinephrine reuptake inhibitor (SNRI) venlafaxine. Sanz et al. noted 17 cases of venlafaxine-related neonatal withdrawal, but there is limited clinical evidence as to whether venlafaxine is as hazardous as paroxetine to newborns. The other SNRI in common usage, duloxetine (Cymbalta), has, as yet, insufficient data to reach a clinical conclusion about its usage in pregnancy. It remains category C and should be used in individual patients when the benefits outweigh possible risks.

Will my child be bipolar? Genetics and family history

A question frequently raised in the course of treating an adult with elevated mood or bipolar disorder is, "What is the likelihood that my child will also develop elevated mood or bipolar disorder?" Although our knowledge of the genetics of mental illness is growing rapidly, there is no genetic "litmus test" or known genetic abnormality that will code for an increased vulnerability to bipolar disorder or elevated mood. Although such an individual gene marker may ultimately be found, it is more likely that an aggregate of combined genetic abnormalities will be shown to provide a vulnerability to bipolar disorder.

The clinician may still assist patients in determining the relative risks. A detailed family history of the given psychiatric disorder, such as bipolar disorder, is the best predictor of development of psychiatric illness (48). Using a strict definition of bipolar disorder, the current estimate in the general population is between 1% and 5% for both bipolar I and bipolar II disorders. Using empiric data derived from studying family members of affected individuals, the relative incidence of risk for a first-degree relative of an individual with bipolar disorder is between 4% and 15%. With biological relatives who are more removed than the first-degree relatives, the relative risks are less certain (49,50). If both parents carry a diagnosis of bipolar disorder, the probability rates for a child developing bipolar disorder are between 20% and 50% (51). These risks are entirely based on probabilities and may be higher or lower for individual patients and families. Using these relative rates as well as other factors such as age, gender, age of onset (earlier age associated with greater genetic loading), number of affected family members, and degree of biological relatedness, a clinician can estimate which patient's children are at the higher or lower end of the risk spectrum.

Providing even such limited estimations of risk can be a two-edged sword. On the one hand, some patients will be helped significantly in making decisions about marriage and childbearing (including possible pregnancy termination). It may also decrease the stigma associated with mental illness and give emotional respite to individuals who may have grossly overestimated the risk of having a child with bipolar disorder. On the other hand, some individuals who have an elevated risk of disease may be inappropriately anxious regarding their children's welfare, leading to increased attention being paid to small details of the child's behavior. Parents with bipolar disorder may develop an excessively keen eye for dissecting their children's emotional reactions and be all too ready to label small changes or problematic behaviors in school as related to bipolar disorder. Other parents, in denial, will miss obvious elevated mood symptoms or abnormal behaviors that are quite apparent to others.

Helping a parent assess their child's behavior

A useful paradigm for the clinician is to suggest that the parents take a broad view of their child, looking at several areas of functioning including peer relations, academic performance, interfamilial relationships, and day-to-day activities including sleep patterns, activity levels, appetite and eating, and sexualized behavior, if any. If an abnormality is noted, even in one area while other areas show adequate or superior functioning, a "watch-and-wait" approach is the best. If there are multiple areas of dysfunction across a broad spectrum of behaviors and activities, further evaluation by a child psychiatrist may be indicated, particularly if such abnormalities and behaviors are long-lasting and intrusive in the child's life.

Geller has identified specific behaviors, which when present, are potentially indicative of elevated mood (see Table 14.1). The presence of one or more of these symptoms should alert the parents and clinician to a significantly higher risk of bipolar disorder or elevated mood. In general, these symptoms do not overlap with attention deficit/attention-deficit hyperactivity disorder and should be considered red flag symptoms of a potential mood disorder. A family history of affective disorder, when present, also supports this conclusion but is not essential to helping parents evaluate the possibility of a mood disorder. In some cases, a clinician might suggest the completion of a screening form such as the ten-item Conners Abbreviated Parent Questionnaire (54,55).

The bottom line

- The risk of elevated mood and depression in susceptible individuals during pregnancy is high.

TABLE 14.1
Factors that may indicate elevated mood in youth (52,53)

- Elation
- Grandiosity
- Flight of ideas
- Racing thoughts
- Decreased need for sleep
- Hypersexuality (in the absence of sexual abuse or overstimulation)

- Medication risks, although not insignificant, may not be as great to the mother and child as untreated mood disorder.
- Each pregnant woman will require an individual approach to assessing and treating any elevated mood that occurs.
- The postpartum period is an exceptionally vulnerable one for mood exacerbations.
- Breast-feeding of infants has advantages to the mother and child, despite the fact that psychotropics taken during lactation do appear in breast milk in small amounts.

REFERENCES

1. Viguera AC, Cohen LS, Baldessarini RJ, et al. Management of Bipolar Disorder during pregnancy: Weighing the risks and benefits. *Can J Psychiatry*, 2002; 47(5):499–507.
2. Viguera AC, Cohen LS, Bouffard S, et al. Reproductive decisions by women with Bipolar Disorder after pre-pregnancy psychiatric consultation. *Am J Psychiatry*. 2002;159:2102–2104.
3. Altshuler LL, Hendrick V, Cohen LS. An update on mood and anxiety disorders during pregnancy and the postpartum period. *Prim Care Companion J Clin Psychiatry*. 2000;2(6):217–222.
4. Moldin S. NIMH human genetics initiative: 2003 update. *Am J Psychiatry*. 2003; 160:621–622.
5. Cohen LS, Sichel DA, Robertson LM, et al. Postpartum prophylaxis for women with Bipolar Disorder. *Am J Psychiatry*. 1995;152:1641–1645.
6. Yonkers KA, Wisner KL, Stowe Z, et al. Management of Bipolar Disorder during pregnancy and the postpartum period. *Am J Psychiatry*. 2004;161:608–620.
7. Teissedre F, Chabrol H. Detecting women at risk of postnatal depression using the EPDS at 2 to 3 days postpartum. *Can J Psychiatry*. 2004;49:51–54.
8. Hannah P, Adams D, Lee A, et al. Links between early postpartum mood and postnatal depression. *Br J Psychiatry*. 1992;160:777–780.
9. Yamashita H, Yoshida K, Nakano H, et al. Postnatal depression in Japanese women: Detecting the early onset of postnatal depression by closely monitoring the postpartum mood. *J Affect Disord*. 2004;78:163–169.
10. Adewuya AO. Early postpartum mood as a risk factor for postnatal depression in Nigerian women. *Am J Psychiatry*. 2006;163:1435–1439.
11. Blackmore ER, Johnes I, Doshi M, et al. Obstetric variables associated with Bipolar affective puerperal psychosis. *Br J Psychiatry*. 2006;188:32–36.
12. Buist A. Treating mental illness in lactating women. *Medscape Womens Health*. 2001;6(2):1–9.
13. Wilson IT. Determinants and consequences of drug excretion in breast milk. *Drug Metab Rev*. 1983;14:619–652.
14. Chen Y, Yu S, Li W, et al. Artificial feeding and hospitalization in the first 18 months of life. *Pediatrics*. 1988;81:58–62.
15. Schou M, Goldfield MD, Weinstein MR, et al. Lithium and pregnancy, l: Report from the register of lithium babies. *Br Med J*. 1973;2:135–136.
16. Edmonds LD, Oakley GP. Ebstein's anomaly, and other congenital heart defects (letter). *Lancet*. 1974;2:594–595.

17. Jacobsen SJ, Jones K, Johnson K, et al. Prospective multi-center study of pregnancy outcome after lithium exposure during pregnancy. *Teratology*. 1990;41:551–552.

18. Cohen LS, Friedman JM, Jefferson JW, et al. A reevaluation of risk of in utero exposure to lithium. *JAMA*. 1994;271:146–150.

19. Schou M. What happened later to the lithium babies? A follow-up study of children born without malformations. *Acta Psychiatr Scand*. 1976;54:193–197.

20. Ananth J. Side effects in the neonate from psychotropic agents excreted through breastfeeding. *Am J Psychiatry*. 1978;135:801–805.

21. Schou M, Amdisen A. Lithium and pregnancy, 3: Lithium ingestion by children breast-fed by women on lithium treatment. *Br Med J*. 1973;2:138.

22. Goldfield MD, Weinstein MR. Lithium carbonate in obstetrics: Guidelines for clinical use. *Am J Obstet Gynecol*. 1973;116:15–22.

23. Yonkers KA, Wisner KL, Stowe Z, et al. American Psychiatric Society. Management of Bipolar Disorder during pregnancy: The postpartum period. *Focus*. 2005;3: 266–279.

24. Newport DJ, Viguera A, Beach A, et al. Lithium placental passage and obstetrical outcome: Implications for clinical management during late pregnancy. *Am J Psychiatry*. 2005;162(11):2162–2170.

25. Kennedy D, Koren G. Valproic acid use in psychiatry: Issues in treating women of reproductive age. *J Psychiatry Neurosci*. 1998;23:223–228.

26. Omtzigt J. The disposition of valproate and its metabolites in the late first trimester and early second trimester of pregnancy in maternal serum, urine and amniotic fluid: Effect of dose, co-medication, and the presence of spina bifida. *Eur J Clin Pharmacol*. 1992;43:381–388.

27. Jager-Roman E. Fetal growth, major malformations, and minor anomalies in infants born to women receiving valproic acid. *J Pediatr*. 1986;108:997–1004.

28. Crawford P, Appleton R, Betts T, et al. Best practice guidelines for the management of women with epilepsy. *Seizure*. 1999;8:201–217.

29. Goldstein DJ, Corbin LA, Fung MC, et al. Olanzapine-exposed pregnancies and lactation: Early experience. *J Clin Psychopharmacol*. 2000;20:399–403.

30. Stones SC, Sommi RW, Marken PA, et al. Clozapine use in two full-term pregnancies. *J Clin Psychiatry*. 1997;58:364–365.

31. Jones KL, Lacro RV, Johnson KA, et al. Pattern of malformations in the children of women treated with carbamazepine during pregnancy. *N Engl J Med*. 1989;320:1661–1666.

32. Rosa FW. Spina bifida in infants of women treated with carbamazepine during pregnancy. *N Engl J Med*. 1991;324:674–677.

33. Scolnick D. Neurodevelopment of children exposed in utero to phenytoin and carbamazepine monotherapy. *JAMA*. 1994;271:767–770.

34. American Academy of Neurology. Practice parameter: Management issues for women with epilepsy (summary statement): Report of the quality standard subcommittee of the American Academy of Neurology. *Neurology*. 1998;51:944–948.

35. Calabrese JR, Shelton MD, Rapport DJ, et al. Long-term treatment of Bipolar Disorder with lamotrigine. *J Clin Psychiatry*. 2002;63(Suppl 10):18–22.

36. Mackay F, O'Brein T, Hitchcock A. Safety of long-term lamotrigine in epilepsy. *Epilepsia*. 1997;38:881–886.

37. Aarskog D. Association between maternal intake of diazepam and oral clefts (letter). *Lancet*. 1975;2:921.

38. Heinonen OP, Slone D, Shapiro S. *Birth defects and drugs in pregnancy.* Littleton, MA: Publishing Sciences Group, 1999.
39. McElhatton PR. The effects of benzodiazepines use during pregnancy and lactation. *Reprod Toxicol.* 1994;8:461–475.
40. Dolovich LR, Addis A, Vaillancourt JMR, et al. Benzodiazepine use in pregnancy and major malformations or oral cleft: Meta-analysis of cohort and case—control studies. *BMJ.* 1998;317:839–843.
41. Briggs G, Freeman R, Yaffe S. *Drugs in pregnancy and lactation.* Philadelphia, PA: Lippincott Williams & Wilkins, 2002.
42. Slone D, Siskind V, Heinonen Op, et al. Antenatal exposure to the phenothiazines in relation to congenital malformations, prenatal mortality rate, birth weight, and intelligence quotient score. *Am J Obstet Gynecol.* 1977;128:486–488.
43. Ernst CL, et al. The reproductive safety profile of mood stabilizers, atypical antipsychotics and broad spectrum psychotropics. *J Clin Psychiatry.* 2002; 63(suppl 4):42–55.
44. McKenna K, Koren G, Tetelbaum M, et al. Pregnancy outcome of women using atypical antipsychotic drugs: A prospective comparative study. *J Clin Psychiatry.* 2005;66:444–449.
45. Field T. Infants of depressed mothers. *Infant Behav Dev.* 1995;18:1–13.
46. Malm H, Klaukka T, Neuvonen PJ. Risks associated with selective serotonin reuptake inhibitors in pregnancy. *Obstet Gynecol.* 2005;106:1289–1296.
47. Hallberg P, Joblom V. The use of selective serotonin reuptake inhibitors during pregnancy and breast-feeding: A review and clinical aspects. *J Clin Psychopharmacol.* 2005;25:59–73.
48. Sanz EJ, De-la-Cuevas C, Kiuru A, et al. Selective serotonin reuptake inhibitors in pregnant women and neonatal withdrawal syndrome: A database analysis. *Lancet.* 2005;365:482–487.
49. Finn CT, Stoler JM, Smoller JW. Genetics and genetic disorders. In: Stern TA, Fricchione GL, Cassam NH, et al., eds. *Massachusetts general hospital handbook of general hospital psychiatry.* St. Louis, MO: Mosby, 2004.
50. Finn CT, Wilcox MA, Korf BR, et al. Psychiatric genetics: A survey of psychiatrists' knowledge, opinions and practice patterns. *J Clin Psychiatry.* 2005;66(7): 821–830.
51. Austin JC, Honer WG. The potential impact of genetic counseling for mental illness. *Clin Genet.* 2005;67(2):134–142.
52. Geller B, Williams M, Zimmerman B, et al. Pre-pubertal and early adolescent bipolarity differentiate from ADHD by manic symptoms, grandiose delusions, ultrarapid and ultradian cycling. *J Affect Disord.* 1998;51:81.
53. Geller B, Zimerman B, Williams M, et al. DSM-IV mania symptoms in a pre-pubertal and early adolescent Bipolar Disorder phenotype compared to attention deficit hyperactive and normal controls. *J Child Adolesc Psychopharmacol.* 2002; 12:11.
54. Rowe KS, Rowe KJ. Norms for parental ratings on Conners' Abbreviated Parent-teacher questionnaire: Implications for the design of behavioral rating inventories and analyses of data derived from them. *J Abnorm Child Psychol.* 1997;14:425–451.
55. Tillman R, Geller B. A brief screening tool for a pre-pubertal and early adolescent Bipolar Disorder phenotype. *Am J Psychiatry.* 2005;162:1214–1216.

Appendix

INTERNET RESOURCES FOR PATIENTS

URL	Description
www.dbsalliance.org	The patient-directed Depression and Bipolar Support Alliance (DBSA)
www.nimh.nih.gov/publicat/bipolar.cfm	The National Institute of Mental Health (NIMH)
www.nami.org	The National Alliance on Mental Illness (NAMI) is helpful for patients and families; the website is organized by the state.
www.nmha.org	Mental Health America (formerly known as the National Mental Health Association)

There are also a number of useful textbooks and materials for laypeople about bipolar disorder, which can be recommended to patients and their families for further education about bipolar disorder.

Several of these include the following:

- *Bipolar Disorder—A Guide for Patients and Families* by Francis Mondimore, MD
- *New Hope for People with Bipolar Disorder* by Jan Fawcett, MD
- *The Bipolar Disorder Survival Guide* by DJ Miklowitz, PhD
- *Bipolar Disorder Insight for Recovery* by Jane Mountain, MD

Index

Note: Page numbers followed by *f* indicate figures; those followed by *t* indicate tables.